QUALITATIVE
RESEARCH
METHODS

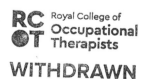

To our children

Zoe Sanipreeya Rice
Emma Inturatana Rice
Timothy Hugh Ezzy
Emily Ruth Ezzy

QUALITATIVE RESEARCH METHODS

A HEALTH FOCUS

Pranee Liamputtong Rice
and Douglas Ezzy

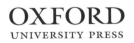

OXFORD
UNIVERSITY PRESS

OXFORD
UNIVERSITY PRESS

253 Normanby Road, South Melbourne, Victoria, Australia 3205
Oxford University Press is a department of the University of Oxford.
It furthers the University's objective of excellence in research, scholarship,
and education by publishing worldwide in

Oxford New York

Athens Auckland Bangkok Bogotá Buenos Aires Calcutta
Cape Town Chennai Dar es Salaam Delhi Florence Hong Kong Istanbul
Karachi Kuala Lumpur Madrid Melbourne Mexico City Mumbai Nairobi
Paris Port Moresby São Paulo Singapore Taipei Tokyo Toronto Warsaw

with associated companies in Berlin Ibadan

National Library of Australia
Cataloguing-in-Publication data:

Rice, Pranee Liamputtong, 1955– .
 Qualitative research methods: a health focus
 Bibliography.
 Includes index.
 ISBN 0 19 550610 3

 1. Health—Research—Methodology.
 2. Research—Methodology.
 I. Ezzy, Douglas. II. Title.

610.72

Edited by Raylee Singh
Cover design by Modern Art Production Group
Index by Geraldine Suter
Typeset by Desktop Concepts Pty Ltd, Melbourne
Printed by Kin Keong, Singapore

Contents

List of Boxes, Figures and Tables

About the Authors

Pranee Liamputtong Rice is a senior lecturer in the School of Public Health, La Trobe University, Melbourne. Pranee has previously taught in the School of Sociology and Anthropology and worked as a public health research fellow at the Centre for the Study of Mothers' and Children's Health, La Trobe University. Her particular interests are in issues related to the cultural and social influences on childbearing, childrearing and women's reproductive and sexual health, and she has published several books and papers in these areas. Three of her books have been used widely in the health area: *My 40 Days: A Cross-Cultural Resource Book for Health Care Professionals in Birthing Services* (1993); *Asian Mothers, Australian Birth* (ed. 1994); and *Maternity and Reproductive Health in Asian Societies* (ed. with Lenore Manderson, 1996). Her main approaches in conducting research are those of qualitative research methods, particularly ethnography, focus groups, in-depth interviews, life histories and unobtrusive methods.

Douglas Ezzy is a lecturer in sociology in the School of Sociology and Social Work, University of Tasmania, Hobart. Douglas previously taught sociology in the School of Sociology and Anthropology, La Trobe University, and was a research fellow in the National Centre in HIV Social Research, at the Centre for the Study of Sexually Transmissible Diseases, La Trobe University. The focus of his research is the social construction of meaning and worth by individuals and organisations. His substantive interests include HIV/AIDS, mental health, the sociology of work and unemployment, and religion. His articles have appeared in journals such as *Social Science and Medicine*, *AIDS Care*, *Qualitative Sociology*, *Sociology*, and the *Sociological Quarterly*. His research typically consists of long life-history interviews, supplemented with survey research, focus groups and unobtrusive methods.

Preface

This book is written in an attempt to demystify the process of qualitative research, particularly qualitative health research. We have produced an easy-to-follow textbook that includes both practical guidance as well as a theoretically informed discussion of some major issues in qualitative research. The text aims to enable researchers embarking on a qualitative research project to carry their endeavour through—from writing a proposal, conducting the research and analysing the results, to writing up for publication.

Biomedicine has produced many significant achievements in the twentieth century. It has radically changed the modern experience of illness and health. However, we believe that many of the fundamental problems of our time cannot be solved by biomedicine alone. This is because many of the health problems of late modernity are fundamentally problems of meaning and interpretation. For example, we have a reasonably clear biomedical understanding of how HIV/AIDS is transmitted. While there can always be improvements in our biomedical understanding, HIV/AIDS remains with us mainly because of social factors, because so few people understand the implications of their actions, and governments remain unwilling or confused about how to respond to the crisis.

Qualitative research methods focus on meanings and interpretations. They provide a sophisticated research strategy to understand how, and why, people act in particular ways. Further, qualitative research methods can provide important policy direction, and a detailed understanding of the implications of particular policies. Qualitative methods are often seen as an easy option, or as an adjunct or precursor to 'hard' statistical methods. However, in our view, qualitative methods are important in their own right. They enable researchers to begin to engage with the complexities of meaning that are often emotionally, politically, and technically a very difficult challenge. The challenge to understand the complexities of meanings and interpretations, of culture, multiculture, and globalised culture, are at the centre of modern health debates. Our hope is that this book will contribute to the ongoing need for a well-informed public health practice into the twenty-first century.

This book would not have been possible without the assistance of a number of people. Our gratitude is extended particularly to Professor Allan Kellehear, who not only always believes in our work but also encouraged us to write this book. Our thanks are also due to Dr Rosalie Aroni for her initial contribution in the development of the proposal for this book. Pranee is indebted to Dr Christopher Peterson, who read many chapters, and to Assistant Professor Susanha Yimyam, who initially helped her with technical management, particularly in managing the data and presenting the final form of the chapters. Douglas would also like to particularly thank Professor Sandy Gifford, who encouraged him to continue teaching qualitative methods.

We are indebted to Jill Lane for her faith in us, and for her dedicated hard work in producing this book, and to Oxford University Press for bringing it to life.

The following authors and publishers are also thanked for granting permission for the use of their work in this book: D. Karp and Oxford University Press, New York, for extracts from *Speaking of Sadness*, 1996; Trinh T. Minh-Ha and Routledge for extracts from *When the Moon Waxes Red*, 1991; Blackwell Publishers for extracts from J. Kitzinger, 'The Methodology of Focus Groups', *Sociology of Health and Illness*, vol. 16, no. 1, 1994; Harper & Row for extracts from E.L. Webb et al., *Unobtrusive Measures*, 1966; Elsevier Science for extracts from P. Clark and A. Bowling, 'Qualityof Everyday Life in Long Stay Institutions for the Elderly. An Observational Study of Long Stay Hospitals and Nursing Homes', reprinted, with permission from Elsevier Science, from *Social Science and Medicine*, col. 30, no. 11, pp. 1201–10, copyright 1990, and from 'D.L. Klinman and L.J. Cohen, 'The Decontextualisation of Mental Illness: The Portrayal of Work in Psychiatric Drug Advertisements', reprinted, with permission from Elsevier Science, from *Social Science and Medicine*, vol. 32, no. 8, pp. 867–74, copyright 1991; Verso, London, for extracts from F. Haug, *Female Sexualization*, 1987; Public Health Association of Australia for extracts from S. Kippax, 'Memory Work', in J. Daly and E. Willis (eds), *The Social Sciences and Health Research*, 1990; M. Hammersley and P. Atkinson and Routledge for extracts from *Ethnography*, 1995; American Anthropological Association for extracts from R.A. Hahn, 'Divisions of Labour', *Medical Anthropology Quarterly*, vol. 1, no. 3, 1987; Dr Muhammad Anisur Rahman and University Press for extracts from *People's Self-Development*, 1993; Professor Mildred Blaxter for extracts from 'Criteria for the Evaluation of Qualitative Research Papers', *Medical Sociology News*, vol. 22, no. 1, supplementary, 1996; John Wiley & Sons, Inc., for extracts from R. Bogdan and S.J. Taylor, *Introduction to Qualitative Research Methods*, 1975. Excerpts from *The Ethnographic Interview* by James P. Spradley, copyright ©1979 by Holt, Rinehart & Winston, reprinted by permission of the publisher.

Introduction

Qualitative inquiry cultivates the most useful of all human capacities—the capacity to learn from others. (Patton 1990, p. 7)

Ways of understanding are integrated works of art created by many minds, like cathedrals, as much masterpieces of the human spirit as the Greek tragedies or the paintings of the Renaissance. Human beings construct meaning as spiders make webs—or as appropriate enzymes make proteins. (Mary Catherine Bateson 1994, in Ely et al. 1997, p. 63)

WHAT IS QUALITATIVE RESEARCH?

Trying to write a guide book for qualitative research is something like trying to write a guide book for writing poetry. There are certain rules and conventions, pitfalls to be avoided and good examples to study. However, in the end, the best qualitative research depends on the creativity and insight of the researcher themselves. The researcher must find the best way of studying how meaning and interpretations are constructed in their particular substantive research area.

In general, qualitative research draws on an interpretative orientation that focuses on the complex and nuanced process of the creation and maintenance of meaning. Qualitative research aims to elicit the contextualised nature of experience and action, and attempts to generate analyses that are detailed, 'thick' and integrative (in the sense of relating individual events and interpretations to larger meaning systems and patterns). However, qualitative research cannot be described in terms of a set of theories and techniques that always apply. Rather, qualitative research draws on a variety of theoretical perspectives and practical techniques, including theories such as phenomenology, symbolic interactionism, cultural studies, psychology, and feminism, and techniques such as interviewing, narrative analysis, ethnography, and focus groups.

Qualitative research is more flexible and fluid in its approach than quantitative statistical methods. Some people seem to think that this makes qualitative research less worthwhile because it is not governed by clear rules. Positivist researchers have argued that the interpretative nature of qualitative data makes it 'soft' science, lacking in reliability and validity, and of little value in contributing to scientific knowledge in general and health care in particular (Baum 1995; Denzin and Lincoln 1994a; Guba and Lincoln 1994).

However, the interpretative and flexible approach is necessary due to the focus of qualitative research on meaning and interpretation (Rice 1996a). According to Hammersley (1992, p. 45), qualitative data are reliable because they 'document the world from the point of view of the people studied ... rather than presenting it from the perspective of the researcher'. Most qualitative research assumes that, in order to understand people's behaviour, we must attempt to understand the meanings and interpretations that people give to their behaviour. Unlike measures of disease epidemiology or clinical test results, meanings and interpretations cannot be measured and dealt with statistically. Metaphors, meanings and interpretations require the more fluid, but no less rigorous, methods employed by qualitative research.

For example, psychological studies have demonstrated that unemployed people are more depressed than people who are working (Winefield et al. 1993). Statistics are an excellent way of proving that unemployment and depression are linked together. However, when the authors of these same studies attempt to examine *why* unemployed people are depressed, they do not seem to be able to discover much more than that unemployed young people tend to watch more television (Winefield et al. 1993). The problem with such studies is that the research has changed from asking questions about the relationship between employment status and various psychological statistical measures, to asking questions about the way unemployed people construct meaning. However, the researchers continue to use a quantitative methodology that does not allow them to examine the interpretative process.

It is not simply television that is the problem for young unemployed people, but, as Seabrook (1982) notes, the fact that unemployed people live in a culture where money is essential to be able to buy the consumer goods (as advertised on television) that enable a person to feel comfortable participating in their community. Going to a bar or nightclub with your friends is very awkward if you cannot afford to buy any drinks or you are not wearing the correct clothes. Watching television programs about groups of friends going to a bar, or advertisements for alcoholic beverages, only reinforces the unemployed person's separation from society. Unemployment leads to social isolation, watching television and to depression. To attempt to blame unemployed people's depression on watching television misunderstands the meaning of television watching. Television watching *per se* is not the problem. Rather, the problem lies in the way television contributes to the interpretations and meanings that young unemployed people give to their life. Only a qualitative study, such as Seabrook's, can describe the interpretative process through which television watching reinforces the social isolation and depression of unemployed people.

There are particular kinds of people who are very good at quantitative methods, who seem to enjoy statistics. One of our colleagues is an outstanding quantitative researcher. He reads books on statistics for pleasure and of his own free will works through the maths of a particular statistical procedure with a paper and pencil so that he thoroughly understands its intricacies. He appears to relish it. While we admire him, and we have been known to perform the odd factor analysis and logistic regression ourselves, we will not emulate his behaviour. The story does, however, suggest an interesting question: what would such a person look like if they were interested in qualitative methods? There are some parallels in that it is possible to perform some aspects of qualitative analysis on a computer, and you could imagine someone doing it by hand first, so that he or she understood the procedure first. There are also texts that describe the techniques of qualitative methods in detail (Strauss and Corbin 1990, for example), and you could imagine such a person reading these texts with pleasure. You could also imagine such a person studying the logic of the various esoteric searching capabilities on some of the qualitative data analysis programs. However, while such techniques are important to qualitative data analysis, the person who has become obsessed with techniques has missed the point of qualitative research.

The qualitative counterpart of our colleague who finds pleasure in statistical technique would be a person who finds pleasure in understanding people. The difference here is not simply in the subject of study: statistics compared to meaning. Rather, the difference is in the method of going about the study. People, and the meanings they give to things, *cannot* be examined using standardised techniques in the way that survey results can be examined through statistics. The reason for this is that the statistical methods used to investigate the results of survey research generally ignore the interpretative process. Qualitative methods, on the other hand, place the interpretative process at the centre of their practice. The interpretative process refers to the way that people interpret and give meaning to events and things.

David Karp's (1996) moving study of depression provides an excellent example of both good qualitative research and the motivation behind qualitative research that we are referring to. When he was asked by family or friends about the research he was working on, he says he would usually say something like this:

> I'm not primarily interested in explaining what causes depression or how to cure it because I don't think anyone can answer those questions. Instead, I'm interested in how depressed individuals make sense of an inherently ambiguous life

situation. I'm interested in how a depression consciousness unfolds over time, how people think about psychiatry and medications, and how they deal with family and friends. (Karp 1996, p. 189)

Karp was interested in the interpretative process. He was interested in the way that people make sense of, and give meaning to, depression.

Having said that the interpretative process cannot be examined through standardised techniques, it is important not to make the opposite mistake. One of us once heard an apocryphal tale about a leading American qualitative researcher whose first action when a new student was assigned to him was to ask them what they were interested in studying. If they said 'illness', for example, without any further discussion of the topic, methodology or goals, he would send them off to begin their empirical observation at, for example, a hospital. We suspect the story is exaggerated, but its moral is worth contemplating. While the standardised techniques of statistical analysis cannot be applied in qualitative methodology, there are a number of methods, procedures and practices that should be systematically considered and planned as part of any qualitative study. Alongside the requirement for creativity and innovation is the requirement for rigour, consistency and integrity. The careful study and review of existing qualitative research methods and theory is an integral part of doing qualitative research.

WHY USE QUALITATIVE RESEARCH METHODS?

In the past decade, qualitative methods have been increasingly accepted as providing valuable information for health researchers. Social scientists have argued for the value of interpretative data in a variety of health-related areas (Baum 1995; Daly et al. 1992; Holman 1993; Morgan 1991; Yach 1992). Baum (1995) argues for the appropriateness of qualitative methods to public health since they 'are well suited to studying such complex situations and offer much to the study of public health'. Qualitative methods are particularly relevant to the new public health, given its emphasis on the need to both describe and understand people. Qualitative methods provide an insight into how people make sense of their experience that cannot be easily provided by other methods (see Rice 1996a, 1996b, for example). Qualitative methods can also play an important role in facilitating the dissemination of research findings. Duhl and Hancock (1988, p. 7) call for the use of qualitative stories about a city's health because, 'unless data are turned into stories that can be understood by all, they are not effective in any process of change, either political or administrative'.

Qualitative methods are also often useful as an exploratory phase of research. McDonald and Daly (1992, p. 213), for example, assert that qualitative data analysis is particularly essential when the researchers have little knowledge about the area of investigation and 'where the social contexts of people's lives is of critical significance'. Even though quantitative statistical data can be very useful in explaining public health issues, especially the cause and extent of disease, they may mask people's interpretations and understandings, and their interactions with others. Qualitative data are more 'powerful in allowing an understanding of the context issues that have become the concern of public health in recent years' (Baum 1995, p. 463). Within the public health arena, Baum contends that qualitative information can be used in three ways:

> to explain the economic, political, social and cultural factors which influence health and disease; to gain an understanding of how communities and individuals within them interpret health and disease; and to study interactions between the various players who are relevant to any given public health issue. (Baum 1995, p. 464)

Similarly, Holman (1993) suggests that qualitative information can greatly contribute to the study of chronic illness. Holman suggests that patients' views are 'better indicators of outcomes than common medical measures' and that they may also 'provide better explanations of events which occurred' (p. 33).

Qualitative data can also be used to explain the results of quantitative research. It is often difficult to know what people *mean* when they rate themselves on particular scales or indicators, and qualitative research can provide information about meanings and interpretations that can be used to assist in the interpretation of statistical data. In investigating the diagnosis of cardiac normality, Daly and her colleagues (1992), for example, clearly illustrate how qualitative data can be used to address problems in medical contexts that cannot be satisfactorily resolved by conventional quantitative techniques in medical research.

Most health care research has focused on generating quantitative statistical data (Daly and McDonald 1992). To criticise health research for focusing on quantitative data does not mean that we think such data are not useful. Quantitative data provides extremely useful information, both on their own and in conjunction with qualitative data. However, we argue that in health care it is crucial to understand people's health agenda and experience from their perspective. In this way we may be able to work more accurately and effectively with people. The qualitative methods and the interpretative data generated from them are therefore invaluable. Indeed, qualitative data yield great benefits to the development of scientific understanding, as Holman (1993, pp. 33–5) puts it: 'Unravelling and modifying the individual sequence is the essence of good medical care … When qualitative methods are clearly established in our research repertoire, the advance of medical knowledge will be greatly accelerated.'

USEFUL BOOKS ON QUALITATIVE RESEARCH IN HEALTH

This book, *Qualitative Research Methods*, provides a practical guide to the various techniques and methods used in qualitative research, with a focus on health-related research in Australia. This focus makes the text unique, as far as we are aware. There are, however, a number of other useful texts that the qualitative researcher might consult, though these have different emphases and uses. Three that we have found particularly useful are described below.

Denzin and Lincoln's (1994) edited collection, *Handbook of Qualitative Research*, provides a broad-ranging overview of qualitative research, with a focus on theoretical and philosophical issues, particularly the implications of post-modernist and poststructuralist thought for qualitative research. However, it does not discuss the practical, political and ethical implications of adopting such research strategies in health care settings. It is also a very expensive text and may be best consulted in the library.

Colquhoun and Kellehear's edited volumes (1993, 1996), *Health Research in Practice*, focus predominantly on debates among practitioners around current health care issues. The chapters provide useful detailed discussion of a selection of methods and issues. However, they do not provide an overview of the variety of qualitative research methods, and do not address the pedagogical needs of developing researchers.

Daly, Kellehear and Gliksman's (1997) well-written *The Public Health Researcher* is focused, as the title suggests, on the needs of public health researchers. It provides a particularly thorough overview of recent research in public health. Its strength is also its weakness: it may not be relevant to health professionals from all fields.

There are a large number of other excellent texts that tend to concentrate on specific forms of qualitative research, such as ethnography (Fetterman 1989; Hammersley and Atkinson 1995), participatory action research (de Koning and Martin 1996; Wadsworth 1991), unobtrusive methods (Kellehear 1993a), in-depth interviewing (Minichiello et al. 1995), focus groups (Dawson et al. 1993; Morgan 1997), or modes of analysis (Corbin and Strauss 1990; Dey 1993; Kelle 1995; Miles and Huberman 1994; Tesch 1990).

ABOUT THE AUTHORS

Good qualitative research requires expertise in *doing* qualitative research. While theoretical knowledge is important and useful, it is essential to understand the way that real life intrudes into the often idealised models and recipes for research methods. Both of the authors have turned to qualitative methods in our health research because we found that they were and still are the most rewarding tools to work with. We have both undertaken large and small studies that have taught us a great deal about the exigencies of doing qualitative research in the real world, where we could test out our reading of the texts that we used when we were novices. These research experiences confirmed our faith in the utility of qualitative methods as an effective mode for understanding health and illness. In addition, we are often approached by health researchers employed in community health centres, hospitals and health bureaucracies who wish to engage in research projects using qualitative methods but who have no practical skills or knowledge in such methods. Even though there have been moves to separate teaching and research in the academic world, our experiences in both have led us to conclude that there is much to be gained by engaging in both activities in an ongoing fashion. Our personal research experiences have informed a more robust teaching model and our teaching experiences have enabled us to ask clearer questions in our research. Aside from this, we both have taught qualitative methods to undergraduate and postgraduate students and have learnt a great deal from them—they have often taught us nearly as much as we have taught them.

ABOUT THE BOOK

First, we introduce the history and philosophy of qualitative research methods (Chapter 1), including a discussion of ethnography, phenomenology, symbolic interactionism, feminism, hermeneutics and postmodernism. Chapter 2 examines the issues of rigour (our preferred word for the issues of validity and reliability), the various methods of sampling, the relationships between researchers and researched, and the ethics and politics of the research process. Chapters 3 to 9 describe some of the more commonly used qualitative research methods, including in-depth interviewing, focus groups, unobtrusive methods, narrative analysis and life history, memory-work, ethnography, and participatory action research. The emphasis in these chapters is on methods of data collection, although data analysis is also discussed as it is integral to some of the methods reviewed, such as narrative analysis, memory-work and participatory action research. Each chapter also provides extended examples of research that has utilised the particular method. Chapter 10 discusses the process of data analysis and includes a review of the various modes of analysis, as well as an overview of issues that arise in computer-aided analysis. Chapters 11 reviews the writing of qualitative research proposals for funding, and Chapter 12 outlines how to write for publication and considers the problem of dissemination and evaluation of qualitative research findings. In the Conclusion, we bring together our thoughts on what qualitative research methods have to offer as a means of gaining a closer understanding of people's perspectives in relation to health.

As you would expect, some parts of our book will be more useful to some readers and other parts will be less interesting. We have tried to provide an introduction to the various research methods that will allow new researchers to begin to conduct research themselves. However, we have also discussed some more complex, innovative and resource-intensive methods that will be of more interest to advanced researchers, although new researchers should also be aware of these methods even if they are not in a position to make use of them immediately. Across the chapters, therefore, we have tried to provide:

- a practical and philosophical analysis of the range of qualitative methods;
- a discussion of each method in detail, with practical examples provided;
- a discussion of when and where to use such methodology in the health sphere;
- a discussion of the political and ethical influences and implications internal and external to the health domain;
- a discussion of current research drawn from refereed journals to illustrate shifts in the use of qualitative methods in the domain of primary, secondary and public health research;
- illustrations drawn from Australian and international studies, and a focus on both classical and contemporary debates;
- tutorial exercises for students to carry out; and
- further reading suggestions for more information on each topic.

1

Theory in Qualitative Research: Traditions and Innovations

Introduction

Theory ... *is always in active relation to* practice: *an interaction between things done, things observed and (systematic) explanation of these. This allows a necessary distinction between theory and practice, but does not require their opposition. (Williams 1976, p. 317)*

Theory is useful; it enables, it helps us better to understand what we already know, intuitively, in the first place. But theory is always plural, theories, and multicentred ... This is the way social theory works. It depends on enthusiasm, passion, suspicion, scepticism, tolerance, patience and judgement. (Beilharz 1991, p. 1)

Theory is integral to the practice of qualitative research in health. Theory is useful in this sense when it informs, and is informed by, practical, empirical qualitative research. This chapter examines some of the theoretical traditions that have informed and influenced qualitative research. There is a long tradition of constructive and vigorous interchange between the more general theoretical traditions and specific health-related empirical research. This chapter continues this tradition of dialogue and debate.

The chapter begins with a review of the role of theory in empirical qualitative research. We argue that different research projects make use of theory in different ways, and that it is important to recognise and accept the variable significance of theory in qualitative research. The rest of the chapter provides an introduction to some of the theoretical orientations that have informed and influenced qualitative methods. These introductions are not sufficient in themselves. They are designed to help a researcher begin to think about which theory might be most appropriate for his or her research. Each section examines one or two key ideas or concepts used in the theoretical orientation, contrasts the theory with other perspectives, and provides a short example of how the theory has been used in empirical health research.

There are a large variety of theoretical traditions and orientations (Denzin 1997; Vidich and Lyman 1994). We have selected several that are the most commonly used and have been the most influential in qualitative research. If none of these fits your particular research goals, there is probably another more relevant theory awaiting your discovery. The theoretical traditions we discuss are: positivism, interpretative ethnography, phenomenology, symbolic interactionism, feminism, poststructuralism and postmodernism, and, finally, hermeneutics.

THE FIRST QUESTIONS IN QUALITATIVE RESEARCH

There are three interrelated sets of questions that need to be clearly addressed at the outset of any qualitative study:
1 What is the theoretical framework within which the study is being conducted?
2 What is the substantive issue being researched?
3 What are the desired outcomes of the research?
While these questions follow logically on from each other, in practice much research begins with the second or third question and works from there to the other questions. The three questions are interrelated and all need to be clearly addressed. However, one question may take priority over the others, and just how these questions are answered will depend on the particular goals of the research.

Douglas' research among unemployed people developed out of a theoretical framework that integrated symbolic interactionism and narrative theory (Ezzy 1996). The research was designed to facilitate the development of a particular theory of narrative identity that drew on these theoretical frameworks. The substantive issue of unemployed people's narratives about job loss takes a secondary role behind the primary (theoretical) aim of developing a theory of narrative-identity.

In contrast, a study of transitions in and out of work among people living with HIV/AIDS was designed to provide various government and community sector organisations with information that could be used to improve the services they provide (Ezzy et al. 1999). The substantive issue of employment transitions was integral to the research and the theoretical framework utilised was selected to best facilitate the research goal. A theory that emphasised the role of unconscious forces or explored the role of the global labour market in the work experience of people living with HIV/AIDS would not have been very useful in this research. Rather, a theoretical framework was developed drawing on studies of illness, symbolic interactionism and gay cultural theory. While theoretical innovation did occur, the theory was employed to serve the more practical goals of the research.

A theory is a set of propositions about relationships between various concepts. Different theoretical frameworks direct attention to different aspects of a phenomenon. For example, rational choice theory is a theoretical framework that assumes that people's behaviour can be explained with reference to rational choices on the part of the individual. Psychoanalytic theory points to the role of the irrational and unconscious in shaping behaviour. Symbolic interactionism emphasises symbolically generated intersubjective interpretations. There are, of course, many other theoretical frameworks. The point is simply that the general theoretical framework fundamentally shapes the sorts of things that the research focuses on and, therefore, also fundamentally shapes the method and techniques required for the research.

Some theoretical frameworks are better suited to some research problems than to others. A theory that emphasises the embodied nature of social life will probably be more useful in a study of women's experiences of breast screening than in a study of the way doctors interpret new information about breast screening in medical journals. This is not to say that such a theory would not be useful or interesting in such a study. The important point is to match theoretical frameworks with the substantive issue being investigated and with the main goal of the research.

Sometimes theoretical frameworks may be derived from the particular research tradition that the person has chosen to work within. Many qualitative studies, for example, begin with a claim to be doing 'grounded theory' within the symbolic interactionist tradition. However, even the symbolic interactionists are divided among themselves over theoretical issues (for more on this debate, see the later section on poststructuralism and postmodernism).

Some researchers may be more concerned with dealing with a particular research question, for example, the understandings of Vietnamese women in Australia about breast screening. When qualitative research is conducted without reference to theoretical frameworks, the researcher effectively takes for granted a particular framework without acknowledging it. This may not be a problem if there is an established research tradition in the field where such issues have been worked through. It may be that an established set of techniques have been used before to examine similar problems and the researcher only seeks similar sorts of answers. For example, there may be an established literature on Vietnamese women and on breast screening among cultural minorities in Australia. However, it should be noted that to not examine the theoretical assumptions of the research limits the extent to which new insights can be discovered.

On the other hand, some people become obsessed with theory. While it is important to recognise the place of theory in qualitative research, the complexities of the theoretical task should never stop a researcher from asking empirical questions. One of the contributions of the symbolic interactionist and pragmatist heritage of early qualitative researchers was to put some of the more complex theoretical questions on hold, or to work with solutions that were not perfect, and to still conduct empirical research.

Once the researcher has identified a theoretical tradition or traditions, chosen an empirical or substantive focus for the study, and clarified the desired outcomes of the research, the methodology must then be carefully constructed. The rest of this chapter examines in more detail the role of theoretical orientations in qualitative research, and outlines some of the more important theories.

POSITIVISM

Positivism has influenced qualitative research because, in many ways, it is the opposite of qualitative research. It is not a theory, so much as a general perspective that includes a number of theories that typically reject qualitative research methods. In social research, positivism refers to a belief that social science can be scientific in the same way as the physical sciences such as physics or chemistry. Positivists usually prefer quantitative methods, to measure things, using structured questions and constructing scales that can be analysed with statistics. Positivists also prefer structuralist explanations and avoid interpretivist explanations that refer to human intentions and emotions (Giddens 1974; Mills 1959; Williams 1976).

Like physical scientists, positivists in the social sciences prefer a methodology that is standardised and repeatable, and that tests a pre-existing hypothesis. They believe that this methodology will lead to true and objective results. Positivists attempt to remove or prevent interpretations influencing the research process in order to ensure objectivity. They may, for example, require an interviewer to always ask the same questions in the same way, to not express any emotion while asking the questions, and to distance themselves from the person they are interviewing (Bergen 1993; Prus 1996).

Qualitative researchers have argued that positivists are wrong in attempting to study people in the same way as physical things. People, they argue, are fundamentally different to things because of the centrality of meanings and interpretations to human social life. In order to understand why people do things, you must understand their interpretations of events and actions (Berger and Luckmann 1967). The attempt to understand meanings and interpretations is at the heart of qualitative research.

ETHNOGRAPHY

Ethnography is a methodology that incorporates a variety of theoretical traditions (see Chapter 8 for a fuller discussion of ethnographic research methods). The point of this section is to contrast the theoretical assumptions of one of the main theoretical traditions of ethnography with those of other theoretical traditions in qualitative research. The later chapter focuses more generally on ethnography in health research. This section takes a specific look at one ethnographic theoretical tradition.

Ethnography is more closely associated with anthropological research than with sociological research. In fact, ethnography is sometimes defined as what anthropologists do (Geertz 1973). Ethnography is also increasingly common in psychology and sociology, but is often referred to by different terms, such as 'community studies' (Whyte 1955).

Clifford Geertz (1973) is one of the most influential proponents of interpretative ethnography in anthropology and we will focus on his analysis as illustrative of the theoretical orientation of ethnography. However, it should be emphasised that there are a variety of theoretical traditions within ethnography, and Geertz's interpretative theory is only one of these (see Rosaldo 1989). Geertz argues that ethnography is not defined by the techniques it employs, such as participant observation and interviews, but by a particular kind of intellectual effort he describes as 'thick description' (p. 5). Thick description focuses on detail and background information. It aims to explain people's pattern of life by describing the patterns of meaning that inform their actions, so as to rend them accessible and 'logical'. Another word for these patterns of meaning is 'culture', which Geertz argues consists of 'socially established structures of meaning in terms of which people do … things' (p. 12).

Ethnography, or at least the interpretative ethnography described by Geertz, focuses on the culture of a group, the webs and patterns of meaning that make up a culture and that guide and make sense of people's actions. Ethnography focuses on discovering the cultural frameworks, analysing their structure and content, and using this as a basis for explanation of particular social phenomena. It should be emphasised, following Geertz (1973, p. 20), that cultures are never finally mapped out. Rather, ethnographic studies are always partial and incomplete guesses at explanations.

For example, Renato Rosaldo (1989) studied head-hunting among the Ilongots in the Philippines. He learnt their language, participated in their social life, interviewed people, and observed their patterns of action in order to try to understand the practice of head-hunting. The Ilongots often told him that 'rage in bereavement could impel men to head-hunt' (p. 3). Stated so simply, this does not really explain their actions, it is too 'thin', and at first Rosaldo dismissed it as an explanation. However, after the death of his wife because of an accident, he began to 'comprehend the force of anger possible in bereavement' (p. 7). Rosaldo describes this experience using 'thick description'. He describes the 'powerful visceral emotional states' and the 'deep cutting pain of sorrow almost beyond endurance'. As he analysed his own experience of bereavement, Rosaldo began to understand the complexity and depth of emotions associated with the Ilongots' experience of rage in bereavement. He describes in detail the intricacies of bereavement and links this to cultural patterns of meaning, providing a thick description of 'rage in bereavement' that in turn makes sense of the Ilongots' practice of head-hunting.

Rosaldo's study makes two important points about ethnography. First, ethnography focuses on describing in detail the systems of meaning and emotions that make up a culture and that can account for particular actions. Second, the pre-existing understandings, experiences and theoretical traditions used by the researcher are integral to what they are able to analyse and describe. Without his own experience of bereavement Rosaldo would not have been able to describe in the same depth the experience of rage in bereavement that leads to head-hunting. The significance of the researcher as a positioned subject will be discussed in further detail later in the chapter.

Another way of thinking of 'thick description' is as 'analytical' or 'theoretical' description. That is to say, the research aims to analyse theoretically social processes and systems of meaning. 'These descriptions must remain close to the concrete reality of particular events, but at the same time reveal general features of human social life' (Hammersley 1992, p. 12). However, as Martyn Hammersley (1992) points out, the relationship between theory and description is more complex than it might first seem. Early debates focused on whether theory should be developed prior to, or after, empirical description. More recent ethnographers use a more complex understanding of the simultaneous interplay of theory and description (Clough 1992; Denzin 1997; Jackson 1989).

Ethnography is distinct as an approach in that it attempts to interpret and present its findings from a cultural perspective. Ethnography searches out the patterns of meaning and emotions that make up culture and how these make sense of actions in everyday life. At the heart of ethnography is good or 'thick' description, typically obtained through an immersion in the everyday life of the group or a given social setting (Van Maanen 1982, p. 103). The theoretical traditions of ethnography are most commonly used in the ethnographic method (Chapter 8). Focus groups (Chapter 4) and in-depth interviews (Chapter 3) are also often part of ethnography and influenced by its theoretical traditions.

PHENOMENOLOGY

Phenomenological theory is more influential on qualitative research than is suggested by the small number of empirical qualitative studies that use it as their guiding theory (Moustakas 1994; Taylor 1993). The European phenomenology of Edmund Husserl (1859–1938), Alfred Schutz (1899–1959), and Martin Heidegger (1889–1976), among others, forms the philosophical background to many of the more familiar theories and methods in qualitative research. After a brief discussion of the concept of the 'life-world', the following section examines one central concept from each of these philosophers to indicate their significance in qualitative research. These summaries are not intended as, and cannot possibly be, representative of the thought of these philosophers. They are simply intended as a reminder of the importance of the phenomenological philosophers, to indicate some of the phenomenological origins of some of the terms used in qualitative research, and to encourage further research. For a more detailed analysis of phenomenological philosophers, see Macann (1993) or Mackie (1985), and for a more detailed analysis of phenomenological qualitative research methods, see Becker (1992) or Moustakas (1994).

Becker (1992, p. 7) puts it simply and clearly: 'Phenomenologists study situations in the everyday world from the viewpoint of the experiencing person.' In contrast to the emphasis on culture that is characteristic of ethnographers, phenomenology emphasises the individual's construction of a 'life-world'. 'Taken together, the whole of people's unquestioned, subjective experience of their biological worlds can be termed their "life-world" (or *Lebenswelt*)' (Ainlay 1986, p. 43). The life-world is the individual's world of their everyday life. The life-world includes taken-for-granted assumptions about everyday life, such as what clothes should be worn, what the weather will be like, the way you should greet a friend, whether to write from left to right or right to left, and how to deal with embarrassing events. Each individual's life-world is different, and individual's actions can be understood by situating them within the life-world of the actor.

The concept of intentionality is integral to Husserl's phenomenology. As Berger and Luckmann (1967, p. 34) put it, 'consciousness is always intentional; it always intends or is directed towards objects'. This philosophical proposition has important implications for the conduct of research into human action. It means that, if we are to understand why people do things, we have to understand the meaning they give to their actions. The phenomenological concept of intentionality was an early and important influence on the development of qualitative research methods that examined the meanings and interpretations people give to their actions.

Alfred Schutz emphasised the need for sociology to examine in detail the taken-for-grantedness of people's life-world. This focus bypassed a number of philosophical problems and led Schutz on to an examination of the nature of 'typifications' in everyday life (1967, p. 97). Typifications refer to the classificatory systems that people develop as a consequence of their history of interaction. The most important exponents of Schutz's phenomenology in the English-speaking world were Peter Berger and Thomas Luckmann (1967). This emphasis on examining the everyday experience of the life-world and the typifications or classificatory systems of understanding used by people in interaction is an important philosophical backdrop that has helped legitimate empirical qualitative research.

Martin Heidegger (1962) used the German term *Dasein* to refer to the person. He uses it to emphasise that people are beings in the world. He wanted to reject the Cartesian understanding of the person as isolated self-consciousness. *Dasein* literally means 'being there'. That is to say, the starting point according to Heidegger is the person's experience in their everyday life and shared social practices. Methodological individualism starts with the isolated individual. Heidegger rejects this and refers to 'being-in-the-world' to emphasise this rejection. 'To separate person and world is false; to be a person is to be in a world' (Becker 1992, p. 13). Although the influence of Heidegger's philosophy is reflected in some current qualitative research, the implications of his thought are still being assimilated into the practice of empirical qualitative research (Denzin 1986). The full impact of Heidegger's philosophical innovations is seen in the development of various postmodern and poststructuralist innovations in qualitative methods discussed later in the chapter.

Along with the phenomenological philosophers, there is also a well-developed empirical phenomenological research tradition that aims to describe the essences of everyday experience, or individuals' life-worlds. Phenomenologically oriented researchers study everyday events from within the life-world of the person experiencing them. 'The aim is to determine what an experience means for the persons who have had the experience and are able to provide a comprehensive description of it' (Moustakas 1994, p. 13).

Phenomenological theory was utilised by Corin and Lauzon (1992) to study the experience of sufferers of schizophrenia in the community. They observe that psychiatry has not systematically studied the construction of interpretations and meanings by sufferers of schizophrenia. Open-ended interviews were conducted with sufferers of schizophrenia that sought to understand 'the rehabilitative strategies and specific forms of being-in-the-world associated with an ability to remain in the community' (p. 266). Traditional approaches to schizophrenia view withdrawal from the community, such as inactivity and lack of involvement, as an indicator of a negative prognosis. In contrast, on the basis of their interviews, Corin and Lauzon argue that withdrawal is understood by the sufferers as a positive, or intentional, strategy that ensures non-rehospitalisation: 'It is characterized by a position at a distance from social roles and social relationships, combined with various strategies for keeping more tenuous links with social environments.' This study demonstrates the usefulness, and importance, of using a phenomenological method to understand an experience from the perspective of the participant.

Phenomenologists focus on the social construction of the life-world, emphasising that people's actions can only be understood when they are situated in the taken-for-granted meanings and routines that constitute their everyday world. Further, phenomenologists emphasise that people's actions should be explained with reference to their conscious intentions, and with references to the typifications, or categories of understandings, that people develop. Phenomenological studies often utilise in-depth interviews (Chapter 3). More generally, phenomenological theory is an important influence on most of the qualitative research methodologies described later in this book.

SYMBOLIC INTERACTIONISM

Symbolic interactionism has its roots in American sociology, in contrast to the European philosophical focus of phenomenology, and the anthropological origins of ethnography. Symbolic interactionists examine how people make sense of their experiences through a common set of symbols. Symbolic interactionists emphasise that these symbols are developed and find meaning through and in interaction. While early interactionists were influenced by philosophical considerations, interactionism has been characterised by a strong empirical focus.

Arguably the most important symbolic interactionist was George Herbert Mead (1863–1931). At the time Mead was developing his thought, psychological behaviourists argued that, although minds and meanings may exist, they were irrelevant in explaining what people do. The behaviourists believed that only observation of behaviour could explain behaviour. In contrast, Mead (1934) argued for the importance of meanings and symbols for understanding human behaviour. Human beings construct action on the basis of the meanings of the objects they encounter. This insight is best expressed in Thomas' (1928, p. 584) dictum that 'if people define situations as real they are real in their consequences'.

Mead takes this analysis of meaning one step further when he describes way that the self becomes an object to itself. Through the process of role-ta a person imagines how they themselves appear to others, thus beco symbolic object to themselves (1934, p. 137). People then respond selves on the basis of the meanings they give to their actions through of role-taking. Herbert Blumer (1969) extended Mead's argument the 'in-process' nature of meaning. Meanings are continually cr and modified in interaction, 'on the fly'. This leads to a con very different to the Cartesian idea of a solid self-substance: a solid given entity that moves from one situation to process, continuously created and recreated in each s enters, held together by the slender thread of memor

Symbolic interactionism was a widely used p 1960s; during the 1970s it became less fashion recent resurgence in popularity, championed (1989b, 1997). There are a number of impo including Howard Becker, Erving Goffman important research in health-related areas, including studies of student doctors (Strauss et al. 1961), mental patients (Goffman 1961), and a number of other empirical studies on health-related topics (see Maines 1991b for a bibliography of Strauss' work).

Goffman's description of the process of internment of mental patients illustrates clearly the powerful way in which social relationships shape the self concept. Goffman describes the various stages of movement towards internment that involve a continual decline in status until not only interactions with relatives, doctors and friends, but also the physical settings, suggest to the patient that they are considered to have a non-viable self. Changes in the environment and in the way the individual is treated by others lead to changes in their self-conception, such that they come to think of themselves as mentally ill when they previously had not thought of themselves in such a way. Once inside the hospital, the patient is required to participate in 'confession', either in private or in group psychotherapy, where they must 'insightfully come to take, or affect to take, the hospital's view of [them]' (Goffman 1961, p. 143). The hospital demands that the patient recognise that they are mentally ill, because only then can the hospital begin to set itself to the business of 'straightening up'.

Symbolic interactionists argue that experiences take on meaning as they become symbolically significant through shared interaction. They study the interactional sources and development of these shared symbol systems and explain actions with reference to them. One of symbolic interactionism's most ~~nt~~ contributions to qualitative methods was the development of ~~discussed~~ in detail in the next chapter. Symbolic interactionist ~~utilised~~ methodologies such as in-depth interviews ~~~nter 4~~), unobtrusive methods (Chapter 5) and

king,
ning a
to them-
the process
emphasising
~~ted~~, recreated
~~eption~~ of the self
The self is [not] …
~~n~~other. It is rather a
~~o~~cial situation that one
(Berger 1975, p. 124).
~~r~~spective up until the late
~~ab~~le, but it has experienced a
~~b~~y the work of Norman Denzin
~~ant~~ other symbolic interactionists,
~~and~~ Anselm Strauss. Each conducted

of feminist thought
~~wa~~ys in which feminist
~~ist~~, feminist thought
the value and legiti-
and subjectivity of the
politicised the research
objective, feminists have
~~c~~ure of the whole research
~~se~~arch reports. Finally, femi-
~~se~~arch encounter, underlining
~~th~~e part of the research process.

While these aspects of qualitative research methods predate feminist research, feminism has accelerated their acceptance and examined their implications in considerable depth.

Denzin (1997, p. xiii) argues that 'ethnography is a gendered project'. Qualitative research cannot produce a gender-neutral story about the real world. As Dorothy Smith (1987, p. 152) puts it, 'it has been argued extensively that, until recently, established sociology had a concealed gender subtext, that it was thought, investigated, and written largely from the perspective of men'. Smith points out that this feminist critique has two foci. First, feminists highlighted the absence of women from both the topics being studied and the research reports. 'However, a second major theme in the critique has questioned established sociological methods.' The second theme pointed to how traditional positivist sociological methods objectify social processes, treating people as passive rather than actively constituting their social world. The sociological emphasis on organisational processes, concepts and variables has ignored or elided the 'actualities of a naturally existing world', and particularly ignored and made invisible roles and activities performed by women that are integral to these social organisations (Smith 1987, p. 153).

Sands (1996, p. 167) puts in succinctly when she says that, 'during the 1980s, feminist literature proposed the existence of a silent, tongue-tied "different" woman who craves to exercise her own voice'. Feminist theorists advocated research methods that enabled women to express their experience from their own perspective, contrasting this with positivist methodologies that claimed to be objective but which were constructed, conducted and analysed from the perspective of men. 'To enlarge our understanding as women of how things come about for us as they do, we need a method beginning from where women are as subjects' (Smith 1987, p. 153). Qualitative research methods that examined interpretations and meanings were thus very important to early feminist researchers. While feminism was important in facilitating the growth of qualitative methodologies, more recent feminists have argued that feminist research can be both qualitative and quantitative, depending on the research problem (Jayaratne and Abibail 1991).

Feminist theorists did not simply argue for the introduction of new topics, focusing on 'women's issues', into sociological research, or for a more interpretative and qualitative approach to sociological research. They also highlighted the role of political and social processes in the development of understandings about social life, both by society and by the sociologists who have studied social processes. In short, they argued that much of social research is androcentric, developed from the perspective of men to serve their political interests.

Dorothy Smith (1987, p. 154), for example, is unashamedly political, arguing that feminist social research is a form of 'consciousness raising' and that it attempts to identify how private experiences of oppression may by understood as part of a general system of oppression that shapes women's experience. Smith here echoes C. Wright Mills' (1959) well-known distinction between private troubles and public issues. However, Smith goes further than Mills in her specifically feminist argument that many of women's private troubles are not recognised as shared public issues because of established sociological methods that systematically ignore the experience of everyday life in general, and of women in particular. Bergen (1993, p. 202) makes a similar point when she argues that 'considering the consequences (on both a personal level and in terms of policy implications) of the research for the participants is essential to the work of feminists as their goal is the liberation of all women'. Mies (1991, p. 63) takes this argument a step further when she argues that the motto of a feminist approach could be: 'In order to understand a thing, one must change it.'

There are some problems with Smith's analysis, particularly as a product of her insistence that feminist theory offers a more accurate account, or science, of empirical reality. Drawing on postmodern perspectives, Clough (1994, p. 74) criticises Smith for not developing an 'analysis of how text-mediated discourse is related to unconscious desire, subjectivity, and production of the reality of experience'. Nonetheless, Smith's work is important because it exemplifies two significant impacts of feminist thought on sociological research. She focuses on the political dimensions of the research process, and on a methodology that attempts to understand experiences from the standpoint of those being studied. Feminist researchers, and particularly poststructuralist feminists, have highlighted this issue of reflexivity and the role of the researcher in the research process (Clough 1992; Sands 1996). This issue is discussed in more detail in the chapter on interviewing methods.

Raquel Bergen (1993) utilised feminist theory in her study of marital rape survivors. Her main research method was in-depth interviews. She states that feminism influenced her study not only through her choice of topic, but also the way in which she conducted the interviews. Bergen rejected the traditional interviewer role as distanced, emotionally neutral and disinterested. Rather, she become 'consciously partial', in the sense that she attempted to make the interview interactive, discussing her own biographical history and interacting on a 'personal level'. In particular, when some of her respondents became distressed when recounting their experiences, she did not attempt to be detached and 'objective'; rather, she 'spent a long time offering support' (p. 208). She argues that this provided her with important insights that would otherwise have been missed. This conscious partiality is consistent, Bergen argues, with feminism's goal of forming 'nonexploitative relationships' with research subjects.

Feminism has had a significant impact on qualitative research. Feminists helped to establish qualitative research as a legitimate methodology. Further, they have highlighted the political and reflexive nature of all social research. Feminist research has used a wide range of methodologies, including all of those described in the methods chapters of this book. Researchers using memory-work (Chapter 7) and participatory action research (Chapter 9) are more likely to draw on feminist theory than on other theoretical traditions.

POSTMODERNISM

Poststructuralism, postmodernism, cultural studies and deconstruction refer to a group of ideas and theories that have had a broad impact on the social sciences and humanities (Harvey 1989; Lemert 1997; Lucy 1997). While some of the postmodernist texts are difficult to understand, we believe that the insights they can provide are worth the effort. There are a number of themes in the postmodernist literature of relevance to qualitative methods that are not discussed here, including debates around the nature of subjectivity (Cadava et al. 1991) and different forms of writing (Richardson 1997). We will limit our discussion to a few examples of the way in which qualitative research has been influenced by postmodernist approaches, focusing on debates about the nature of 'reality'.

The implications of postmodernism and related theories for qualitative research are still being worked out, and are often associated with strongly expressed emotions (Richardson 1997, p. 127). This is clearly illustrated in the debate surrounding Denzin and Lincoln's *Handbook of Qualitative Research* (1994a). Snow and Morrill (1995, p. 341) criticised the book for 'privileging the postmodern perspective', arguing that the usefulness of postmodernism for qualitative research still needs to be demonstrated. In reply, Denzin and Lincoln (1995, p. 352) argue that innovation is at the heart of qualitative research: 'The open-ended nature of the qualitative research methods project leads to perpetual resistance against attempts to impose a single umbrella-like paradigm over the entire project.' Both observations are correct, but are used selectively by the authors to argue for different practices among qualitative researchers. Snow and Morrill are arguing for the value of tradition and tried-and-proved methods in qualitative research. Denzin and Lincoln, on the other hand, are arguing for the value of innovation and experimentation that characterise postmodernist qualitative research.

One of the first premises of the postmodernist perspective is that simple summaries or recipes (grand narratives) are not very good explanations. They argue for descriptions of the world that are complex, overlaid with competing and perhaps contradictory understandings. It is therefore rather difficult to briefly summarise the ideas of postmodernism when one of the assumptions of the theory is that simple summaries are not very useful. However, it is possible to illustrate some of the central assumptions that guide postmodernist thought.

Norman Denzin (1997, p. xiii) argues that 'the worlds we study are created, in part, through the texts that we write and perform about them'. What does this mean? Does Denzin mean that reality does not exist and that there are only texts and interpretations? Some qualitative researchers think that postmodernism involves a form of extreme scepticism and relativism that denies the existence of reality (Faberman 1992; Prus 1996). However, Faberman and Prus appear to have misunderstood what the postmodernists are saying. Faberman and Prus could be paraphrased as arguing that either reality exists independently of our interpretations, or it does not exist at all. Postmodernists, such as Denzin, refuse to accept this two-way choice. As we understand it, the point of much postmodernist theory is not to deny the existence of reality, but to point out that reality is as much constructed in talking and writing as it is 'out there'. However, it must be acknowledged that there is considerable diversity of opinion among postmodernists and some appear to advocate an approach that borders on the form of scepticist relativism criticised by Prus and Faberman, while others clearly do not.

The postmodernist analysis of 'reality' is difficult to understand. This is, in part, a consequence of the difficult language that many postmodernists use. However, they are also difficult to understand because they are talking about qualitative research in a very different way, and this difference in perspective is difficult to understand. In the next few paragraphs we will examine a quote from a postmodernist and then try to translate and reinterpret the meaning of the text.

Trinh is a film-maker who has developed a critique of contemporary ethnography derived from her analysis of modern cinema (Denzin 1997). The following extract is taken from her (1991) book *When the Moon Waxes Red*. While her thought is more complex than is represented in this short quote, it indicates some of her central ideas:

> The task of inquiring into all the divisions of a culture remains exacting, for the moments when things take on a proper name can only be positional, hence transitional. The function of any ideology in power is to represent the world positively unified. To challenge the regimes of representation that govern a society is to conceive of how politics can transform reality rather than merely ideologize it. (Trinh 1991, p. 2)

What does this very dense quote mean? Let us examine the first sentence. One of the reasons that postmodernist approaches are so threatening, and generate such heated debate, is that postmodernists do not simply argue for a different approach or for the usefulness of a particular kind of theory; they argue for a fundamental shift in the way that research and theorising are practised. The reference to 'positional and hence transitional' indicates Trinh's postmodernist approach. This means that things (including illness, doctors, or the moon) do not have any intrinsic definition, meaning or 'proper name'. Rather, their significance depends on the position of the person naming them, and may change as a consequence of changed social situations (hence they are transitional).

As Denzin (1989b, p. 74) puts it, Trinh 'seeks to undo the entire realist ethnographic project'. Terms such as truth, reality and facts come to have very different meanings in the postmodernist project. They no longer refer to taken-for-granted understandings of things 'out there'. Rather, they refer to social processes that are integrally part of the construction of facts, truth and reality. Trinh does not, however, believe that all interpretations are equal, or that there are no criteria by which analyses should be judged. She suggests that any study of culture (including ethnography and much of qualitative research) is demanding, or 'exacting'. In other words, postmodernists are not trying to avoid the issues of rigour that make qualitative research worthwhile (see Chapter 2).

The chapter from which the above quote is taken includes a number of stories about the moon. To illustrate her argument, Trinh reviews the way in which the meaning of the moon changes depending on historical period and social location of the person observing. For example, the Asian autumnal festival of the full moon involves street dancing, food and music, and can be understood, and valued, as a celebration of the 'feminine beauty and the carnal presence of the loved woman' (Trinh 1991, p. 3). However, these same celebrations of the moon were understood, and denigrated, by Chinese revolutionaries as symbols of counter-revolutionary Chinese feudalism. Similarly, Trinh points out how the colour changes of the moon are understood to symbolise impending calamity in some cultures, but have now been demystified and commodified by scientists who even so find them 'undeniably lovely' (p. 8).

Trinh also points out how the way in which the moon is understood is part of a broader societal culture and worldview. The repression of the festival of the full moon in revolutionary China is consistent with a more general attempt to remove the influence of feudalism from China's social organisation and culture. We understand Trinh's references to an 'ideology in power' and to 'regimes of representation' as referring to these more general cultural practices, such as revolutionary China's rejection of anything associated with feudalism. The world is 'positively unified' in the sense that the understandings of the moon are forced to be consistent with these more general cultural practices. The moon festival could not be tolerated by the revolutionary Chinese as it was not consistent with their desire to leave behind feudalism.

In her final sentence, Trinh says that 'to challenge the regimes of representation that govern a society is to conceive of how politics can transform reality rather than merely ideologize it' (p. 15). Trinh does not want to simply exchange one particular cultural formation with another. She wants to 'challenge' the way social and cultural formations are constructed and used. She wants people to recognise that the way things are described (including the moon, illness and doctors) are political acts that both reflect and change the nature of things, including the organisation of society. Trinh's title of her own book, *When the Moon Waxes Red*, draws on the imagery of the coloured moon as an indicator of impending calamity, suggesting that she has a broader conception of society as headed towards calamity, or at least as in crisis. This crisis is, in part, a product of the realisation that there is no correct way of understanding the moon. We should not attempt to find a correct way of understanding the moon, or, more generally, a final solution to all our health and social problems. Rather, postmodernists, such as Trinh, argue that we must recognise that all truth is partial and benefits some people and disadvantages others. In short, she could be paraphrased as arguing that qualitative researchers must stop pretending that we have final and correct answers.

Michel Foucault's (1967) study of mental illness provides a good example of how postmodernist insights have been applied to issues in health. One of the central themes of Foucault's work is that the treatment of madness since the Enlightenment reflects an Enlightenment emphasis on the importance of logic and reason (Samson 1995). Since the Enlightenment, truth has been understood to be discovered through logical reason. Thoughts, ideas and people who did not use logical reason were denigrated and silenced as not truthful. Prior to the Enlightenment, the mad and mentally ill were at liberty to wander and were not excluded from society. Following the Enlightenment, people who were mad were understood as being irrational, to be separated off from society in institutions. In other words, the silencing and repression of the mentally ill in institutions that began in the eighteenth century was a product of a particular post-Enlightenment culture that silenced and repressed anybody or anything that could not be subjected to logic and reason.

Postmodernism and poststructuralism have generated considerable debate among qualitative researchers. One of the themes of postmodernism is that specific understandings and interpretations reflect more general cultural patterns and understandings that are integrally political. Further, interpretations, and cultural patterns of meaning, are not fixed, but continually changing and transforming under the influence of the power of vested interests. Postmodernist qualitative researchers try to present analyses that acknowledge the situated and political nature of their particular analysis. Postmodernist and poststructuralist studies have used a range of methodologies, but they tend to favour unobtrusive methods (Chapter 5), often focusing on secondary analysis of existing data, or on historical analysis. Participatory action research (Chapter 9) is also consistent with this approach as a consequence of its integration of political action.

HERMENEUTICS

Hermeneutics is the 'critical theory of interpretation' (Rundell 1995, p. 10). It focuses on meanings and interpretations. Early Biblical hermeneutics examined Biblical texts. More recent hermeneutics has argued that human action can be interpreted like a text. The hermeneutic method is applied to social life. One of the central arguments of hermeneutics is that the tradition of interpretation influences how a text or set of events is understood. Positivists describe interpretations as uncertain, variable and dependent on the observer, and contrast interpretation to truth, which is certain and invariable. Hermeneutics turns this understanding on its head, by pointing out that truth is not as certain and invariable as it seems and by exploring the way in which interpretations and interpretative contexts make truth meaningful.

The implication of this hermeneutical analysis is that there is never any truth independent of interpretation. Every researcher brings assumptions, a tradition of understanding, to their research. These assumptions shape how the research is conducted, what is done and what is found. Positivists attempt to avoid, or deny, the effect of these assumptions, arguing that they can study reality independently of their interpretations. On the other hand, some postmodernists argue that there is no independent reality, or at least that the facts of what actually happened are irrelevant (Linde 1993, p. 14). Hermeneutics attempts to chart a middle ground between these two extremes. It acknowledges that our understandings of reality are always influenced by interpretations, that there is no independent truth. However, hermeneutics argues that our understandings of reality are also influenced by what happens in the world, providing us with historical information. It attempts to accept the influence of pre-existing interpretations and to examine how these shape the research process. These points are illustrated in the discussion below.

There are many similarities between phenomenology and hermeneutics. Some of the philosophers previously discussed in the section on phenomenology are sometimes considered as part of the hermeneutical tradition, particularly Heidegger. Phenomenology focuses on the detail of everyday life, or the 'life-world'. Hermeneutics, on the other hand, takes a broader view, with a fuller analysis of both the past and the future, and broader cultural factors (Rundell 1995, p. 12). Perhaps the most important current hermeneutical philosopher is Hans George Gadamer (1975). However, arguably, the person who has done the most to provide a bridge between philosophical hermeneutics and applied qualitative research is Paul Ricoeur (1984, 1985, 1988, 1992). Specifically, Ricoeur's concept of 'narrative-identity' provides an analytic bridge between philosophical hermeneutics and the empirical concerns of qualitative research.

Ricoeur (1988) argues that self-identity is not something that people are born with, that remains unchanged throughout life. However, neither is self-identity an illusion, as some of the poststructuralists have suggested. A person creates a sense of self-identity through telling a story, or narrative, about their life. This story provides a sense of continuity, of self-sameness, through their life. However, the story also changes as the person has new experiences and as new events occur. The story a person tells about themselves shapes how they understand and experience events, and events, in turn, also shape the self-story or narrative-identity. New events shape new self-stories and new self-stories lead to new actions and events. Life is an ongoing cycle of actions and constructing and reconstructing self-stories.

Douglas (Ezzy 1998) has used Ricoeur's hermeneutic theory of narrative-identity to examine the experience of living with HIV/AIDS. He identifies two self-stories told by 'Scott'. The first is a narrative-identity that assumes that HIV/AIDS means that Scott only has a short time to live. This identity develops as a result of events such as a serious illness and a positive HIV test. The narrative-identity also leads to particular actions, including changes in employment and lifestyle. The second narrative is of hope for a longer life with HIV/AIDS. This narrative-identity develops as a result of the event of new treatments for HIV/AIDS and Scott's taking up of these treatments.

Hermeneutics examines the cycle of interpretations as lived experience and storied interpretations continually influence each other. Hermeneutics provides a sophisticated philosophical response to some of the issues raised by the post-modernists, but it also suggests an alternative way of avoiding the problem of relativism that focuses on the hermeneutic circle of interpretations. As the above example suggests, narrative method (Chapter 6) is particularly consistent with hermeneutic theory, although hermeneutic theory can also be used to inform a variety of other empirical methods.

SUMMARY

Many of the theories outlined above make similar points. This is because they are all broadly consistent with the emphasis of qualitative research on under-standing meanings and interpretations. However, each has a long tradition with distinctive emphases. Each theory will be more useful in some research projects and less relevant to others. The qualitative researcher should attempt to identify the theoretical tradition that best suits their research topic and explore this theory in detail. Useful theoretical traditions can often be identified by review-ing which theories other researchers have used in similar studies. However, new insights and understandings can also be obtained by applying a new theoretical tradition to an old research topic. Good qualitative research depends on a combination of careful research and some imagination and intuition on the part of the researcher in deciding which theory and methodology will provide the best results for the particular topic under study.

Qualitative methods are currently in a liminal or transitional state (Denzin 1997). Positivist, interpretative and postmodernist theory, methods and evalua-tion criteria coexist. There is no singular, authoritative and agreed-upon set of methods for conducting qualitative research. 'Until consensus about this new form of textuality occurs, each position is obliged to clarify the standards and programs that organize its practices' (Denzin 1997, p. 21). That is to say, qualitative researchers should not assume that the particular theory and research method used in their project will be understood by all other qualitative researchers. If a piece of research is to be meaningfully understood and assessed by other qualitative researchers, the researcher must explicitly state the theoretical tradition and methodological criteria employed.

Tutorial exercise

Existing research suggests that many teenagers engage in brief sexual encounters when they are on holiday and that they are less likely to use condoms when they do so. Public health authorities are concerned about an outbreak of sexually transmitted diseases such as chlamydia, herpes, hepatitis B and HIV. Imagine that you have been commissioned to do some research on the processes that lead teenagers to be less likely to use condoms when they are on holiday. What might be some of these reasons? Can you suggest how using feminist theory might facilitate your examination of some reasons but not others? How would this differ if you drew on symbolic interactionist theory?

Further reading

Ethnography
Geertz, C., 1973, *The Interpretation of Cultures*, Basic Books, New York.
Rosaldo, R., 1989, *Culture and Truth*, Routledge, London.
Phenomenology
Becker, C., 1992, *Living and Relating: An Introduction to Phenomenology*, Sage, Newbury Park.
Moustakas, C., 1994, *Phenomenological Research Methods*, Sage, Thousand Oaks.
Symbolic interactionism
Blumer, H., 1969, *Symbolic Interactionism, Perspective and Method*, Prentice-Hall, Englewood Cliffs, NJ.
Denzin, N., 1989, *Interpretive Interactionism*, Sage, Newbury Park.
Feminism
Clough, P., 1994, *Feminist Thought*, Blackwell, Oxford.
Smith, D., 1987, *The Everyday World as Problematic: A Feminist Sociology*, Open University Press, Milton Keynes.
Postmodernism
Clough, P., 1992, *The End(s) of Ethnography*, Sage, Newbury Park.
Trinh, T. Minh-ha, 1991, *When the Moon Waxes Red: Representation, Gender and Cultural Politics*, Routledge, New York.

Hermeneutics

Ricoeur, P., 1992, *Oneself as Another* (trans. K. Blamey), University of Chicago Press, Chicago.

Rundell, J., 1995, 'Gadamer and the Circles of Hermeneutics', in D. Roberts (ed.), *Reconstructing Theory: Gadamer, Habermas, Luhmann*, Melbourne University Press, Melbourne.

2

Rigour, Ethics and Sampling

Introduction

The ultimate test of a study's worth is that the findings ring true to people and let them see things in new ways. In this case, I hope those personally familiar with depression recognize themselves in the words of my respondents and feel that my analysis illuminates their life situations. Aside from the scientific worth of what I have done, such a response is important to me because I believe that knowledge and understanding are the fundamental preconditions for positive change. (Karp 1996, p. 202)

We can never fully know what consequences our work will have on others. We cannot control context and readings. But we can have some control over what we choose to write and how we write it. At this point in my life, for example, I could not do a community study like Street Corner Society *[Whyte 1955]. I wouldn't want to take responsibility for how I brought the 'community' into my text (theory, debates, and so on); I wouldn't want to 'give voice' to real, live people who know each other and could identify each other in my text. For me, it might be 'text'; for them, it is life. (Richardson 1997, p. 117)*

David Karp and Laurel Richardson highlight the two main aspects of qualitative research that are dealt with in this chapter. First, Karp highlights the importance of following correct procedure, a rigorous methodology and a purposive sampling strategy. These are important, not simply because they ensure the 'scientific worth' of a study but also because a research report based on a rigorous and well-designed study is the foundation for positive change.

Second, Richardson highlights the importance of the qualitative researcher never losing sight of the ethical, political and very real consequences of their research. It is no longer acceptable to hide behind a vague claim to be doing 'objective' research, the political consequences of which are someone else's concern. Whatever one may think of poststructuralism and postmodernism, they are certainly correct when they demonstrate the inherently political nature of even the most 'objective' of research. Social research reports in general, and qualitative research reports in particular, are inherently moral and political documents that must be weighed in these terms. As Richardson so piquantly puts it, while for the researcher it may be just another report, 'for them, it is life'.

This chapter focuses on specific procedures that are the foundation of rigorous and ethical research practice. Rigorous methodological procedures are essential if the research is to be accepted as reliable and useful research by other qualitative researchers. However, as we argue in the chapter, the detailed following of procedures alone will never ensure that a study is rigorous and ethical. Procedures and rules must be situated within the broader ethical and political frameworks of the lives of the people being studied, the audience of the report and the researcher(s) themselves.

The chapter is divided into four sections. First, we provide a theoretical introduction to the problem of rigour that addresses many of the philosophical and epistemological issues raised by the postmodernists. Second, we cover a number of specific aspects or techniques for ensuring rigour, including theoretical rigour, methodological rigour, interpretative rigour, triangulation, evaluative rigour (including ethical and political considerations), and rigorous reflexivity (which examines the role of the researcher in the research). Third, we review a number of different sampling strategies that are commonly used in qualitative research and comment on the problem of the generalisability of qualitative research findings. The final section provides a short discussion of theoretical sampling, a concept that is regularly referred to in qualitative research but often misunderstood.

THEORETICAL APPROACHES TO RIGOUR

We use the term *rigour* to refer to the issues that are raised by the terms *validity* and *reliability*. Validity can be defined as a concern with the questions: Does the instrument or measurement strategy actually measure what the evaluator purports to measure? Does it yield data that accurately represent 'reality'? Reliability refers to 'the consistency or dependability of the instrument or measurement strategy' (Goodwin and Goodwin 1984, p. 417). As is obvious from the language of the definitions, these terms derive from experimental and quantitative research methodologies. There are clearly a number of problems in applying them to qualitative research methods. However, they still indicate issues that need to be addressed by qualitative researchers.

The concepts of validity and reliability have two functions. First, they are used to assess whether statistical and experimental studies are worthy of being trusted as a basis for further research (Mason 1996; Mishler 1990). Second, if a study has validity and reliability, this says something about the relationship of the research findings to the object of the study (Altheide and Johnson 1994). We do not believe, even after we have encountered postmodernism, that this latter concern should be abandoned. However, we also do not accept a simplistic positivist framing of these issues. We therefore use the term 'rigour' to indicate that we think the issues raised by the concepts of validity and reliability are important in qualitative research, but that they need to be conceptualised differently. Rigorous qualitative studies are more trustworthy and useful than others. Rigorous qualitative research also attempts to provide information that is related to events that happen in the world.

At the heart of the problem with the concepts of validity and reliability in qualitative research is the relationship between the observer and observed 'reality'. Is observed reality independent of the observer? At the other extreme, some postmodernists appear to argue that there is no such thing as observed reality, we are all observers. In between these two extremes is a more sophisticated approach, which addresses the complex interplay of the observer and the reality of what they observe. We will address this issue through a discussion of four approaches: naive realism, interpretative realism, relativism, and hermeneutics.

Naive realism and rigour

> Naive realists assume that there is a real world, independent of human interpretation. (Altheide and Johnson 1994, p. 490)

According to naive realists, to be rigorous is to ensure that the research describes what is actually there in the real world (validity), and that this can be done repeatedly (reliability). This can be done by following set methods and procedures.

Positivists are naive realists. At the heart of positivist understandings of social research is the belief that what is being studied is external to the observer, does not change with time and is not influenced by simply being observed (Denzin 1989b, p. 24). They believe that there is a real world out there and that our understandings of it are not, or should not be, influenced by the social and historical location of the observer. The concepts of validity and reliability, as defined above, only make sense if these assumptions are accepted.

Can naive realism be used in qualitative research? While a rock may stay the same no matter what the cultural background of the scientist observing it (although some would argue even with this), the assumptions of naive realism are more problematic in studies of people's beliefs and actions. For example, it was previously thought that 'culture' was something objective, that could be observed and measured, like a natural object. All that was required, argued traditional positivist approaches, was correct questioning techniques, and people would reveal their 'culture' to the researcher. However, recent anthropological critique of the concept of culture suggests that this approach ignores the 'fragmentary, contested and partial' nature of culture. It also ignores the complex variations in the way people experience culture (McEwan 1993, p. vii). For example, part of the 'culture' of modern Australia is the belief that physical illness should be treated by a doctor, and not by a priest alone. However, some Australian churches still practise faith healing, and many seriously ill people are prepared to experiment with such practices, although they may not tell you that they have done so unless some level of trust has first been established. Unlike 'things' such as rocks or chemicals, culture changes depending on its social and historical location and who is observing.

The assumptions made by positivists about the research process are in direct conflict with the practice and methodology of qualitative research (Mishler 1990). Qualitative researchers typically do not study things, but people. They study the way people interpret their experiences, their shared understandings or culture, their patterns of behaviour. The researcher is also a person who is part of the society they are studying. Understandings and interpretations change, and may be different in different social locations and may even differ from time to time for the same person in the same social situation. Further, the actions of social researchers can also change what they observe. There is an apocryphal story that Douglas once heard about a social researcher who interviewed a woman working in a factory. She was asked: 'Do you ever think about going on holidays?' She replied: 'No, never.' However, some years later she was talking about this question to another social researcher, and she said: 'You know, ever since I was asked that question, I haven't stopped thinking about going on holidays.'

Interpretative realism and rigour

> Interpretive realists assume reality exists, but can only be known imperfectly due to reality's interpreted nature.

According to interpretative realists, rigour involves the careful study of social relations, taking into account the influence of subjectivity but attempting to minimise its effects. One tradition of interpretative realism derives from Weberian and phenomenological sociology, which argued that social researchers should attempt to be 'value free' and 'bracket' their assumptions about the world during their research. Berger (1977, p. vii) describes this approach succinctly when he says:

> Sociology is a systematic attempt to see the social world as clearly as possible, to understand it without being swayed by one's own hopes and fears. This ideal of lucidity (one could even call it selfless lucidity) is intended by what Max Weber called the value-freeness of the social sciences.

Interpretative realism is the most common approach to the problem of rigour in qualitative methods. It has also been called 'postpositivism' (Guba and Lincoln 1994). Interpretative realism corresponds to the modernist phase in ethnography (Denzin 1997, p. 17). As Denzin points out, this phase is characterised by an attempt to formalise the methods of qualitative research in a manner that parallels the methods of the physical sciences, but takes into account the interpretative nature of human activity studied by qualitative methods (Kirk and Miller 1986).

Postmodernism, relativism and rigour

Postmodernist relativism argues that there is no 'real' world, only interpretation.

Postmodernists either reject the idea of rigour or reconceptualise it as involving the demonstration of the absence of a clear relationship between reality and a study's findings (Lather 1993). Rigour may also be reconceptualised as a moral and ethical task focused on emancipation and political action, particularly when postmodernism is combined with either feminist or socialist ideals (Beilharz 1994; Clough 1992).

According to postmodernist understandings, there is no independent knowable phenomenal reality. All knowledge is based on assumptions and interpretations that do not just shape what is seen but also actually create what is seen. If pursued, this leads to a form of extreme relativism and scepticism. Extreme relativism is the idea that all beliefs and interpretations are equal, since there is no objective reality against which they can be compared. Tyler (1986, p. 138), for example, argues for a 'post-modern ethnography'. He suggests that 'no object of any kind precedes and constrains the ethnography. It creates its own objects in its unfolding and the reader supplies the rest' (p. 138). Similarly, Hammersley (1992b, p. 48) criticises relativist postmodern ethnography for abandoning any attempt to represent an 'independent reality'. This leads, he suggests, to a form of relativism where all accounts are equal.

It is important to note that many postmodernists do not subscribe to radical relativism, that to accuse them of this is a simplification of the various postmodernist positions, and that in some senses it grossly oversimplifies a complex set of ideas. For example, 'standpoint epistemology' is a predominantly feminist, postmodernist alternative to positivism and interpretative realism (Mason 1996, p. 151). Eschewing the idea that ethnography can be objective, feminist standpoint theorists argue that each ethnographer studies and speaks about the world from their own 'standpoint'. 'The world of human experience must be studied from the point of view of the historically and culturally situated individual' (Denzin 1997, p. 87).

One of the problems with some forms of postmodernism and poststructuralism is that their focus on multiple interpretations is not very useful. Lather

(1993, p. 674) is a self-confessed feminist poststructuralist. She explains her decision to conduct empirical research as a result of the extravagances of post-modernist methodologies. She describes her empirical research among women with HIV/AIDS as 'an opportunity to wrestle across the deconstructive excesses and extreme forms of social constructionism characteristic of some poststructuralisms via the political responsibility to real bodies and political rage entailed in such a study' (p. 684).

Postmodernist and poststructuralist approaches should not be dismissed out of hand. They have examined a number of central, and systematically ignored, problems in qualitative research, including the role of the researcher in the research, the multiple and contradictory nature of interpretations, the problematic nature of 'reality', and the politically infused nature of all interpretations (Denzin 1997). However, it is also important to recognise the potential problems with postmodernist frames, including the difficulty of using the approach in some of the concrete research tasks performed by qualitative researchers.

Hermeneutic realism and rigour

> Hermeneutic realism argues that there is a real world, and our experience of it is always and already interpreted. (Ezzy 1998)

According to hermeneutic realism, rigorous research both provides information that is related to events that happen in the world, and considers the political and socially constructed nature of the research findings. This approach is similar to the 'analytic realism' of Altheide and Johnson (1994) and Hammersley's (1992b) 'subtle realism'. These approaches develop out of a response to the problems raised by the postmodernists and poststructuralists, but do not accept all of their conclusions.

Hermeneutic realism rejects the (modernist) idea shared by both naive realism and scepticism that 'knowledge must be defined as beliefs whose validity is known with certainty' (Hammersley 1992b, p. 45). Hermeneutics, like pragmatism, is not particularly interested in continuously debating philosophical problems. It is prepared to live with uncertainty, with human finitude, with the reality that we always know imperfectly. However, hermeneutics is also concerned with conducting empirical research and confronting the concrete methodological and political issues that research raises.

These approaches assume that there are independent knowable phenomena, but our knowledge of them is always shaped by culture and socially constructed. The interpreted nature of human existence has to be accepted, but this does not mean there is no such thing as objectivity or valid knowledge. These concepts are utilised, but their political and problematic nature is explicitly acknowledged. Altheide and Johnson (1994, p. 489) summarise the argument clearly:

The applicability of the concept of validity [or rigour] presented here does not depend on the existence of some absolute truth or reality to which an account can be compared, but only on the fact that there exist ways of assessing accounts that do not depend entirely on the features of the account itself, but are in some way related to those things that the account claims to be about.

TECHNIQUES FOR ENSURING RIGOUR

This section reviews a number of specific aspects or techniques for ensuring rigour in qualitative research. Theoretical rigour refers to sound reasoning and argument and the choice of methods appropriate to the research problem. Methodological or procedural rigour refers to clear documentation of methodological and analytic decisions. Interpretative rigour examines the problem of interpreting data, with an extended discussion of the practice of inter-rater reliability checks. Rigour can also be enhanced through triangulation or data sources, methods, researchers and theories. The ethical and political aspects of qualitative research are considered in the section on evaluative rigour. Finally, rigorous reflexivity refers to honest reporting of the role of the researcher in the research.

Theoretical rigour

A study has theoretical and conceptual rigour if the theory and concepts are appropriately chosen so that the research strategy is consistent with the research goals. Theoretical rigour is an extension of the issues discussed in the previous chapter. It ensures that a study integrates the research problem with the method it utilises and the concepts it employs. Theoretical rigour is also a product of soundly constructed arguments and analysis. Points should follow on from one another and be clearly supported with evidence from previous research and literature. One of the ways that this is assessed is through the peer review process through publication, where external peers and other relevant audiences evaluate the trustworthiness of a particular study (Goodwin and Goodwin 1984; Mishler 1990).

Another reason a study may lack theoretical rigour is if it applies concepts to experiences or events that do not properly describe them. Mason (1996, p. 90) observes that this issue is related to sampling strategies: 'For each sampling decision, therefore, you should ask whether this person, or these people, or this or these documents, or this or these instances or experiences, can potentially tell you what you want to know.' For example, imagine a study of why some groups of people do not seek medical advice when they experience symptoms related to sexually transmitted diseases. A set of focus groups about health beliefs may seem an obvious research strategy. However, it may not be the most useful tool in a study. If the researcher uses a health beliefs theoretical orientation, they have already assumed that the units of analysis are the individual and the problem is located in people's understandings. The problem may be related to lack of access to medical services, as is the case in many rural communities, and may have little to do with health beliefs. In this case, the units of analysis should be communities, not individuals. The conceptual shift from health behaviours to health beliefs shifts the focus of the research from access and structurally generated inequalities to a framework focused on the individual that potentially blames the victim.

Methodological or procedural rigour

Qualitative research reports should provide an explicit account of how the research was conducted by the researcher (Burgess 1984; Sliverman et al. 1990; Willms et al. 1990). As Ratner (1996, p. 319) puts it, 'procedural rigour' involves carefully documenting the means of arriving at qualitative research findings in order to avoid unwarranted overgeneralisation and 'unsubstantiated conclusions'. Altheide and Johnson (1994, p. 493) suggest that such an account could address problems such as: how access was obtained to organisations and individuals; how the researcher approached and presented himself or herself to participants; the development of trust and rapport; how mistakes and surprises were dealt with; how the data was collected and recorded; the method of data coding and analysis; and the production of the report. An explicit account of refusals to participate may also be kept.

Maintaining and reporting an audit trail of methodological and analytic decisions allows others to assess the significance of the research. As Stevens and Doerr (1997, p. 525) put it, the dependability of their study's findings 'were ascertained by keeping an audit trail of methodological and analytic decisions'. This will enhance credibility and allow other researchers to decide whether the research is worthy of being relied upon as a basis for decision making and conducting future research.

Interpretative rigour and inter-rater reliability

Mason (1996, p. 149) observes that 'many researchers encounter crises of confidence about the validity of their own interpretations'. We would add that this is, perhaps, a particularly common problem among new researchers. An account has interpretative rigour if it accurately represents the understandings of events and actions within the framework and worldview of the people engaged in them. While postmodernists have argued that there are no final grounds for accepting interpretations as 'accurate', this does not mean that all interpretations are equal or will be equally acceptable to participants in a study.

One way that interpretative rigour can be ensured is to demonstrate clearly how the interpretation was achieved. This is an aspect of methodological rigour described above. Mishler (1990, p. 437) argues that the trustworthiness of interpretations in a qualitative study can be improved by including substantial parts of, or complete, primary texts in the research report, or by making them available to other researchers. Plenty of direct quotes and complete interviews provide the reader with a clearer sense of the evidence on which the analysis is based. Making the primary text available allows other researchers to 'inspect it and assess the adequacy with which the methods and interpretations represent the data'.

The complexity of demonstrating interpretative rigour is illustrated in the debates surrounding the issue of inter-rater reliability in qualitative research. Daly and others (1992, p. 204), for example, use a number of independent observers to address 'the problem of research bias'. The observers read transcripts of clinical encounters between cardiologists and their patients and graded them on an agreed set of categories. The authors then report that 'statistical analysis showed that inter-observer agreement between the independent gradings of the cardiologist and the sociologist researchers was good' (p. 204). The strategy in this research clearly draws on a modernist realist-interpretivist framework. The researchers assume that interpretations generated by 'independent' observers will result in accurate interpretations of an objective reality.

On the other hand, researchers who have rejected the notion of one objective and independent reality may still want to 'demonstrate that [their] interpretation is indeed valid, without resorting to claims to ultimate truth and objectivity' (Mason 1996, p. 150). Armstrong and his associates (1997) conclude their analysis of the role of inter-rater reliability in qualitative research arguing that the interpretative processes inherent in qualitative research create a number of problems for modernist or realist-interpretative frameworks. They argue that claims to objectivity in qualitative research based on inter-rater reliability checks make the same mistake as traditional statistical methods, assuming that there is one true meaning to a text, uninfluenced by the beliefs and understandings that the researcher brings to the research task. Armstrong and his associates found that independent observers identified similar themes but interpreted them in a variety of ways, reflecting their different general frameworks of understanding based on geographical location, disciplinary training and biographical history.

Inter-rater reliability may be a useful rhetorical tool to convince positivist researchers of the rigour of qualitative research, and this is how Daly and her associates use it. However, if a researcher rejects the modernist and positivist assumption that there is one true objective interpretation, inter-rater reliability can still be a useful tool to provide a more complex and nuanced understanding of the possible interpretations of texts. It does not, however, guarantee the reliability or validity of interpretations. We contend that validity and reliability are not established simply through following procedures that ensure findings validly and reliably reflect 'reality'. Rather, the social and interpretative process is integral to establishing rigour. Knowledge is legitimised when external peers, the people studied and other relevant audiences agree that interpretations and conclusions are accurate reflections of the phenomenon (Atkinson et al. 1991).

Triangulation

Triangulation, or the use of multiple methods, involves using a combination of methods, researchers, data sources and theories in a research project. Advocates of triangulation recognise that different results will be obtained by using different research methods and different researchers, informed by different theoretical traditions (Denzin 1970, p. 298). Research methods are not neutral tools that will produce the same results regardless of the method. Triangulation addresses this problem.

Early advocates saw triangulation as a strategy that would enable researchers to rise above 'the personalistic biases that stem from single methodologies' (Denzin 1970, p. 300). However, more recent qualitative researchers have cautioned against seeing triangulation as a way of discovering what is actually going on by comparing one method against another and deciding which one represents the truth (Mason 1996, p. 149). Rather, triangulation allows the research to develop a complex picture of the phenomenon being studied, which might otherwise be unavailable if only one method were utilised (Flick 1992; Lucchini 1996).

There are four distinct types of triangulation:
- Data Source Triangulation involves the use of multiple information sources. For example, in his classic study of mental asylums, Goffman (1961) obtains information from medical staff, patients, administrative staff, and written notes and files.
- Methods Triangulation involves the use of multiple research methodologies. Goffman (1961) utilised long interviews, participation observation, documentary analysis, and unobtrusive observation.
- Researcher Triangulation involves the inclusion of a variety of researchers in the research process. In their study of women living with HIV/AIDS, Lather and Smithies (1997) explore the different perspectives that the two main researchers bring to the research. They also include their participants as co-researchers to obtain yet another perspective.
- Theory Triangulation involves drawing on multiple theoretical perspectives to provide new insights. Lather and Smithies (1997), for example, utilise a combination of feminism and postmodernism to inform their research.

Evaluative rigour: ethics and politics

> To a greater or lesser extent, 'politics' suffuses all sociological research. (Punch 1986, p. 13)

The ethical and political aspects of qualitative research have two main dimensions. First, ethics and political aspects must be addressed procedurally. This involves obtaining ethical approval from the various organisational bodies that may have jurisdiction over the particular research project. In some cases, there may be a number of ethics committees that require an ethics application, including universities, hospitals and other professional and bureaucratic bodies. Following correct procedure may also involve adequate consultation with relevant community leaders and representatives. Second, a simple completion of the tasks required by procedural ethics does not address the more general issue of considering the political and social consequences of the research for the participants. As Punch (1986) suggests, politics, moral issues and ethics infuse the research process in a way that procedural ethics can never address.

One of the concerns of ethics committees is the potential of qualitative studies to cause distress to participants. Researchers often arrange with appropriate agencies to provide counselling to participants if they consider they require professional assistance with the issues raised in a qualitative interview (Lather 1993; Punch 1986). However, sensitively conducted qualitative research typically docs not disturb pcoplc to thc cxtcnt that thcy rcquirc counsclling, cvcn if the issue is potentially distressing. Grafanaki (1996) notes that qualitative research often promotes reflexivity, self-awareness and empowerment among the parties involved. This is primarily due to the nature of qualitative methods, which 'allow subjects to tell stories in their own words … [that can be] cathartic and therapeutic in itself' (p. 329).

Most ethical codes require the confidentiality of participants be maintained. As Bulmer (1982, p. 225) puts it: 'Identities, locations of individuals and places are concealed in published results, data collected are held in anonymized form, and all data are kept securely confidential.' Sometimes complex strategies are used by researchers to ensure the anonymity of participants, such as combining various parts of different participants' responses to make a composite picture (Lincoln and Guba 1985). Whether subjects should be assured of anonymity is still debated in the methodological literature (Lofland and Lofland 1984, p. 29). In some places, research data may be subpoenable and guarantees of confidentiality may be very costly to sustain. If research is to be conducted that may involve activities of a legally ambiguous nature, the researcher should carefully consider the possible consequences of their research and the significance of their assurances of confidentiality.

Ethics committees also typically require assurances of informed consent associated with a clear statement of the nature of participation in the research. While researchers must address the issues raised by their ethics committee, the complex, and often intimate, nature of much qualitative research makes it difficult to set a general set of abstract guidelines (Madak 1994). While participants can typically be informed about the goals and general nature of most research projects, qualitative research is often exploratory, with a concomitant lack of clarity about the consequences of the studies' findings (Ramos 1989). Within this context, researchers should ensure that all aspects of their study are handled in a way 'which is respectful of the human rights, and needs, of the participant' (Batchelor and Briggs 1994, p. 949).

The requirement of informed consent can be broadly interpreted as implying 'a responsibility on the sociologist to explain as fully as possible, and in terms meaningful to participants, what the research is about, who is undertaking it and financing it, why it is being undertaken, and how it is to be disseminated' (Hornsby-Smith 1993, p. 63). Research that involves deceiving participants about the nature and intentions of the research is generally considered unethical, because of the potential risk of harm to the participant and the emphasis placed on informed consent (Goode 1996). However, there is considerable debate about the ethical nature of research involving deception. For example, should researchers repeatedly inform participants of the nature of the research (Punch 1986, p. 37)? Jack Douglas (1976, p. 57) argues that many of the arguments for informed consent are inconsistent and that covert research is an acceptable research practice in many situations. He suggests that problems of misinformation, lies and deception are integral to most research projects and are not as easily addressed as is suggested by some of the ethical codes arguing for informed consent.

Ethical issues often arise as part of the research process, unanticipated during planning. For example, a research project on sexual practice may find that one of its interviewers is uncomfortable asking some of the questions. The resolution of ethical issues often has consequences for the research process, in this case requiring the recruitment and training of a new interviewer. Batchelor and Briggs (1994) point out that open and easy communication between a research coordinator or director and the researchers actually conducting the research tasks will help to ensure that many ethical dilemmas are identified and addressed early in the process.

Most professional associations with members who conduct qualitative research have codes or guidelines for ethical behaviour in research, and the guidelines relevant to a particular research process should be carefully reviewed. In Australia, the National Health and Medical Research Council has a regularly updated *Statement on Ethical Conduct in Research Involving Humans*. Michael Hornsby-Smith (1993, p. 63) observes that most organisations are moving away from restrictive codes of conduct to more general guidelines for ethical practice: 'These recognise that, in the last analysis, it is the individual researcher who must take responsibility for the methods he or she uses and that rigid codes are too restrictive and cannot be applied to every conceivable research situation.'

Rigorous reflexivity

Qualitative research should also be reflexive. Mason (1996, p. 6) argues that 'this means that the researcher should constantly take stock of their actions and their role in the research process, and subject these to the same critical scrutiny as the rest of their "data" '. Reflexive research acknowledges that the researcher is part and parcel of the setting, context and culture they are trying to understand and analyse. That is to say, the researcher is the instrument of the research. Altheide and Johnson (1994, p. 493) argue that 'a key part of the ethnographic ethic is how we account for ourselves. Good ethnographies show the hand of the ethnographer.' This point could be symbolised by the practice of writing ethnographies with or without using the word 'I'. Qualitative research reports that avoid the pronoun 'I' are, in some senses, attempting to disguise the role of the researcher in the research. Rigorous qualitative research is honest about the role of the researcher in the project.

Reflexivity is, in one sense, at the heart of Lather's (1993) postmodernist conceptualisation of rigour. Lather provides a useful overview of four different ways that validity can be reconceptualised within a postmodernist frame. Her main point is to demonstrate that there is no final arbiter of truth. For example, she suggests that to define 'validity as simulacra/ironic validity' shifts the focus of research from describing social reality to demonstrating that it is very difficult to identify social reality (p. 679). Her final postmodernist frame of 'voluptuous validity/situated validity' incorporates a feminist commitment to emancipation and an attempt at 'blurring the lines between the genres of poetry and social science reporting' (p. 683). That is to say, validity is achieved through reflexively understanding the integral role of our political commitments in shaping the way research is conducted. According to Lather, research that pretends it is not political is not rigorous.

Rigour: a summary

We see the opportunity to conduct qualitative research as a privilege. Douglas and Pranee have often come away from a long interview with a deep sense of gratitude and debt to the person who has just shared many intimate details of their life with an interviewer whom they do not know and will probably never see again. Within this context, the onus is on the researcher to deal with their participants with integrity, honesty and fairness.

SAMPLING STRATEGIES FOR QUALITATIVE RESEARCH

This section examines the place of sampling in qualitative research. Issues addressed include: the objective of sampling, including a discussion of the nature of the generalisability of the findings from qualitative studies; the units to be sampled; types of sampling strategies; the sample size; and rigour in sampling.

Sampling and generalising findings

The objective of sampling in qualitative research is fundamentally different from that in quantitative research such as surveys, epidemiological studies or case control studies. The goal in these methods is to ensure that the sample is statistically representative and that the findings can be confidently generalised to the population from which the sample is taken.

Sampling in qualitative research is not concerned with ensuring that the findings can be statistically generalised to the whole population. Rather, sampling in qualitative research is *purposive*. The aim is to describe the processes involved in a phenomenon, rather than its distribution. A sample will aim, for example, to identify the cases that will provide a full and sophisticated understanding of all aspects of the phenomenon. The aim is to select information-rich cases for studying in depth. Qualitative research typically uses nonprobability sampling techniques. The aim is not to generalise about the *distribution* of experiences or processes, but to generalise about the *nature* and interpretative processes involved in the experiences.

For example, Karp's (1996) study of clinical depression is based on a small sample of fifty people. The aim of the study is to describe the experience of being clinically depressed by focusing on the processes involved, such as diagnosis, coping with treatment regimes and adapting to symptoms. Many people use a variety of medications and continue to use them for many years. The aim is not to describe how long the average clinically depressed person is likely to use medication after their diagnosis (this is a quantitative question), but to describe why people often continue to use drugs. The focus of the research is on describing in depth the experiences and meanings. Karp's study does not tell us what percentage of people continue to use medication five years after their initial diagnosis. However, it does suggest why people might continue to use medication for such long periods. The aim is to provide generalisations about social processes and typical patterns of meanings.

Inexperienced qualitative researchers often confuse the two sampling strategies of qualitative and quantitative methods. We have seen proposals for qualitative research that attempt to include some quantitative aspects, such as scales for measuring some facet of the phenomenon under investigation, or that suggest very large samples. While it can be appropriate to include scales in some qualitative research, the reason that researchers want to include them is often a product of confusion about the goal of the study. The aim of qualitative research is not, for example, to measure the mental health of people with HIV/AIDS, but to understand the interpretative process through which these people come to be depressed or hopeful. While it may be useful to include a scale to measure a respondent's mental health, the main purpose of scales is to allow statistical comparisons between groups of cases, and this is not done in qualitative research.

People are typically, but not necessarily, the units of analysis in qualitative research. Other sampling units might include settings or places (beaches, beats, cities, hospitals), events (meetings, carnivals, drinking), things or artifacts (newspaper headlines, advertisements, garbage). A sampling frame is a list or account of all the possible people or things that might be sampled for the project. Some examples of sampling frames include: all people clinically diagnosed with depression; everyone between the ages of 20 and 50 years who has lost a job in the last year; or all people who have received a terminal diagnosis in the last three months. A qualitative research project should first define its sampling frame and then explain what sampling method or selection criteria will be used to select from the sampling frame.

Sampling methods

While qualitative samples do not attempt to be statistically representative, this does not mean that sampling in qualitative research proceeds without any guidance. Purposive sampling, for example, aims to select information-rich cases for in-depth study to examine meanings, interpretations, processes and theory. Theoretical sampling (discussed below) selects cases on theoretical grounds derived from the analysis of cases already examined.

Convenience sampling is the least desirable form of sampling within qualitative research and should be avoided if at all possible. A study of hospitalised stroke patients may begin by sampling from a nearby hospital to which the researcher has easy access (a convenience sample). However, if it is a private hospital in an expensive suburb, the sort of people attending the hospital are likely to have a distinctive experience and some other sampling technique would be required to provide a sample that represents all types of experiences of stroke. While convenience may provide a good place to begin, it is better to use theoretical or purposive sampling.

There is a wide range of strategies for selecting samples. The following list is drawn from various sources but relies heavily on the list provided by Patton (1990, p. 169), who describes a rich variety of qualitative sampling strategies under the general heading of purposeful sampling.

Extreme or deviant case sampling
Cases are selected that are unusual or have distinctive characteristics that illustrate the processes being examined. The aim is to elicit rich and detailed information that provides a new perspective on more typical cases. For example, Browne's (1987) *When Battered Women Kill* uses extreme responses to domestic violence to provide an insight into the effects of domestic violence and the processes and structure of experiences involved.

Maximum variation sampling

This sampling strategy aims to select cases that provide for wide variations in the experience or process being examined. For example, comparing people who recover extremely quickly with those who take inordinate amounts of time to recover may provide some important insights into the recovery process.

Homogeneous group sampling

In this instance, the sample is selected to minimise variation and to maximise homogeneity in order to describe the experience or process in as much depth and detail as possible. Focus group participants are often selected along these lines (see Chapter 4).

Typical case sampling

'The case is specifically selected because it is not in any way atypical, extreme, deviant or intensely unusual' (Patton 1990, p. 173). This strategy is often used when the units of analysis are large, as for example in studies of villages in developing countries. Selecting a typical village allows the research to illustrate the general process that occurs. This strategy is particularly useful if the research report will predominantly be read by people who are unfamiliar with the area of research.

Critical case sampling

Cases are selected that illustrate processes where these processes would be thought least likely. Bloor (1986) employs this strategy in a study of therapeutic communities. The aim of Bloor's research is to refute Sharp's (1975) claim that all therapeutic communities manipulate their clientele, preventing dissent and minimising autonomy in order to control them. Bloor selected the critical case of a therapeutic community almost exactly the same as the one originally studied by Sharp, demonstrating that staff also provoke, tolerate and orchestrate dissent and autonomy.

Criterion sampling

All cases that meet a set of criteria are selected. In criterion sampling it is important to select the criteria carefully, so as to define cases that will provide detailed and rich data relevant to the particular research problem. For example, all former clients of an intensive care unit who return to intensive care with the same complaint within three weeks may constitute a sample for in-depth, qualitative study. These criteria would facilitate a study of the effectiveness of after-care programs attached to intensive care units.

Stratified purposive sampling

This sampling strategy is drawn from quantitative research where cases are selected from previously identified subgroups. Trost (1986) describes this technique as a kind of 'statistically nonrepresentative stratified sampling' because, while it is similar to its quantitative counterpart, it must not be seen as a sampling strategy that allows statistical generalisation to the large population. For example, a qualitative study of the use of treatments among people living with HIV/AIDS in Australia would probably want to interview women and men, both in and outside of Sydney. These dimensions would be used to stratify the sample because previous research indicates that these are major dimensions along which the experience of living with HIV is shaped (Ezzy et al. 1998). Nickel and her associates (1995) produce a type of stratified purposive sample, using a combination of the statistical methods of cluster analysis and random sampling to select twenty respondents to participate in long interviews from a larger quantitative sample of 1500 respondents.

Snowball or chain sampling

An initial respondent, or group of respondents, is asked to suggest other people who may be willing to participate in the research (Biernacki and Waldorf 1981). This method of sampling may be useful when the people being studied are well networked and difficult to approach directly, or when the focus of the study is social networks (Bernard 1988, p. 98). It is also often used to access hidden populations such as drug users or the homeless. Spreen and Zwaagstra (1994) argue that the results from a snowballing methodology can be improved if the analysis of the structure of friendship networks is made an explicit part of both the study's methodology and theory. However, the sample that results may have distinctive characteristics that should be taken into account. The characteristics of the initial respondent or respondents will shape the structure of the sample. For example, if a study of people living with HIV/AIDS began with a group of men in inner-city Melbourne and the rest of the sample was recruited through snowballing, the sample could easily exclude women, Aboriginal people, injecting drug users, people who do not speak English and people living in rural areas. That is to say, snowball sampling often results in a homogeneous sample.

Opportunistic sampling

Many qualitative studies include, as an aspect of their design, the assumption that the full dimensions of the research will not be known until the study is completed. New opportunities to recruit participants or to gain access to a new site may develop after the fieldwork has begun. Opportunistic sampling takes advantage of these junctures. Unexpected opportunities that occur during the research may be used to facilitate sampling. A researcher studying heart attacks may, for example, meet a cardiologist while interviewing one of his or her patients. The cardiologist may suggest how the researcher can contact other cardiologists who would be willing to refer clients to the researcher.

Convenience sampling

'Finally, there is the strategy of sampling by convenience: doing what's fast and convenient. This is probably the most common sampling strategy—and the least desirable' (Patton 1990, p. 180). Convenience sampling is cheap, easy and quick. However, while efficiency and budget constraints need to be considered in most qualitative research, they should not be the first considerations. Convenience samples are often biased in systematic ways and will probably tend to provide a homogeneous sample. While for some studies this may be acceptable, the researcher who employs convenience sampling should address the potential problems that may arise as a consequence. Convenience sampling is not purposive sampling, because it fails to theorise the sample.

Volunteer sampling

Samples are often drawn through advertising, requesting people to volunteer to participate in the study. This can be particularly useful when potential participants are dispersed throughout the community or difficult to contact directly. However, volunteer samples are typically biased in particular ways. For example, a volunteer sample of people living with HIV/AIDS will systematically be biased to exclude people who are denying or ignoring their HIV status.

Triangulated sampling

The above sampling strategies can be combined in a multitude of ways to suit the particular needs of your research project. Karp (1996, p. 197), for example, utilised a number of strategies in his study of depression. He began with friends and acquaintances whom he knew suffered from depression. He followed this convenience sample by snowballing from this group. He then advertised in local newspapers and recruited through a self-help group and an internet support group, all forms of volunteer recruiting.

Sample size

Many people become concerned about how many cases constitute a large enough sample for qualitative research. The answer to this question is simple: when the researcher is satisfied that the data are rich enough and cover enough of the dimensions they are interested in, then the sample is large enough. In quantitative methods, required sample sizes can be calculated on the basis of the type of analysis that is anticipated. In qualitative analysis, it is difficult to predict accurately what the sample size will be. However, the sample size is determined in a similar way. The sample is large enough when it can support the desired analyses. As the focus of the analysis is qualitative, the criteria for the sample size are also qualitative.

While many qualitative studies contain around forty respondents, and those with over 200 respondents are uncommon, the number of participants is less important that the richness of the data. Charmaz (1991, p. 271), for example, began with a sample of thirty-five people who had a serious chronic illness. However, this sample was derived from referrals from doctors, and she was concerned that the doctors had selected particular types of patients that they thought she 'ought to see'. She therefore sought additional participants from other sources, including those who might have avoided the medical system, resulting in a final sample of ninety people. The important point to note, however, is not the number but the rationale given by Charmaz for her sampling technique, which relates to theoretical criteria. Her sampling strategy was truly purposive.

Lincoln and Guba (1985, p. 202), following grounded theory, advocate sampling to the point of redundancy. Purposive sampling aims to create rich, in-depth information. 'The sampling is terminated when no new information is forthcoming from new sampled units; thus *redundancy* is the primary criterion.' Additional data can always be found if the researcher allows the topic of the research to expand unchecked. The researcher has to decide how much detail, and how much breadth, is required in the research, balance this with the resources of time and money available, and make a judgment about when additional sampling would be redundant. Most qualitative studies have fewer than 100 participants because it becomes very difficult to manage and analyse data from transcribed long interviews with more than 100 people, unless the questions you are asking are relatively simple and the interviews short and you have ample financial resources.

Researchers often have to provide detailed plans and costings for their research. In this environment, Patton (1990, p. 186) suggests specifying 'minimum samples based on expected reasonable coverage of the phenomenon given the purpose of the study'. However, this has the potential to limit the sample size as funds will only be obtained for the minimum sample size. Research proposals should therefore probably allow for a slightly larger sample than the minimum possible.

THEORETICAL SAMPLING

Theoretical sampling is part of the qualitative research methodology of grounded theory (Glaser and Strauss 1967; Strauss and Corbin 1990). Grounded theory is one of the more influential research methodologies utilised in qualitative research (see Chapter 10 for a more detailed discussion). In health research, it has been widely taken up, particularly in nursing research. The work of Charmaz (1990, 1991, 1995) provides a particularly sensitive and useful introduction, overview and illustration of the application of the methods of grounded theory to health and illness research issues. Lincoln (1992, p. 375) argues that qualitative methods, and grounded theory in particular, 'exhibits greater utility, power, and synergism with emerging concepts in health research ... and provides more stakeholder-based policy analysis and evaluation studies'. (Grounded theory, as a method of data analysis, is described in detail in Chapter 10.)

As defined by Corbin and Strauss (1990, p. 9), 'theoretical sampling' involves a process where the 'representativeness of concepts, not of persons is crucial'. The aim is not simply to generalise the findings to the broader population, but to construct a theoretical explanation by specifying the conditions and process that give rise to the variations in a phenomenon. That is to say, the units of analysis are concepts, and the representativeness is of the theoretical complexity of the phenomenon being described. As Strauss (1970, p. 52) succinctly summarises it, 'in theoretical sampling, the basic question is: What groups or subgroups does one turn to next in data collection? And for what theoretical purpose? Since possibilities of choice are infinite, choice is made according to theoretical criteria.'

The sample size is determined on theoretical as opposed to statistical grounds. Specifically, Strauss and Corbin (1990, p. 188) suggest that the important criterion for the ending of fieldwork is 'theoretical saturation', which they define as occurring when:

(1) no new or relevant data seem to emerge regarding a category; (2) the category development is dense, insofar as all of the paradigm elements are accounted for, along with variation and process; (3) the relationships between categories are well established and validated.

Grounded theory is grounded in the sense that it is inductively derived from observation. It attempts to systematically represent the reality and experience of the people being studied so it makes sense to them. However, it also attempts to be abstract enough to include variations and be applicable in other contexts. Emerging theory guides what to look for and where to go to find it.

In theoretical sampling, the sample design must be flexible in order to evolve with the study, the sample units are selected serially, the sample is adjusted continuously in relation to the development of theory, sample selection continues to the point of saturation, and sampling includes looking for negative cases.

CONCLUSION

In this chapter we have outlined some of the ethical and political issues that must be dealt with when conducting qualitative research. While procedural ethics must be followed, the ethical and political concerns that cannot be dealt with through rules and procedures must also be carefully addressed. We have also reviewed a variety of sampling methodologies. Snowball and convenience sampling are the most common sampling strategies in qualitative research and also the least desirable. Finally, the methodology of theoretical sampling was discussed, with particular emphasis on its link to grounded theory.

Tutorial exercise

Hepatitis C has been identified as a major health problem in Australia. While there are other transmission routes, most people acquire hepatitis C through sharing needles. However, symptoms of infection may not emerge until some years later, when some people have stopped injecting while others continue to inject. Imagine that you have been commissioned to conduct a qualitative study of how people respond to their initial diagnosis of being hepatitis C positive. The study is to include both long interviews and focus groups. Can you suggest some different responses you might anticipate? What sampling strategies would you employ? How would you recruit people who deny or ignore their diagnosis? What ethical issues could you envision arising during the research? After you obtained their address or phone number, how would you go about contacting people, given that some may not have told others they are living with, including their partners, about their diagnosis or their injecting past?

Further reading

Altheide, D. and Johnson, J., 1994, 'Criteria for Assessing Interpretive Validity in Qualitative Research', in N. Denzin and Y. Lincoln (eds), *Handbook of Qualitative Research*, Sage, Thousand Oaks.

Daly, J., McDonald, I. and Willis, E., 1992, 'Why Don't You Ask Them? A Qualitative Research Framework for Investigating the Diagnosis of Cardiac Normality', in J. Daly, I. McDonald and W. Willis (eds), *Research Health Care: Designs, Dilemmas, Disciplines*, Routledge, London.

Flick, U., 1992, 'Triangulation Revisited: Strategy of Validation or Alternative?', *Journal for the Theory of Social Behaviour*, vol. 22, pp. 175–97.

Goode, E., 1996, 'The Ethics of Deception in Social Research', *Qualitative Sociology*, vol. 19, no. 1, pp. 11–33.

Goodwin, L., and Goodwin, W., 1984, 'Are Validity and Reliability "Relevant" in Qualitative Evaluation Research?', *Evaluation and the Health Professions*, vol. 7, pp. 413–26.

Lather, P., 1993, 'Fertile Obsession: Validity after Poststructuralism', *Sociological Quarterly*, vol. 34, pp. 673–93.

Lincoln, Y., 1992, 'Sympathetic Connections between Qualitative Methods and Health Research', *Qualitative Health Research*, vol. 2, pp. 375–91.

Mishler, E., 1990, 'Validation in Inquiry-Guided Research: The Role of Exemplars in Narratives Studies', *Harvard Educational Review*, vol. 60, pp. 415–42.

Patton, M., 1990, *Qualitative Evaluation and Research Methods*, 2nd edn, Sage, Newbury Park.

Trost, J., 1986, 'Statistically Nonrepresentative Stratified Sampling: A Sampling Technique for Qualitative Studies', *Qualitative Sociology*, vol. 9, pp. 54–7.

Willms, D., Best, J., Taylor, D., Gilber, J., Wilson, D., Lindsay, E. and Singer, J., 1990, 'A Systematic Approach for Using Qualitative Methods in Primary Prevention Research', *Medical Anthropology Quarterly*, vol. 4, pp. 391–411.

3

In-Depth Interviews

Introduction

I interview because I am interested in other people's stories. (Seidman 1991, p. 1)

One of the ambiguities I experienced while conducting long intensive interviews was that the mutual trust developed during the interview had no place in an ongoing relationship. Interviewees often revealed quite personal feelings about their experiences and some cried as they discussed particularly painful events in their past. My feelings of incongruence were sometimes exacerbated by the isolation and distress that some people described as their experience of unemployment. Similarly, at the end of the interview, I left with 'the data' and the interviewee was left with the memory of a conversation. However, several people explicitly commented that they found the interview useful and worthwhile because it helped them to understand and come to terms with some aspects of their experience. For example, after I had asked Judy what her plans were she spent some time attempting to describe her hopes and thoughts about the various possibilities. Then she said:

Judy: *That is helpful. I didn't know that until now.*

Doug: *What do you mean?*

Judy: *Well, I guess in terms of realising that I am thinking quite a bit about what direction should I go. (Ezzy 1996, p. 88)*

A good interview is like a good conversation. Good conversation is a two-way affair. One person talks, while the other listens, responds and encourages. In a good interview, the person who does most of the talking is the interviewee. While the interviewer asks questions and may talk a little about themselves, most of the time the interviewer listens, and the focus of the conversation is the experience of the interviewee. There are different ways of listening. Have you ever had those conversations where the other person does not really hear what you are saying? They seem to have their minds elsewhere? The good interviewer may not say much, but they are working hard at listening to what is being said. Careful listening will lead to the interviewer asking good questions that make the interviewed person think, exposing what the person does and how they understand it. That person will feel like they have been heard, and may comment that the interview allowed them to talk through the issue or subject of the interview in a depth that they have not done before.

In-depth interviewing is a privilege. There is something deeply rewarding and satisfying about talking to another person for an hour or more in such a way that you come to understand a particular part of their life 'in depth'. In Douglas' interviews with unemployed people, some cried as they described the struggle of being without work and talked about their inability to find work no matter how hard they tried. Others spoke with courage and hope about finding work that was meaningful and worthwhile (Ezzy 1996). Similarly, in Pranee's interviews with migrant women, often she wept with the women as they described the difficulties of living in a new land. We often find it surprising, and humbling, that people are prepared to share so much of their lives with someone they may have never met before and are unlikely to meet again.

Judy's comments, in the extract above, demonstrate that interviews involve the co-construction of biographies, by interviewer and interviewee, as much as they involve the description of pre-existing biographical narratives. Interviews are not merely an opportunity to discover information that already exists. Meanings and interpretations predate interviews and continue on after them. However, to varying degrees, these meanings are created, recreated and transformed during an in-depth interview. Part of the pleasure of doing in-depth interviews is participating in the process of people making sense of their lives!

WHAT ARE IN-DEPTH INTERVIEWS?

In-depth interviews are also variously described as focused interviews, unstructured interviews, non-directive interviews, open-ended interviews, active interviews, and semi-structured interviews (Fontana and Frey 1994; Holstein and Gubrium 1995; McCracken 1988). These terms can be used interchangeably to mean the same thing. However, there are some differences in emphasis, and we prefer the terms *focused interview* or *in-depth interview*. Some authors suggest that in-depth interviews can be seen as part of a continuum, with the structured interviews characteristic of survey research methods at one end and completely unstructured, conversational interviews at the other end (Minichiello et al. 1995). Semi-structured, or focused, interviews sit somewhere between the fixed questions and forced responses of surveys and the open-ended and exploratory unstructured interviews with no fixed interview schedule.

However, we would suggest that it is not very useful to describe qualitative interviews as semi-structured, an open-ended version of fixed response survey interviews. This implies that the important issues in qualitative interviews are a watered-down version of structured interviews. Under the influence of positivism both structured interviews and semi-structured interviews have been conceptualised as a behavioural event rather than a linguistic and interpretative one (Holstein and Gubrium 1995; Mishler 1986). This means that great emphasis is placed on administering questions in the same way every time because it is assumed that a consistent stimulus behaviour is required for reliable responses. Bowling (1997, p. 277), for example, suggests that interviewers for structured interviews need to be trained so that 'they always ask the question using the exact words printed on the questionnaire, and in the exact order they are in on the questionnaire, to minimise interviewer bias'. This model of research is strongly influenced by positivism and limits the results that may be obtained from qualitative research (see Chapter 1). Structured interviews may yield worthwhile results in large quantitative surveys. However, in-depth interviews aim to explore the complexity and in-process nature of meanings and interpretations that cannot be examined using positivist methodologies. In-depth interviews are more like conversations than structured questionnaires. In-depth interviews stand in 'stark contrast' to structured interviews (Taylor and Bogdan 1998, p. 88).

Our understanding of interviewing as like a conversation is perhaps best described in Mishler's (1986) analysis of interviews as speech events in which meanings are negotiated and reformulated, in Holstein and Gubrium's (1995) work on *The Active Interview*, and in some recent feminist analysis of interviewing (Clough 1992; Oakley 1981). Interviewers should not be passive and distanced but actively involved in encouraging the respondent to talk, to converse, about the research issue under discussion. The negotiation of meaning in interviews means that 'the relation of teller to listener is as important as the content and structure of the tale itself' (Brooks 1994, p. 50). In other words, the influence of the interviewer on the production of the interview narrative cannot be ignored. The interviewer is a co-participant in the discourse (Mishler 1986, p. 82):

> Where the standardised approach attempts to strip the interview of all but the most neutral, impersonal stimuli, the consciously active interviewer intentionally, concertedly provokes responses by indicating—event suggesting—narrative positions, resources, orientations, and precedents for the respondent to engage in addressing the research questions under consideration. (Holstein and Gubrium 1995, p. 38)

This method of interviewing might be criticised as intentionally introducing bias into the interview. However, such a criticism is based on three incorrect assumptions (Mishler 1986). First, it assumes that it is possible to avoid bias, perhaps through quantitative methods. However, a structured questionnaire does not eliminate the problem of bias, it just changes its form. Similarly, in-depth interview styles that attempt to be non-interventionist have an equally powerful 'biasing' influence on the interview narrative. Second, it assumes that the in-depth interviewers are not aware of this problem. However, the method of the active interview grows out of an attempt to constructively respond to the problem of subjectivity in interviews rather than to pretend it can be avoided. Finally, it presumes that there is only one correct answer or version of events, and anything that differs from this needs to be eliminated as a problem created by, for example, interviewer bias (see Bowling 1997, p. 275). However, in-depth interviews in qualitative research draw on an interpretative theoretical framework that emphasises that meanings are continually constructed and reconstructed in interaction (see Chapter 1). As Holstein and Gubrium (1995, p. 4) put it, 'respondents are not so much repositories of knowledge—treasuries of information awaiting excavation—as they are constructors of knowledge in collaboration with interviewers'.

Bowling (1997) is right to point out that an in-depth interviewing methodology that attempts to be more conversational and engaging requires greater skill and experience. As Daly and her associates (1997, p. 101) note, the level of skill required means that 'it is common for interviews to be conducted by the researchers themselves rather than by research assistants'.

Most qualitative research is both inductive as well as deductive. In other words, it is assumed that all relevant questions are not known prior to the research. It makes use of some of the assumptions of grounded theory that attempts to build up understandings of general patterns and important issues through the process of interviewing (see Chapter 2). Quantitative structured interviews assume that all the questions and possible answers are known prior to the questions being asked. In structured interviews there is typically very little opportunity for the research to discover that a particular question does not make very much sense to particular participants or that an important response category has been left out.

In-depth interviewing can involve a single half-hour interview with each participant, or it may involve several sessions each of two hours' duration or up to twenty-five sessions in some cases (Taylor and Bogdan 1998). Rosenwald and Wiersma (1983) found that their first interview was like a 'press release' and that quite different stories were obtained in their second and third interviews. However, most in-depth interview studies seem to consist of single interviews of approximately ninety minutes, and these are the main focus of this chapter.

THE ART OF A GOOD INTERVIEW

Creative interviewing, as we shall see throughout, involves the use of many strategies and tactics of interaction, largely based on an understanding of friendly feelings and intimacy, to optimize cooperative, mutual disclosure and a creative search for mutual understanding. (Douglas 1985, p. 25)

How are we to think of an in-depth interview? An in-depth interview is like the half of a very good conversation when we are listening. The focus is on the 'other person's *own* meaning contexts' (Schutz 1967, p. 113). Good interviewing is achieved not only through technique and method, but also out of a fascination with how other people make their lives meaningful and worthwhile. It is this inquisitiveness that motivates the in-depth interviewer who uncovers new and exciting insights. 'The great creative interviewers, those discoverers of the uncharted truths about human life and the soul, find the exploration of human beings very exciting in itself and a source of joy in accomplishing something very difficult' (Douglas 1985, p. 28).

'The hardest work for most interviewers is to keep quiet and to listen actively' (Seidman 1991, p. 56). One of the most important skills to learn in interviewing is that of keeping silent. When a respondent struggles to answer a question, the interviewer is often tempted to jump in and suggest the sort of responses that may be given. These suggestions shift the focus from the participant's contexts of meaning and interpretations to the interviewer's contexts of meaning. This reduces the quality of the information obtained. When the participant struggles to respond to a question or does not respond immediately, the interviewer should focus on the non-verbal cues. Some participants like to think about their responses for some time and, if they appear comfortable, it is preferable to give them this time to think. However, other participants may be uncomfortable with the question or not understand what is intended. Facial expressions will often indicate confusion or doubt, and an appropriate response may be to suggest putting the question in different words, if the participant wishes.

Another related skill in in-depth interviewing is to not interrupt the participant while they are talking. If the interviewer is thinking about the interview, an interesting question may occur to them while the respondent is talking. It is tempting to interrupt with the new question. However, the full response to the previous question is then lost. It is important to practise keeping quiet, allowing the respondent to talk and remembering your question. It may help to write notes on the theme list to remind yourself of these ideas.

Listening can be divided into two main tasks. First, the interviewer must listen to the content of what is being said. The names of other participants, the sequencing of events, the emotions described may be important clues that suggest further questions or probes. Second, the interviewer must be aware of the process of the interview, as well as the content (Seidman 1991). Questions about process include: What topics on the interview schedule are yet to be covered? How much time is left? What do non-verbal clues, such as the participant's body language, suggest about how comfortable they are with particular questions, or how tired they feel? 'This type of active listening requires concentration and focus beyond that we usually do in everyday life' (Seidman 1991, p. 57). As an extension of this, many interviewers keep a journal that they write in immediately after each interview, with reflections both on how to improve their interviewing style and on emerging theories about the topic being studied (Holstein and Gubrium 1995; see also the section on grounded theory in Chapter 10).

Some books advise researchers doing in-depth interviews to strive for 'strict neutrality' (Bowling 1997, p. 340). Interviewers who try to be 'neutral' or non-interventionist do so through not giving any opinions at all on the topics discussed, remaining somewhat distanced from the person being interviewed and generally trying to 'minimise their own, potentially biasing, role, limiting their interactions to encouraging nods and expressions and non-directive, neutral probes' (Bowling 1997, p. 340). In our experience this non-interventionist style of interviewing reflects the residual influence of positivism and often results in more superficial data. Similarly, Chambron argues that non-interventionist styles tend to result in simplified characterisation and linear plots, whereas openly dialogical interviews in which both interviewer and interviewee are 'given a space of interpretation' tend to achieve a narrative of greater complexity and 'polyphonic authoring' (1995, p. 135).

What is it like to be interviewed by an expert? Maines (1991b) provides a revealing insight into what it was like to be interviewed by Anselm Strauss, one of the leading figures in qualitative sociology in the second half of the twentieth century. Not long after he completed his doctorate, Maines had his first encounter with Strauss. As he was driving over to meet him Maines planned the conversation, thinking of questions he would ask as he interviewed this great man. Not long into the conversation Maines noticed that Strauss was asking the questions and Maines was doing most of the talking, which was not at all as he had planned:

> It was only afterwards that I realized that Anselm had interviewed me! A bit frus-
> . trated with myself, I took comfort with the fact that I had just talked with a master
> interviewer, one who conveyed sincerity, interest, and curiosity and who kept inter-
> viewing tactics in the back recesses of his discourse. (Maines 1991b, p. 8)

INTERVIEW TECHNIQUES

Conducting a good in-depth interview is an art that cannot be achieved by following rules or particular methods. However, this is only half the story. There are many skills, techniques, rules of thumb, and practical guidelines that, if followed, will also facilitate a good interview.

Interviewees will often say things like: 'My experience is very different to other people's and may not interest you', or 'You will probably think I'm crazy'. These types of statements are a form of 'face work' designed to avoid embarrassment by the participant (Goffman 1967). They should be seen as cues for the interviewer to provide positive and encouraging feedback with comments such as: 'We are interested in everyone's experience of living with HIV/AIDS, no matter how different it is', or 'Not at all, I think that experience is quite common'. The response should be designed to reassure the respondent that they are 'OK' and that their experience, whatever it may be, is what the interviewer is interested in.

Some researchers suggest that interviewers should be of similar age, gender, race, class, and sexual orientation to the people being interviewed (Tagg 1985). However, this is not necessarily the case. Sennet and Cobb (1972) identify themselves with the educated upper middle class, but managed successfully to interview people from the working class. They note that people were quite reserved at first, but became more open as they built up trust and a sense of genuine interest: 'The greatest mark of trust we received, however, was when … people felt they could express anger to us about the barriers they felt between people in our class and theirs' (p. 38). While differences in social background can often be overcome, in some cases it may be appropriate to select particular types of interviewers. Jack Douglas (1985) reports that in his study of beautiful women he decided that the best types of interviewers were mature men or women, who typically were less likely to be perceived as having other motives for the interview. Similarly, in a team study of people living with HIV/AIDS, Douglas Ezzy found that the gender and sexual orientation of the interviewer was not particularly important if the interview focused on working life, but that it was more appropriate for a gay man to interview other gay men about their sexual practice, rather than a female or a heterosexual male interviewer (Bartos et al. 1998).

Some feminists have pointed out that it may be appropriate to offer emotional support in interviews, particularly when the interview is about a difficult topic, such as women's experiences of marital rape (Bergen 1993). The skills and experience of the interviewer, the topic of the interview, and the appropriateness of offering support all need to be considered in these situations. When interviewing people about sensitive issues we have often arranged with relevant community groups for them to be referred on to trained counsellors if they felt that they needed to talk further about the issues raised in the interview. Similarly, while we generally prefer to interview people by themselves, requesting that other people leave the room, sometimes it may be appropriate for a friend or relative to be present for support when the interview is on a sensitive topic. This was the case in Douglas' team study when we interviewed one HIV-positive woman whose child had died of AIDS (Bartos et al. 1998).

Finally, informed consent is typically required by ethics committees. However, it should be noted that when interviews are taped consent can be rbally and the participant may not need to sign a consent form. This is particularly useful if the study participants are from difficult-to-access communities such as homeless people or prostitutes, who may be distrustful of signing official documents (Minichiello et al. 1990), and some ethnic communities who are similarly suspicious (Rice 1996c).

WORDING 'QUESTIONS'

One of the practical consequences of an understanding of interviews as linguistic events involving the negotiation of meaning is that in-depth interviews do not use fixed format questions. Subjects often have different vocabularies and the questions need reinterpretation to make sense to each subject. For example, some American studies suggest that men are more reluctant to talk about their feelings than women (Gergen 1992). This would suggest that questions about emotional responses to particular events would need to be worded quite differently for men than for women. While an interview schedule is typically used (see below), questions are reformulated as understandings emerge during the interview. As Denzin (1989a, p. 42) puts it, 'the phrasing of the questions and the order in which they are asked are altered to fit each individual. Open-ended interviewing assumes that meanings, understandings, and interpretations cannot be standardized.'

While questions are not prescribed beforehand, the general topics and themes of the interview are typically already decided upon. How should an interviewer ask questions about these topics or themes? According to Anderson and Goolishian (1992), dialogue is best enabled through a questioning strategy they describe as 'not-knowing'. Understanding is best gained, they argue, through 'questions born of a genuine curiosity for that which is "not-known" about that which has just been said' (Anderson and Goolishian 1992, p. 37).

Questions should be open-ended. Such questions establish the topic or issue to be discussed, but they do not suggest how to respond. The participant is encouraged to take up the topic and talk about it in their own terms. Seidman (1991, p. 63) says that, after asking about what happened at an event, he often uses the question: 'What was that like for you?' The aim is to elicit the participant's experience in their own words.

Questions that are best avoided include those that appear to be a test of knowledge (Morse and Field 1995). Try not to ask questions that begin with 'What do you know about this?' Rather, start with something that invites people to share, such as: 'Tell me about that.' It is also best to avoid technical phrases. Tagg (1985) suggests that it is not a good idea to ask participants to rely on their memory. They are less likely to remember things if they are specifically asked to remember. As far as possible, questions should be asked using the participant's own language. Taylor and Bogdan (1998, p. 99) point out that 'in-depth interviewing requires an ability to relate to others on their own terms'.

CONSTRUCTING A THEME LIST

Although in-depth interviews are 'open' and often exploratory, a *theme list* or inventory of important topics is typically used. This ensures that all relevant issues are discussed and that the interviewer is free to concentrate on the ongoing interaction (McCraken 1988, p. 25). However, such lists do not prevent the contingent nature of the interview being exploited, with new lines of information being pursued as they arise and subsequently integrated into the theme list where appropriate.

Theme lists are best kept to one page. This ensures that it can be referred to without having to flip pages over, which can be very distracting. It may also be appropriate to use a separate list for each interview. We find that the theme list is a useful place to take notes and record questions that should be returned to later in the interview.

At the start of an interview, we typically explain its purpose to the participant and emphasise that we are interested in their story, that they are the expert. We try to stress that the criteria for what is important or relevant are what the participant thinks is important. Douglas (1985, p. 60) describes his first introduction to an interviewee in a similar manner:

I make my first approach to anyone by explaining the basic idea of all such research: 'The world is a serious place where people who are directly involved in it can know completely what it's like. You are that expert and I meekly beseech your help in gaining a more complete—never complete—understanding of it.'

In our experience, this honest approach to people seems to work well.

Towards the end of an interview, it may be worthwhile to reflect back to the participant some of the main themes of the interview, to check that the interviewer has understood the main responses and interpretations that have been described. At the very end, both Pranee and Douglas always ask the participant if there is anything else that they think is important in understanding the issue under discussion, that has not already been covered. This question sometimes produces surprising results, suggesting a completely different approach to an issue or problem. Karp (1996, p. 13) suggests that, at the end of the interview, it may also be useful to reserve time 'for respondents to "process" [the] conversation and to communicate how they felt about the experience'.

'The key to asking questions during in-depth interviewing is to let them follow, as much as possible, from what the participant is saying' (Seidman 1991, p. 59). Theme lists should not so much direct questions as remind interviewers of the topics that need to be covered. After they have answered one question (question B, for example), participants often begin to answer another question further down the schedule (for example, question E). It is best to encourage the flow of conversation by pursuing the response to question E as it arises and return to the intervening questions later on in the interview.

In-depth interviews aim to elicit information about the meanings and interpretations of events for the participant. For example, in Douglas Ezzy's (1996) study of the mental health consequences of unemployment, the main themes were: the significance of the previous job for the individual, the effects on self-evaluations of job loss, and the nature of plans for the future. For each individual, themes and ideas were explored as they arose that impinged both on the subjective significance of work and unemployment and on the objective structures of possibilities. An interview schedule (similar to the one in Box 3.1) was used as a guide and prompt for discussion.

Box 3.1 An interview theme list

The following is a sample interview schedule for an unemployment and mental health study:

1 History of education and employment.
2 Parents' occupations/main activities.
3 The last job.
    Probe for details about period of employment, details about the task, responsibilities, satisfaction, friendships.
4 The event of job loss.
    What happened?
    Was it shared, anticipated, desired, and if so, why?
    Feelings (depression, anxiety?).
    Effects on finances and relationships.
5 Associated events around that time.
    The first encounter with social security.
    The day they finished and what they did.
6 Some of the other activities in their life.
7 Important friends.
    What do they do?
    What do they think of you being unemployed?
8 Can you give me ten answers to the question: 'Who am I?'?
9 What are some of the things that are important to you?
10 Is there anything else that you think is important to understanding your experience of job loss or leaving that we have not discussed?

Source: adapted from Ezzy 1996, p. 86

PROBING

A probe is a follow-up question that aims to elicit information to fill in the blanks in a participant's first response to a question. 'Throughout the interviewing, the researcher follows up on topics that have been raised by asking specific questions, encourages the informant to provide details, and constantly presses for clarification of the informant's words' (Taylor and Bogdan 1998, p. 106). However, probing can go beyond the search for detail and clarification. As the interviewer becomes more familiar with the topic, probes may take the form of comparisons with people who have different experiences, or questions about why a participant does not respond in a way that the theory suggests they should. This sort of probe is more oriented towards theory building (see the section on grounded theory in Chapter 10). People often hold contradictory views about events or experiences and these contradictions may be revealed in the course of the interview (Merton and Kendall 1946). While it can be worthwhile to enquire about such contradictions, it is important not to pursue them too far, as the respondent will often feel threatened and may become uncooperative.

Types of probes

Rubin and Rubin (1995, p. 150) suggest that there are six different types of probes: elaboration, continuation, clarification, attention, completion and evidence probes.

- Elaboration probes ask for more detail:
  'Can you tell me a little more about that?'
  'What did she say to you?'
- Continuation probes encourage the participant to keep talking:
  'Go on.'
  'What happened then?'
  Body language such as a raised eyebrow can also serve as a probe.
- Clarification probes aim to resolve ambiguities or confusions about meaning:
  'I'm not sure I understand what you mean by that.'
  'Do you mean you saw her do that?'
- Attention probes indicate that the interviewer is paying attention to what is being said:
  'That's really interesting.'
  'I see.'
- Completion probes encourage the participant to finish a particular line of thought:
  'You said that you spoke to him. What happened then?'
  'Are you suggesting there was some reason for that?'

- Evidence probes seek to identify how sure a person is of their interpretation and should be used carefully:
  'How certain are you that things happened in that order?'
  'How likely is it that you might change your opinion on that?'

Participants often laugh in response to nervousness or ambiguity rather than simply because something is funny. If this is the case, laughter is often a good cue for a probe or further exploration (Seidman 1991, p. 67).

MANAGING THE INTERVIEW

Once a sampling strategy has been decided upon (see Chapter 2), there are a number of considerations relevant to contacting potential interviewees. First, having someone introduce you is very helpful. If someone the participant trusts introduces you, the process of gaining their trust will have already begun. Second, it may be essential to obtain permission from formal or informal gatekeepers. This sometimes takes the form of seeking ethics approval from, for example, a hospital ethics committee before proceeding with interviews with some of its patients. However, in other cases, it may be necessary obtain approval from the leaders of the community, such as Aboriginal elders or ethnic community leaders (see Rice 1996c; and Chapter 8 in this volume). Extra time taken to obtain these approvals will typically result in much easier access to participants and potentially a higher level of trust in the interviews. Some gatekeepers may wish to discuss the methodology and provide useful suggestions for more appropriate ways of introducing questions or topics for discussion (Daly et al. 1997).

A database of participants can be very useful to ensure that all the appropriate phone calls and confirmations have been completed. In-depth interviewing typically requires a relatively large investment of time and energy in recruiting participants and arranging interviews. Each interview may require a letter of introduction, a personal introduction, consent from gatekeepers, phone calls to schedule the interview, travel arrangements for the interviewer and the interviewee, the booking of an interview room, a letter or a phone call to confirm the interview time, the scheduling in of other appointments around the interview, and a thank you letter after the interview. While many interviews will not require all of these stages, given the amount of time, energy and money that may be invested in one interview, it is very important that every care is taken to ensure that this investment is not wasted. Even with all or most of the above stages, it is our experience that people still regularly do not turn up for interviews.

Deciding where to conduct the interview can be difficult. Most people will feel more comfortable and relaxed in their own homes, particularly if the interviewer has been introduced to them by someone they trust (Taylor and Bogdan 1998). However, some people can feel threatened if the interviewer is not known to them, it may be difficult to find a private space in a shared home, and some people may not want other family members to know or hear what they say in the interview. A neutral location may be less threatening for both interviewer and interviewee. Community organisations often have rooms in their offices that can be used for this purpose. However, if the researcher is associated with a particular organisation, some participants may assume that the request for an interview has a more sinister purpose. This was the case with one of Douglas' respondents who thought that Douglas was trying to expose social security fraud, because the interview was being conducted at a community-based organisation that helped the unemployed to find work (Ezzy 1996).

When the interviewer actually arrives at the interview, an additional task is '"settling" into the interview' (Morse and Field 1995, p. 98). Interviewers are often nervous during their first interview, and at the beginning of interviews. We find that, at the start, it is important for the interviewer to observe their own body language to ensure that nervousness is not being reflected in 'closed' body language, such as crossed arms and legs, that might make the development of trust more difficult to attain.

After an interview we often find that it is important for the interviewer to have an opportunity to debrief with someone else working on the project or someone familiar with the issues dealt with in the project. This is particularly important where sensitive or emotionally charged issues are involved.

TAPE-RECORDED INTERVIEWS

Tape recorders have many advantages (Taylor and Bogdan 1998). They provide a level of detail and accuracy not obtainable from memory or by taking notes. They also allow for greater eye contact than is possible if the interviewer is taking notes. However, tape-recorded interviews are costly, both in terms of equipment and transcribing. They may also provide a greater level of detail than is required if the research has specific and limited aims. Some respondents prefer not to have interviews tape-recorded, and some locations may be too noisy to allow recording.

Taylor and Bogdan (1998) suggest that the tape recorder and the microphone should be small, and the tapes should be long playing. Our experience is that the most important piece of equipment is a small high-quality external microphone. Internal microphones typically pick up a lot of background noise from the tape recorder. Expensive tape recorders do not seem to provide many more benefits. Make sure that the type of tape used by the recorder is consistent with those accepted by the transcriber you will be using. It is also an advantage if the tape recorder has a clear 'on' light that indicates battery level. It is very distracting if the interviewer keeps checking the tape recorder during the interview (and this is hard not to do if you have experienced the pain and anguish of losing one or two interviews due to the failure of a tape recorder). It is also an advantage if the tape recorder automatically changes sides, although make sure that it does not change back again and record over the first part of the interview! We usually carry a second tape recorder, batteries and microphone when interviewing.

The tape recorder should be set up and tested prior to going into the interview. This results in the minimum of distraction created when setting up the tape recorder in the interview. Background noise can be particularly frustrating during transcription, and it may be appropriate to ask the respondent to close a window or turn off a stereo. Tapes should be labelled clearly, and it is safer to use a new tape for each interview in order to eliminate the possibility of recording over a previous interview.

We usually try to position the tape recorder quite a bit closer to the participant that to the interviewer. This is because, in our experience, the participant is more likely than the interviewer to speak very quietly, making transcription difficult. People tend to talk very quietly, or quickly, when they are revealing sensitive or particularly important details. It can be extremely frustrating when transcribing interviews to find that, just at the critical moment, the participant drops their voice and their response is inaudible.

Tapes should be checked immediately after the interview to ensure that the recorder worked correctly. Researchers often underestimate how much can be remembered if a tape fails or a respondent refuses to allow the use of the tape recorder. A great deal of information can be recalled if the interviewer sits down immediately after the interview and takes notes on the conversation. We sometimes use the tape recorder to note additional information after the interview, recording notes about body language, or ideas for further analysis.

TRANSCRIBING INTERVIEWS

It is often useful for interviewers themselves to transcribe the tapes of their first one or two interviews. This is particularly the case for a first-time interviewer but may also be useful at the beginning of new projects for the experienced interviewer. The careful attention to the tape required during transcription sensitises the interviewer to ways in which they could have asked questions differently or to cues that were missed.

There are a variety of transcription methods in use, each designed for a particular type of analysis (Edwards and Lampert 1993). A consistent system is required for recording, for example, the length of pauses, other sounds such as laughter, whether words such as 'um' are to be transcribed (this will increase transcription costs), and how to indicate who is speaking. Some people advocate using all capitals to indicate the words of the interviewer. This has the advantage of clarity, but lines of all capitals are harder to read and we prefer not to use them. Transcripts generally need to be checked through by the interviewer to ensure that technical terms and difficult areas have been correctly transcribed.

If you intend using a qualitative data analysis computer package, consideration should also be given to the distinctive requirements of that package (see Chapter 10). Lewins (1998) suggests some generic rules applicable to most packages, such as the necessity of consistent spelling and speaker identifiers throughout the transcript, and the avoidance of bold, italics or underline for emphasis, as these cannot be processed in most packages. Lewins also suggests that it may be worth actually entering the first transcript into the package before transcribing other tape recordings to ensure that any problems are resolved at an early stage.

IN-DEPTH INTERVIEWS IN HEALTH: SOME EXAMPLES

In-depth interviewing is one of the most commonly used methods in health-related qualitative research. However, explicit and extended discussions about how the interviews were conducted, and about the issues and problems that arose, are more difficult to find. We provide three examples drawn from qualitative studies of cardiography (Daly et al. 1992), chronic illness (Charmaz 1991), and parents with learning difficulties (Booth and Booth 1994).

Daly and her associates (1992) used in-depth interviews to study the use of a particular cardiac imaging test (echocardiography) in the diagnosis of cardiac normality. They suspected that this particular test was used to reassure patients who were anxious, but that it had the unintended consequence of increasing anxiety. Their paper is particularly interesting because they describe how they decided to use qualitative in-depth interviews after considering other possible methods. The research problem was identified as part of a study that was quasi-experimental in design, using forced response questionnaires. They point out that while this quantitative study focused their attention on the problem, it could not provide the answer, because they wanted to understand the social and decision-making processes involved in diagnosis and choice of diagnostic tests. They reviewed the methodologies of a randomised control trial and a survey, as ways of exploring their problem, and found that neither could adequately address their concerns. 'At this point then it became clear that the standard methodological approaches were inappropriate for studying the problem which we had identified' (p. 191). They then suggest that most medical researchers choose between two options: 'To abandon the problem, putting it into the "too hard" basket, or to modify the problem to fit in with methodological preconceptions about the need for quantification' (p. 192).

Daly and her associates decided to utilise the qualitative methodology of in-depth interviews. In-depth interviews with both cardiologists and patients, along with tape-recorded clinical interaction, formed the basis of their approach. Although qualitative methodologies are often seen as not very useful from a medical perspective, Daly and her associates point out that 'the study enabled us to assess the social context of the use of technical investigations in medical practice in a way which no other research design would have done' (p. 205).

Charmaz (1991) in her study of the self in chronic illness also utilised in-depth interviews as her method of data collection. The aim of her study was to examine the relationship between having a chronic illness, the self-concept, and experiencing time. She interviewed fifty-five people, twenty-six of whom she interviewed more than once, and sixteen of whom she interviewed numerous times over a five-year period. In line with her grounded theory approach (see Chapter 10), Charmaz says that her 'interview questions developed in theoretical scope and usefulness during the course of the study' (p. 274). As she began to understand her research problem more fully and her skills as an interviewer developed, her questioning became more focused and theoretically oriented. Later in her interviews she began asking questions that were specifically designed to check her emerging theory about the development of chronic illness over time.

Charmaz captures articulately the central skill that makes for a good interview: 'As a researcher, I sought to have people tell me about their lives from their perspectives rather than to force my preconceived interests and categories upon them. So I listened' (p. 275, emphasis added). She also reports that many of her respondents cried during the interviews. The level of trust built up in interviews was not something Charmaz felt she could take for granted and leave. She argues that it is important for researchers to provide respondents with a level of support when they are forced to confront such sensitive and painful topics as the experience of illness. Along with comments that respondents found the interviews therapeutic, Charmaz reports some remarks that indicate some respondents developed a high level of trust in her: 'Several people commented that they found me easy and safe to tell their feelings to. I told people to call me if they wanted to talk further, and occasionally a few of them did' (p. 275).

Booth and Booth (1994) provide an excellent review of their research procedure, utilising in-depth interviews with people with learning difficulties. Their study of thirty-three parents with learning difficulties involved between one and twenty interviews with each of their subjects, as well as numerous phone calls and short visits. The aim of the study was to 'explore the experience of child-rearing and parenthood by mothers and fathers with learning difficulties as a basis for framing a set of "good practice principles", grounded on parents' perceptions of their own needs, for the guidance of service providers and practitioners' (p. 416).

As they typically used multiple interviews about sometimes sensitive and personal topics, establishing trust and rapport and obtaining consent were seen as integral processes by Booth and Booth (1994). They obtained entree through an introduction by a professional worker who was known to the family being studied. This worker asked if they were willing to meet the researchers, and if they agreed, the researcher was then given their name and contact numbers. This approach provided excellent solutions to some of the problems associated with confidentiality as participants' names were only released with their consent. It also provided a personal introduction, which improved levels of trust in the interviewer and facilitated an easier first interview.

Many qualitative projects involve one-off interviews that could be described as a 'hit and run' approach (Booth and Booth 1994, p. 417). However, Booth and Booth wanted to establish a greater level of intimacy to gain a more sympathetic understanding of the meaning and significance of events for the people themselves. They therefore spent considerable time developing this trust, for example, often devoting the entire first interview to establishing rapport. This paid significant dividends, as some details of some participants' experiences began to emerge only in later interviews when greater trust had been gained. Another result was the higher level of personal involvement with their research participants. For example, they sometimes assisted participants with current demands, such as responding to an overdose in the family or helping to fill out official forms. 'To maintain a detached stance at these times was not possible in human terms nor desirable on research grounds' (p. 418). The more personal nature of the relationships that were established also meant that the researchers had to take more time and care in withdrawing from the relationship.

While many interviewers emphasise the value of using tape recorders, Booth and Booth note that they deliberately chose not to record in some situations. Not recording allowed greater freedom to move around the respondent's house and to continue discussions in noisy environments (for example, while children were playing), as well as providing more scope in the type of discussion. They point out that interviewers should be skilled at taking notes after an interview, so that interviews that are not recorded still yield valuable data.

IN-DEPTH INTERVIEWS: ADVANTAGES AND LIMITATIONS

In-depth interviews typically require less time than participant observation but more time than focus groups (Taylor and Bogdan 1998). Concomitantly, participant observation typically provides a depth of understanding that cannot be gained through in-depth interviews alone (Becker and Greer 1957), but in-depth interviews provide more detail about an individual's understandings and experiences than can be gained through focus groups.

Advantages

- In-depth interviews are an excellent way of discovering the subjective meanings and interpretations that people give to their experiences (Denzin 1989a).

- In-depth interviews allow aspects of social life, such as social processes and negotiated interactions, to be studied that could not be studied in any other way (Daly et al. 1992).
- While it is important to examine pre-existing theory, in-depth interviews allow new understandings and theories to be developed during the research process. That is to say, in-depth interviews work well with an inductive theoretical approach (see Chapter 1), and with grounded theory (see Chapter 10).
- People's responses are less influenced by the direct presence of their peers during in-depth interviews. Participants may be more prepared to discuss sensitive matters, such as sexual practice or strong emotional responses, which they would not otherwise talk about in front of other people, and which could not be examined using methodologies such as participant observation or focus groups.
- People generally find the experience rewarding. Karp (1996, p. 13) observed in his study of people with clinical depression: 'Nearly everyone expressed gratitude for the chance to tell their story, often saying that doing the interview gave them new angles on their life.'

Limitations

- 'Interviewing research takes a great deal of time and, sometimes, money' (Seidman 1991, p. 5). In-depth interviewing requires a considerable investment of time and energy. This investment needs to weighed against the research problem and goals. When detailed data are not required on meanings and interpretations, other less expensive methods may be more appropriate.
- In-depth interviewing takes time (Fontana and Frey 1994). Understandings and experiences are developed from interview to interview. By comparison, in a focus group new ideas can be responded to immediately by all other participants.
- In-depth interviewing is difficult to do well. It requires persistence, and sensitivity to the complexities of interpersonal interaction. It may not always be appropriate to delegate the task of interviewing to research assistants (Daly et al. 1997).

CONCLUSION

One aspect of the conversation or two-sidedness of interviewing is described clearly by Karp, who interviewed people with clinical depression. Karp himself also suffers from clinical depression and he says (1996, p. 21) that 'I know that the wisdom in each of their stories has helped me to live my own life more easily. For that reason I owe those who have shared their time, thoughts, and experiences much more than the usual debt of scholarly gratitude.'

As Karp suggests, most qualitative researchers do not acknowledge the influence of their research on their own lives, preferring to focus on the scholarly results of their research. However, as C. Wright Mills (1959, p. 215) has so astutely observed, 'the most admirable thinkers within the scholarly community ... do not split their work from their lives. They seem to take both too seriously to allow such dissociation, and they want to use each for the enrichment of the other.'

For both of us, part of the joy of interviewing is precisely that it enriches our lives well beyond what we have suggested in our formal publications. As always, such privileges also come with a responsibility. The time, emotional energy, and trust that the participants of in-depth interview studies invest in the project confers a responsibility on the researcher to publish well-written and scholarly works that honour that trust.

Tutorial exercise

Imagine you are working as an in-depth interviewer on a research project examining how people make the decision to go and see a doctor. The researchers are particularly interested in the effects of financial concerns, time constraints imposed by work or study, and how people gauge whether an illness is serious enough to require the attention of a doctor. The interview you will conduct focuses on general patterns in usage of doctors, and particularly, on a recent trip to the doctor (one that the participant is happy to talk about). Spend ten minutes constructing a theme list. Break into groups of two and interview each other using your theme list. Make sure you begin the interview by assuring your respondent of the confidentiality of what they say, and this assurance should be taken seriously. Take short notes on the interview as you proceed. After you have interviewed each other, spend another ten minutes writing up some notes about what was said in the interview, and some reflections on your own skill as an interviewer. Discuss your experiences in the larger tutorial group, but be sure not to disclose any information that the participant might consider confidential. In your discussion focus on your own experience of doing the interview. Were you nervous? Did you have trouble stopping yourself from talking or interrupting? What else did you observe about your own responses to interviewing?

Further reading

Bergen, R., 1993, 'Interviewing Survivors of Marital Rape', in C. Renzetti and R. Lee (eds), *Researching Sensitive Topics*, Sage, Newbury Park.

Booth, T. and Booth, W., 1994, 'The Use of Depth Interviewing with Vulnerable Subjects', *Social Science and Medicine*, vol. 39, pp. 415–24.

Daly, J., Kellehear, A. and Gliksman, M., 1997, *The Public Health Researcher*, Oxford University Press, Melbourne.

Douglas, J., 1985, *Creative Interviewing*, Sage, Beverly Hills.

Holstein, J. and Gubrium, J., 1995, *The Active Interview*, Sage, Thousand Oaks.

Lewins, A., 1998, Basic Text Transcription Guidelines, <http://www.soc.surrey.ac.uk/caqdas/>.

McCraken, G., 1988, *The Long Interview*, Sage, Newbury Park.

Mishler, E., 1986, *Research Interviewing: Context and Narrative*, Harvard University Press, Cambridge, Mass.

Rubin, H. and Rubin, I., 1995, *Qualitative Interviewing: The Art of Hearing Data*, Sage, Thousand Oaks.

Seidman, I., 1991, *Interviewing as Qualitative Research*, Teachers College Press, New York.

4

Focus Groups

In a room near the cafeteria in one main shopping centre in Beijing, a group of 10 workers from a sales department gathered together to discuss issues related to their perceptions and attitudes toward HIV/AIDS. At the same time but in a different room, a group of 8 administrative workers grouped together to talk about the same health issue. (Rice field observations, Beijing, 1995)

In Melbourne, Australia, a number of Australian Aborigines: some were young, some were older; some had breastfed their infants but others had not; some were only pregnant while others had already had their babies; some were health workers and others were mothers, and a group of men gathered together in several focus groups to discuss their perceptions and experiences of infant feeding beliefs and practices. (Holmes et al. 1997)

INTRODUCTION

The two examples cited are from focus group interviews conducted in two different locations. Focus groups have been used for a long time in market research, but it is only in the last decade that they have started to gain popularity as a research method within the social and health sciences (Knodel 1994). Focus group interviews are now extensively employed. Morgan (1996) points out that a review of on-line databases in social science in 1994 alone shows that over 100 papers utilising focus groups as a method appeared in refereed journals. In addition, a content analysis of the materials from Sociological Abstracts indicates that more than 60 per cent of research employing focus groups was done in combination with other research methods in the past decade. Self-contained focus group research has gradually become more common in recent years.

This chapter will discuss the use of focus groups in health. In particular, it will focus on the importance of the focus group interview, its history, and its benefits and pitfalls. The chapter also examines focus groups as a method and provides some examples of health research employing focus groups.

WHAT IS A FOCUS GROUP INTERVIEW?

According to Khan and Manderson (1992, p. 57), a focus group interview is a qualitative method 'with the primary aim of describing and understanding perceptions, interpretations, and beliefs of a select population to gain understanding of a particular issue from the perspective of the group's participants'. Typically, focus group interviews involve a group of people (about 6–10) who come from similar social and cultural backgrounds or who have similar experiences or concerns. They gather together to discuss a specific issue with the help of a moderator in a particular setting where participants feel comfortable enough to engage in a dynamic discussion for at least one to two hours. Accordingly, a focus group interview has several important features:

- It enables in-depth discussions and involves a relatively small number of people.
- It is focused on a specific area of interest that allows participants to discuss the topic in greater detail.
- It is a group discussion that relies heavily on the interaction between participants, rather than a group interview. It is successful only when the participants are able to talk to each other, rather than individually answering the moderator's questions.
- Interaction is a unique feature of the focus group interview. Indeed, this characteristic distinguishes the method from the individual in-depth interview. It is based on the idea that group processes assist people to explore and clarify their points of views. Such processes tend to be less accessible in an individual interview. Indeed, as Morgan (1988, p.12) puts it, the focus group makes 'explicit use of the group interaction to produce data and insights that would be less accessible without the interaction found in a group'. This group interaction has been termed 'the group effect' by recent writers on focus groups (see Carey 1994; Carey and Smith 1994).
- A moderator introduces the topic and assists the participants to discuss it, encouraging interaction and guiding the conversation. The moderator plays a major role in obtaining good and accurate information from focus groups method (see the section on the moderator later in this chapter).
- The participants usually have shared social and cultural experiences (such as age, gender, ethnicity, religion, and educational background) or shared particular areas of concern (such as childbirth, infant feeding, childhood immunisation, diarrhoea, nutrition, mental health, diabetes, contraception, STDs or HIV/AIDS).

The focus group interview method is largely influenced by the hermeneutics tradition. However, depending on the topics and participants, it can also be influenced by feminist and phenomenological traditions (see Chapter 1).

HISTORY OF FOCUS GROUPS

Focus group interviews are not new. They can be traced back to Bogardus, who in 1926 described group interviews in social science research. They were also used during the Second World War when Merton employed the method to examine people's reactions to wartime propaganda and the effectiveness of training materials for the soldiers (Merton and Kendall 1946). In the same period, Lazarsfeld and others introduced focus group methods into marketing research. Since then, focus groups have been popular and used extensively in the applied social sciences, particularly in marketing research (Krueger 1988).

Focus groups have become a well-known method in qualitative research in the social sciences and this is reflected in a number of papers and books (for example, Dawson et al. 1993; Krueger 1988, 1994; Morgan 1988, 1997; Stewart and Shamdasani 1990), as well as in the recent publication of two special journal issues on focus groups (Carey 1995; Knodel 1995). Focus groups virtually disappeared from the social sciences, however, during the three decades from 1950 to 1980. Morgan (1997, p. 4) argues that the main reason for this was that the method was largely neglected, 'both by the technique's original proponents, who turned to other pursuits, and by its potential users, who concentrated on other methods'.

In the early 1980s, focus groups were introduced in the health area through studies of knowledge, attitudes and practices of contraception (Folch-Lyon and Trost 1981; Stycos 1981). Knodel and colleagues (Knodel et al. 1984; Knodel et al. 1987) used focus groups to elicit information about the transition of fertility in Thailand. With the acquired immunodeficiency syndrome (AIDS) epidemic, focus groups were used as a first step to overcome researchers' limited knowledge about the gay community (see also Joseph et al. 1984). Health educators have also used the technique. Basch (1987), for example, utilised the method to improve the effectiveness of intervention programs in public health. In more recent times, focus groups have been popularly employed in public health research. Some of these studies will be discussed in greater detail in later sections (see 'Focus groups in health: some examples').

WHY USE FOCUS GROUPS?

A focus group interview is a useful research tool when the researcher does not have a depth of knowledge about the participants. Stewart and Shamdasani (1990, p. 140) maintain that focus groups provide 'a rich and detailed set of data about perceptions, thoughts, feelings, and impressions' of people in their own words. Focus groups 'represent a remarkably flexible research tool in that they can be adapted to obtain information about almost any topic in a wide array of settings and from very different types of individuals'.

Focus groups are particularly useful when a researcher wishes to explore people's knowledge and experiences. They can be used to find out not only what people think but also how and why they think the way they do (Kitzinger 1995). This is particularly important when the researcher needs to find out about the perspective and experience of people who have different social and cultural backgrounds from theirs, or when there is little information about the group of people under investigation (see, for example, Hughes and Dumont 1993; Irwin et al. 1991; Naish et al. 1994).

Another important issue in using this method is related to its suitability for examining 'sensitive' issues or its use in research involving 'sensitive' populations, because people may feel more relaxed about talking when they see that others have similar experiences or views. Several writers have demonstrated that focus groups can be used to study sensitive issues such as HIV/AIDS (for example, Hull et al. 1996; Irwin et al. 1991; Kitzinger 1994, 1995; Konde-Lule et al. 1993; Seals et al. 1995). There have also been studies that utilised focus group interviews to elicit information from people who are seen as 'difficult subjects' (such as difficult-to-reach and high risk families) (see, for example, Chapman and Hodgson 1988; Jarrett 1993, 1994; Kline et al. 1992; Lengua et al. 1992), or 'high apprehensive' (people who feel anxious about communicating) (see Lederman 1983).

Focus groups have been used to 'give a voice' to marginalised groups such as the poor, minority ethnic groups, women, or those affected by HIV/AIDS. They enable researchers, policy makers and others to 'listen' to people who may have little chance to express an opinion about their health and needs. In early HIV/AIDS research, Joseph and others (1984) employed focus groups as a means to understand gay and bisexual men who were perceived as at-risk groups, yet their health behaviours and needs were not well understood by the researchers and the public. The voice of marginalised groups is essential in participatory action research. Hence, focus groups are used extensively in this type of qualitative research as a basis for empowering marginalised people (Hughes and Dumont 1993; Jarrett 1993, 1994; Kline et al. 1992; Magill 1993; Montell 1995; Nichols-Casebolt and Spakes 1995; Race et al. 1994) (see also Chapter 9).

In health programs, focus groups are invaluable. Dawson and others (1993, pp. 9–10) point out that focus groups are commonly used in the following areas:
- exploratory studies in health issues;
- testing ideas about and acceptances of new programs;
- solving specific program problems; and
- evaluating health programs.

However, focus groups do not suit all research aims and there have been times when they were found to be inappropriate (Agar and MacDonald 1995; Morgan 1995; Yelland and Gifford 1995). For example, focus group discussions may not go into sufficient depth to allow the researcher to gain a good understanding of the participants' experiences. In addition, the participants may not actively participate in group discussion. What, then, can we do to overcome this problem? Morgan (1997, p. 17) asserts that 'the simplest test of whether focus groups are appropriate for a research project is to ask how actively and easily the participants would discuss the topic of interest'. If the researcher suspects that there may be significant barriers to active and easy interaction, they should review some of the detailed procedures described by other researchers who have dealt with the issue (for example, Dawson et al. 1993; Jarrett 1993; MacDougall and Baum 1997; Morgan 1995). If there are still problems, perhaps the researcher needs to look for an alternative method that may be more suitable.

Morgan and Krueger (1993, p. 10) advise that focus groups should not be employed when:

- a group discussion is not an appropriate forum;
- the participants have difficulty in discussing the topic; and
- statistical data are required.

FOCUS GROUPS AS A METHOD

There are three different ways in which focus groups can be used (Morgan 1997, p. 2):

- Focus groups are used as a 'self-contained' method. In this case, they serve as the main primary source of data collection. They can be used to examine research questions from the perspectives of the participants as well as to explore new research areas. The basic argument for using focus groups as a 'self-contained' approach, as opposed to individual interviews, is that they reveal the participants' experiences and perspectives that may not be accessible without group interaction.
- Focus groups are used as a 'supplementary' source of data. Information from them can be used as a source of preliminary data in quantitative research. Most often, focus groups are used to generate survey questionnaires. They may be used for developing a program or intervention. They can also be used to validate the findings of quantitative research methods such as surveys when the results of the survey method cannot provide a deeper understanding of the participants' perspective.
- Focus groups are used in 'multimethod' studies, where a combination of several approaches is used to collect information. They can be used in conjunction with in-depth interviews and participant observation in an ethnographic study, for example. Morgan (1997, p. 3) argues that, 'in these combined uses of qualitative methods, the goal is to use each method so that it contributes something unique to the researcher's understanding of the

phenomenon under study'. The main purpose of this multimethod is the 'mutual enhancement' of the understanding of each method by the other. This is known as 'triangulation' (Miles and Huberman 1984; see also Chapter 2 in this volume).

Focus groups can therefore be used in multiple ways. However, there is a mistaken tendency to see them as only a preliminary or exploratory method, to be backed up by other methods, particularly quantitative ones. Morgan (1997, p. 18) relates that qualitative researchers are more interested in 'understanding the particular than the general' and in 'issues of meaning than in precise numerical descriptions'. Because of this, focus groups can be utilised to 'generate and to answer research questions'.

Nevertheless, in whatever form focus groups are used, there are several points that need to be understood to ensure a successful focus group interview.

FOCUS GROUP INTERACTION

A focus group interview is not a group interview. It is a group of people gathered together to discuss a 'focused issue of concern'. The emphasis is therefore on the interaction between participants in the group. As Morgan (1997, p. 2) puts it, 'the hallmark of focus groups is their explicit use of group interaction to produce data and insights that would be less accessible without the interaction found in a group'. Kitzinger (1994, p. 107) asserts that the intention of focus group discussions is to 'encourage interaction between research participants as much as possible. When group dynamics work well the co-participants act as co-researchers taking the research into new and often unexpected directions and engaging in interaction which is both complementary (such as sharing common experiences) and argumentative (questioning, challenging, and disagreeing with each other).' With this kind of interaction, focus groups 'reach the parts that other methods cannot reach—revealing dimensions of understanding that often remain untapped by the more conventional one-to-one interview or questionnaire' (p. 109). Jarrett (1993, p. 192) argues similarly that, in the focus group interview, 'the primary interaction takes place between respondents. Indeed, it is the presence of others that enhances the intensity of interaction and, ultimately, the richness of the data. The interchange—a dynamic give and take—stimulates respondents to analyze their views more intensely than in an individual interview.'

Khan and Manderson (1992, p. 57) point out that interaction in focus groups occurs because 'the informal setting, relaxed atmosphere and open-ended nature of questions are intended to encourage participants to feel free from the constraints typical of one-to-one interviews, and hence to express their views openly and spontaneously'. Kline and others (1992, p. 448) put forward a similar argument: 'The informality of the group setting is designed to encourage a degree of candidness and spontaneity among participants that is not so readily captured in a more structured one-on-one interview situation.'

How long should it take?

As a rule of thumb, a focus group should not last longer than two hours. Most are conducted within one and a half hours. However, sometimes they can go for three hours depending on the participants. Sometimes the participants find the discussion really interesting and they have many views to contribute, and this makes the discussion hard to stop. However, this is rare. There are a number of reasons why a session should not take too long:

• The participants may find the discussion tiring. To concentrate on a particular issue for two hours is exhausting for anyone.

• Some participants may run out of the ideas to contribute and hence find the discussion boring.

• The participants may have other important matters, such as childcare, cooking, or returning to work, to attend to.

Language issues

Focus groups should be conducted in the native language of the participants, in the same way as other research methods. Problems and difficulties can arise if the researcher and the participants do not share the same language. Usually, a bilingual moderator is used to lead the group discussion. If this moderator is not trained properly, does not have a full understanding of the particular research project or has biased ideas, the quality of information obtained may be distorted. Yelland and Gifford (1995) have documented this problem with their study on Sudden Infant Death Syndrome among some groups of Asian immigrants in Australia. Intensive and proper training of the bicultural moderator can overcome this, however. This is made explicitly clear in Jones' study (1997) on cervical screening among Vietnamese women in Australia.

If the researcher needs to conduct focus groups in another language by themselves, a translator will be necessary. However, the natural flow of discussion will also be affected, and sometimes a focus group discussion may turn into a group interview instead. When Pranee initially conducted focus groups on health issues in Beijing, she needed assistance from an interpreter. Each focus group took longer than anticipated, despite extra time having been allowed for in the planning stage. The natural flow of the group discussion was continually interrupted. However, later on when she trained a Chinese moderator to conduct focus groups, these problems were resolved.

THE PARTICIPANTS

There are several important issues regarding participants in focus groups. As the emphasis is on group discussion, the composition of the group plays a major role in the interaction process. Conventionally, it is argued that participants should have something in common so that maximum interaction within the group can be achieved and individuals dominating or withdrawing can be avoided (Khan and Manderson 1992). In general, there are three points of concern regarding this commonality.

A homogeneous group or a heterogeneous group?

It is usually argued that if the participants come from similar social and cultural backgrounds, they may feel more comfortable talking to each other and also more likely to talk openly. Indeed, as Morgan (1997, p. 35) points out, it is this social and cultural homogeneity that allows for 'more free-flowing conversations' among the participants. Social and cultural backgrounds here include such factors as age, sex, religion, socio-economic background, educational background, occupation, status within the community, and ethnicity. Dawson and others (1993) point out that participants with different backgrounds can restrict the openness and sincerity of the discussion. For example, researchers interested in sexual practices in a project concerned with the prevention of HIV/AIDS should not conduct focus group sessions which mix younger and single women with older and married women. The reason for this is that young and single women may feel that they have to speak about only the 'acceptable' norms within the community, rather than their true experiences and behaviours, in front of older and married women. Sani and colleagues (1990) undertook concurrent focus group interviews with mothers and grandmothers in a study of maternal management of diarrhoeal disease in Thailand. This was to avoid imposition of the values and practices of one group on another.

However, some researchers argue that heterogeneous group composition can sometimes work in a favourable way. Khan and colleagues (1991), for example, point out that heterogeneity can be useful in assessing community attitudes and beliefs and in maintaining the flow of the discussion in some cases. They provide an example from their own research in India, in which younger women had difficulties in the discussion of reproductive issues. However, the problem was resolved when a mother-in-law of one of the participants, who was present in the focus group session, started to talk. The younger women then joined in.

Morgan (1997) points out that researchers need to ask themselves which type of group—homogeneous or heterogeneous—might best serve the purposes of their research. Some research questions are more suited to one than the other.

Morgan argues that careful consideration and commonsense play a vital role in the selection of research participants.

Shared experiences?

Khan and others (1991) assert that focus group participants need to be homogeneous in terms of shared experience. People who have common attitudes towards certain issues or have similar health and illness experiences are more likely to talk openly with each other. The reason for this is simple: they feel that others in the group can understand them better because of the shared experience. For example, researchers interested in issues related to childbearing and childrearing need to recruit, for their focus group sessions, women who have children. If there is also an interest in the attitudes of those who have not had experience of childbearing, a separate group needs to be conducted of women who fall into this category. To combine the two groups in one focus group session might not be successful, as those who have no children may disagree in many ways with those who have.

Even if a group is heterogeneous, but has shared experience, the discussion can be very successful since the participants feel that they have something in common. Hence, it is likely that meaningful discussions will take place because of shared experiences. This was clearly noticeable when Pranee conducted focus group interviews on childhood immunisation with Chinese mothers in Beijing. Because all of the mothers had taken their children for immunisation, they had a shared experience about this health issue and its importance, and this made the group discussion really lively.

Familiar faces or strangers?

Many texts about focus groups advocate having strangers in a focus group session (Krueger 1988; Morgan 1997; Stewart and Shamdasani 1990). Khan and Manderson (1992) point out that an ideal focus group interview is when the participants do not know each other in advance, so that a free dialogue can be facilitated. This is particularly important when the topic for discussion is culturally sensitive (see, for example, Irwin et al. 1991). In this case, Khan and Manderson argue that 'the quality of information is enhanced through anonymity' (p. 61).

There are many situations, though, when using strangers is not permissible or practical. As Khan and Manderson (1992) argue, in these situations familiarity rather than anonymity may be the key to free-flowing discussions. There are situations where women, for example, do not wish to talk openly in front of strangers but are willing to do so with their acquaintances. In rural areas or in small villages and in slums in underdeveloped countries, where most people know or know about each other, strangers can be difficult to recruit (Kumar 1987). For example, in Fuller and colleagues' (1993) study on the effects of household crowding in slums in Bangkok, the authors state that it is difficult to recruit strangers in slums and low-income flats because people tend to know each other. People live in a very close proximity in such areas and gossip is very common. More importantly, in the Thai context, strangers are not trusted and hence people do not wish to talk about family matters with strangers. In their focus groups, the participants were therefore recruited from acquaintances. In Kline and associates' study of intravenous (IV) drug users and HIV-positive women (1992), the participants are drawn from clients who attend the same clinic for treatment. In this case, it is likely that many women know each other by sight. Therefore, anonymity can often be difficult to achieve. Similar experiences occurred in Pranee's focus group interviews about HIV/AIDS with patients and doctors from a teaching hospital in Beijing. Most of the doctors know each other through their work and the patients know each other by sight through their stay in hospital.

On the other hand, familiarity provides a social context within which people's ideas are formed and their decisions made. Kitzinger (1994), for example, recruited people who know each other in her study on the impact of the media on AIDS in the United Kingdom:

> Although the practice of using existing friendship groups is discouraged by standard market research texts such wariness seemed unjustified in our case. By using pre-existing groups we were able to tap into fragments of interactions which approximated to 'natural occurring' data (such as might have been collected by participant observation). The fact that research participants already knew each other had the additional advantage that friends and colleagues could relate each other's comments to actual incidents in their shared daily lives. They often challenged each other on contradictions between what they were professing to believe and how they actually behaved (e.g. 'how about that time you didn't use a glove while taking blood from a patients?' or 'what about the other night when you went off with that boy at the disco?'). (Kitzinger 1994, p. 104)

Jarrett (1993) argues that focus groups conducted with acquaintances not only allow the participants to share their experiences but also to disclose personal information. The more the participants interact, the deeper the levels of disclosure that can be obtained. Because of this self-disclosure, the participants are able to examine their own views and the views of others in the group more intensely. This enhances the richness of the information gathered.

Whatever choices the researcher may make about the nature of their participants (strangers or acquaintances), one must remember that they generate different group dynamics. Think carefully about the nature and objectives of the research prior to making a decision about group participants.

HOW MANY GROUPS AND PARTICIPANTS ARE ENOUGH?

In general, there are about six to ten participants in one focus group session, but some sessions may have up to twelve people (Morgan 1997; Stewart and Shamdasani 1990). Dawson and others (1993) point out that focus groups work well with four to twelve people. Generally, these numbers are based on the argument that if the number is less than six and if the participants have a low level of involvement with the issue, it may be difficult to generate interest and maintain an active discussion and hence one or two people may try to dominate the discussion. The information gained may not be adequate or rich enough since there are fewer people to interact. On the other hand, a group with more than eight people may be difficult to manage. Some participants may find it difficult to talk in a big group where everyone else is trying to talk. Others may have to wait a long time for their turn and hence may lose interest before their turn finally comes.

An important question that most researchers frequently ask is how many focus groups are needed to ensure adequate coverage. Morgan (1997) argues that, as a rule of thumb, three to five sessions may be enough for each variable of investigation. But this could easily become unmanageable if a researcher wished to examine a number of variables, such as age, gender, class, religion, education, ethnicity, language, sexual orientation, rural or urban residence, and marital status (see, for example, Sittitrai and Brown 1990). If the rule of thumb is followed (three to five sessions for each variable), the researcher ends up with thirty to fifty focus groups. If each focus group contains about ten participants, the researcher has to analyse transcripts with 300–500 participants. Given time and cost constraints, this could be difficult to manage.

Saturation theory can be applied in most situations (Glaser and Strauss 1967). Saturation occurs when additional information no longer generates new understanding. At this point, it is time to wrap up the research (see also Khan and Manderson 1992; Morgan 1997; Scrimshaw and Hurtado 1987; Chapter 2 in this volume). This may happen after only three sessions have been conducted with one group, but it may occur in the fifth or sixth session. Morgan (1997, pp. 43–4) argues that how many focus group sessions will be adequate for saturation depends on the variability of the research participants, both within and across groups. Within groups, research projects that comprise more heterogeneous participants will require more total groups. This is because the diversity in the group makes it more difficult to identify 'coherent sets of opinions'. Across groups, 'projects that compare several distinct populations segments' will need more total groups in order to 'achieve saturation within each segment'.

Another rule of thumb is that a researcher should conduct as many sessions as is required to provide a reliable answer to the research question. However, one needs to take into account time, budget and personnel limitations. Dawson and colleagues (1993) warn us not to get too complicated in the selection process. It is too easy to dive into great detail about group composition. In the end, one may not have enough time, resources or energy to complete all tasks. Lettenmaier and others (1994, p. 96), for example, provide an example from their study in Burkina Faso, in sub-Saharan Africa, where they over-recruited participants. The researchers point out that those extra focus group sessions were not necessary at all since they did not 'enrich the results, but merely prolonged the collection and analysis of the data'.

HOW CAN WE RECRUIT PARTICIPANTS?

As in other qualitative methods, the participants in focus groups are not randomly selected. A 'purposive' sampling method is normally employed (Dawson et al. 1993; Glaser and Strauss 1967; Morgan 1997; Patton 1990). Put simply, the participants need to be selected to suit the investigated issue. They are chosen because the researchers believe that they will provide the best information (see Chapter 2 on reliability). Borkan and colleagues (1995, p. 978) argue that the purposive sampling method 'adds power to qualitative research since it selects "information-rich cases" which can best generate the desired data'. A random sampling method is seldom used in focus group research. Dawson and colleagues (1993) argue that random sampling can be a real disadvantage in focus groups. For example, if a researcher wanted to find out why women do not breastfeed, it would be more 'convenient' to choose women who have young infants and children and their family members. Similarly, if the issue of concern were cervical cancer, it would be more useful to recruit women who have had children and older women. Similarly, Morgan (1997) points out that random sampling is seldom used for focus groups for two reasons. Firstly, a small size sample is not adequate to represent the whole population. Secondly, and more importantly, a random sample cannot guarantee that a shared perspective on the issue of investigation will occur and hence the participants may not interact well to generate meaningful discussions.

What then is the best way to recruit focus group participants? Krueger (1988, pp. 94–6) has a number of suggestions:

- Random telephone screening: participants are randomly selected from a telephone directory.
- Snowball: participants are asked to bring a friend to the discussion.
- Piggyback: participants suggest others who meet the characteristics for focus groups.
- Existing lists: lists of people, such as consumers of health services, are used.
- On the spot: people using a particular service are invited to participate.

In conducting focus groups in a small community or village in underdeveloped countries or in some ethnic communities in a host country, it is essential to follow the local custom (Dawson et al. 1993). Typically, the community leader should be contacted first. After some explanation of the research project, permission to conduct focus groups in the village can then be sought. Following completion of this process, community leaders are generally able to recruit the participants for the researchers (see also Chapters 3, 8 and 9). It may also be necessary to contact local health workers, since they usually know the people in the village and so may be able to assist in the recruitment process.

Gaining access to certain groups of people may pose some difficulties but, with careful preparation and sensitivity, it is possible to do so. Jarrett (1993), for example, provides an example from her focus group research with low-income minority women in the USA. Jarrett made a special attempt to recruit this hard-to-reach group through personal means, by visiting them prior to the interviews and spending time with them in order to establish her relationship with the women. She explicitly made it clear to them that she 'was genuinely interested in hearing about their lives on their own term ... Unlike the usual helping professionals who entered their lives, [she] was there to listen, not to advise' (p. 199). Accordingly, Jarrett successfully conducted ten focus groups with eighty-two low-income African-American women on their contemporary patterns of family life in America.

Gaining access to a community and recruiting participants does not guarantee that they will attend focus group sessions. There are other circumstances that may prevent attendance, for example emergencies, illness (their own or that of family members), or transportation problems. The researcher needs to prepare for such an eventuality before the focus group sessions begin. The best way is to slightly over-recruit for each session. Inviting two more participants is better than having to cancel the session because there are not enough participants.

The key to successful recruiting is to understand the working and living patterns of the participants. It may be necessary to make attendance at sessions easier and, perhaps, to provide incentives. For example, doctors may be more easily recruited if the focus groups are conducted in a hospital where they usually spend their working time; mothers with young infants may attend if the session is organised in a maternal and child health centre where they normally take their young infants for a routine check-up; and poor people in a slum may turn up if the session is set within close proximity to their area and a meal is provided. Stewart and Shamdasani (1990, p. 59) argue that this understanding is essential in the planning of focus groups, since 'it provides a basis for developing a recruitment plan that includes a location that optimizes participation, the identification of ways to eliminate barriers, and provides incentives for participation in a focus group'.

INCENTIVES?

In marketing research, participants are paid. In health research, however, there are debates about this. Some researchers argue that payments are necessary if the researcher needs to recruit those who are 'hard to find' because of their busy schedules, such as high-level administrators, medical practitioners and some bureaucrats (see Krueger 1988; Morgan 1997). Such participants are paid about $100 to $150 per session in compensation for their time. Other researchers argue that payments should also be made to poor people, who may need the money for their survival.

Kumar (1987) argues that in development projects and programs in underdeveloped countries, payments may not be necessary. First, participants tend to suggest friends or family members once they know that participants in focus groups will receive payment, and hence the findings of the focus groups may be biased. Second, payment may encourage participants to attend many focus groups and this is not recommended in focus group interviews. However, Kumar also suggests that payment is essential in some situations to attract participants, but it must be modest.

Stewart and Shamdasani (1990) point out that incentives can be organised in other ways to encourage participation. Although payment is often used, sometimes incentives include free products (for example, condoms or other contraceptives), free transportation and free accommodation. For some people, the focus group itself is an incentive since it offers some enjoyment in talking with others and the chance to talk about something which they may not have such opportunity to discuss outside the focus group. When Pranee conducted focus groups concerning communicable diseases with elderly Chinese in Beijing, the participants were given a pen as a gift. Although the incentive was minimal, the elderly said that they enjoyed meeting others and felt good about having a chance to discuss the health issues which they did not have the chance to do so in their local areas.

It is also recommended that snacks or light refreshment be provided at the end of a session, regardless of the form of incentives to be employed. People tend to feel more relaxed if they have the chance to eat and drink together, and this may also allow the researcher an opportunity to clarify some issues in further discussions.

Nevertheless, Stewart and Shamdasani (1990) warn us, as researchers, that we need to be sensitive to the sacrifice participants make for our research. The incentives they receive mean little compared with the effort they have to make to meet our requirements. This has to be remembered when planning focus groups. 'Researcher arrogance may be the single most important factor in the failure of a focus group: participants are doing the researcher, and his or her

sponsors a favor, regardless of the compensation and other incentives provided'
(Stewart and Shamdasani 1990, p. 59).

THE MODERATOR

One of the key players in a focus group, who has a significant influence on the
collection of rich and valid information, is the moderator (sometimes called a
facilitator). An inexperienced moderator may have an impact on the quality of
data collected. The task of the moderator is to stimulate the participants to
actively engage in the discussion of the topic. The moderator also needs to be
able to control the group to proceed in the direction that the focus group takes.
Hence, the main task of the moderator is as leader. Moderating a focus group
discussion is a demanding task. Anyone can be a moderator, but not everyone
can be a good moderator.

There are a number of characteristics of a good moderator (Dawson et al.
1993; Morgan 1997):
- A moderator needs to be sensitive to the needs of the participants.
- A moderator needs to be non-judgmental about the responses from the
  participants.
- A moderator needs to respect the participants.
- A moderator needs to be open-minded.
- A moderator needs to have adequate knowledge about the project.
- A moderator needs to have good listening skills.
- A moderator needs to have good leadership skills.
- A moderator needs to have good observation skills.
- A moderator needs to have patience and flexibility.

THE NOTE-TAKER

A note-taker is also essential in focus group interviews. The moderator is not
able to take notes, because of the demanding nature of the task of running focus
group sessions. The note-taker records the key issues emerging in the session
and other factors that may be important in the analysis and interpretation of the
results. The note-taker writes down the participants' responses as well as
observes and records non-verbal responses that may assist in understanding how
participants feel about particular issues (Dawson et al. 1993). Non-verbal
responses include facial expressions and body postures, which may convey some
feelings (such as approval, interest, boredom, impatience, resentment or anger).
An example of note-taking during focus group sessions on smoking (taken from
Pranee's field observations in 1995) is provided in Box 4.1.

Box 4.1 An example of note-taking

Moderator asks question about what makes people smoke. Man 1 says, 'I find it relaxing'. Man 2 says, 'I smoke because it helps me to deal with stress better. I tend to forget things if I smoke.' [Several men nod their head—do they agree? One smiles after hearing that remark—why does he smile?] Man 3 says, 'Some women smoke because they work in a bar or nightclub. The work they do makes them smoke.' Man 4 quickly says, 'Only some women, not all of them'. [At this stage, Man 7 frowns a bit—he does not agree, perhaps?].

RECORDING GROUP DISCUSSIONS

Focus group discussions are generally recorded in two ways. First, the note-taker or assistant moderator records the information in written notes (as shown above). Second, the discussions are recorded by a tape recorder. This method is invaluable and generally recommended for all focus groups. Typically, the note-taker will not be able to record everything that is discussed, but this can be overcome with the tape recorder. The recorded discussions are then later transcribed in full for data analysis.

Participants need to be fully aware of the presence of the tape recorder and to understand that its purpose is to capture their comments as accurately as possible. The researcher also needs to obtain permission from the participants. This must be organised before the focus group is started.

FOCUS GROUPS IN HEALTH: SOME EXAMPLES

As mentioned, focus groups can be used as a self-contained method or in combination with other methods. In the United Kingdom, Kitzinger (1994) used focus groups in the AIDS Media Research Project, a three-pronged study of the production, content and effect of media messages about AIDS. Kitzinger (1994, p. 104) points out that focus groups were employed to examine 'the "effect" element in this equation—to explore how media messages are processed by audiences and how understandings of AIDS are constructed'. She was interested not only in 'what people thought but in how they thought and why they thought as they did'. In addition, she attempted to examine 'how diverse identities and social networks might impact upon research participants' perceptions of AIDS and their reactions to the media coverage'. Therefore, Kitzinger argued, her research objectives 'necessitated the use of in-depth work'. A group approach was, however, chosen because of her 'interest in the social context of public understanding'.

In this study, fifty-two focus group sessions were undertaken, with a total number of 351 participants. Each focus group comprised an average of six participants. The participants were drawn from 'general population' groups, including women whose children attended the same playgroup, members of a retirement club, and civil engineers who worked at the same place, as well as some specific groups who might have particular views on AIDS, including prison officers, male prostitutes, IV drug users and lesbians. The focus group discussions lasted about two hours and were tape-recorded.

This study is rather unusual in terms of the number of sessions because the researcher made more extensive use of focus groups than most focus group research. The main reason, Kitzinger (1994) argues, was that the participants covered a wide range of different groups of people in England, Scotland and Wales. More importantly, the groups were chosen to explore diversity, rather than to establish any kind of 'representativeness'.

An interesting aspect of this study is that Kitzinger chose to work with pre-existing groups, including people who knew each other through living, working or socialising together. The reason for this was to find out how people talk about AIDS within the 'various and overlapping groupings within which they actually operate' (p. 105) (see also the earlier section on 'Strangers or familiar faces?').

Focus groups used as a 'supplementary' approach can be seen in a number of studies. In Uganda, Konde-Lule and others (1993) used focus group interviews to examine knowledge of and attitudes to AIDS among various sections of the community in Rakai district. The focus groups were conducted as part of a health education and KAP-sero-epidemiology project in the district. The researchers claimed that focus group discussions were employed because they 'approach sensitive subject matters by a different, often more fruitful method than standardized questionnaires' (p. 679).

In this study, a total of thirty-five focus groups were held: nineteen in trading centres (urban areas) and sixteen in rural areas. Eighteen focus groups were conducted with males, fifteen with females, and two that contained both sexes. Categories of groups included married women or men, manual workers, barmaids, young people, community leaders, police, business persons and traditional healers, who are herbalists practising throughout the district. Interviews with male groups were facilitated by a male moderator and female groups with a female moderator. Each focus group had eight to twelve participants and two facilitators (a moderator and a note-taker). All focus groups were tape-recorded.

The researchers claimed that the focus group results confirmed the earlier survey finding that knowledge about AIDS symptoms and HIV transmission was quite good within the district. However, many unexpected beliefs and attitudes were uncovered during the focus group discussions. Most people no longer feared contact with AIDS patients. However, they blamed spouses of people with AIDS for spreading the infection. Most people did not trust condoms, believing that they could not prevent the transmission of AIDS. Some believed that condoms could be torn while being used and might cause complications in women. The discussion results also revealed that most people did not trust injections for treatment, for fear of AIDS transmission through injection. If it were possible, they would ask for disposable needles and syringes. People did not trust hospitals where AIDS patients seek help and they believed that the patients were intentionally killed off by doctors. One interesting result from the focus group discussions was that sexual behaviours had been modified to some extent, including a reduction in the number of sexual partners. This was particularly marked in rural areas, but the practice of multiple sexual partners was still high compared with people in urban areas. More importantly, the researchers also found the diminished interest in serological results to be unexpected. The results from the survey carried out a year before the focus groups showed that about 85 per cent of all the persons screened indicated that they would be interested in knowing their results. However, during the focus group discussions there was almost no one interested in knowing their HIV serological results. Konde-Lule and colleagues (1993, p. 683) argue that 'it appears from the focus groups, that most people prefer the comfort of ignorance to the uncertain probability of the pain of knowing that they are infected even when mixed with the potential pleasure of knowing that they are not infected'. The researchers claim that the reasons behind many of the various attitudes, beliefs and practices were discovered because of the nature of focus group discussions, which allow participants to speak from their own perspectives.

A third approach in which focus groups can be used is as a 'multimethod'. Several studies fall in this category. Borkan and colleagues (1995) employed qualitative research methods, including focus groups, individual interviews and participant observation, to understand low back pain (LBP) among primary care patients in Israel. The study utilised these three methods because it attempted to 'examine the personal and shared meanings of the phenomenon among primary care LBP patients, to enter their world and explore their embodied knowledge and the nature of their suffering within its context' (p. 978). Ten focus groups were conducted in three distinct geographic locations. The participants were recruited from known LBP patients who were over 18 years of age and had had at least one episode of LBP. In each focus group, there were four to fourteen individuals, and each session lasted about two to three hours. All of the focus group discussions were facilitated by a moderator, with the assistance of a note-taker, and were tape-recorded. Additionally, ten individual interviews and participant observations were conducted, in the clinic or in the participants' homes, with LBP patients from the same geographic areas. Questions used in individual interviews were similar to those in focus groups. Each interview lasted from ten minutes (only one case) to two hours.

The researchers found that their LBP patients had a rich and varied perspective of pain sensation, awareness and meanings. From this, the researchers managed to construct a classification system of back pain, explanatory models and coping strategies among the patients. In their conclusion, Borkan and colleagues (1995) claimed that their findings suggest that LBP in primary care is 'a much more complex phenomenon than the current biomedical conceptualization'. For example, in describing back pain, rather than using a category of 'acute' or 'chronic' pain, the patients described the 'intermittent' characteristics of their pain as 'acute-recurrent' or 'chronic-recurrent'. The patients also employed 'multiple conventional and alternative treatments' which were often based on 'what works'.

In their concluding remarks about having used three different research methods, Borkan and others state that 'use of three data collection techniques overcomes some of the limitations of each method and permits comparison and triangulation of findings' (p. 985). They point out that in focus groups people may be reluctant to express extreme opinions or share intimate experiences. Information from an individual interview 'may fill in potential information gaps by furnishing a setting that engenders more personal accounts'. Lastly, participant observation 'allows a glimpse into actual lived behavior'.

It is interesting that several patients in the study claimed that their LBP symptoms were relieved after attending focus group discussions. In two communities, the patients initiated 'back school' group sessions with a physical therapist following the focus groups. Borkan and others (1995, p. 986) argue that 'focus groups can be hypothesized to legitimize and normalize the experience of LBP and provide a sense of shared experience. Telling one's story has a psychotherapeutic component, allowing a joint "reframing enactment". Information on how others cope may help the participant to reorganize the illness and model different solutions.'

WHAT DETERMINES SUCCESSFUL FOCUS GROUPS?

Successful focus groups occur when their use is consistent with the purposes and aims of the research (Stewart and Shamdasani 1990). However, there are at least four criteria by which success or good quality can be determined (Merton et al. 1990):

- Range: successful focus groups should cover a maximum range of relevant issues, not only providing important issues relevant to the research questions but also revealing some unexpected or unanticipated issues.
- Specificity: focus groups should provide information that is as specific to the participants' experiences and perspectives as possible.
- Depth: focus groups should foster interaction, which enhances the exploration of the participants' perspectives in some depth.
- Personal context: focus groups need to take into account the personal context in the generation of participant responses. In other words, what is it about the person that makes them respond in a particular way? Thus, information

gathered may make sense to the researcher both in the data collection and analysis processes.

In his recent writing, Krueger (1994) points out several factors that can be used to determine the quality of focus groups:

- Clarity of purpose: the purpose of focus groups must be clear and focus groups should not stretch beyond their limits.
- Appropriate environment: this includes both physical and socio-political environment. A proper physical environment, such as the location of focus groups needs to be provided for maximum group interaction. In addition, they need to be organised free of intimidation and possible conflicts between the participants and the sponsors and/or the researcher.
- Sufficient resources: when resources such as time and budget are not realistic, this can affect the quality of focus groups. Always remember that all research takes longer than was planned, and focus groups are no exception. The focus groups researcher may, however, need to be more cautious about this since working with groups is more complicated than say working with an individual person.
- Appropriate participants: it is essential to select the right people for focus group sessions. Participants, therefore, need to be carefully recruited to answer the research question.
- Skilful moderator: moderating a quality focus group interview requires group interaction skills. Without these skills, the quality of information collected can be affected greatly.
- Effective questions: quality focus groups depend greatly on questions asked. If there are too many questions, they are not asked specifically, and if there is no follow-up for clarification, these factors can affect the quality of information gathered.
- Honouring the participant: quality of focus groups can be affected when the participants are not respected or their needs are not taken seriously. If the participants can sense this, they will not willingly provide their experiences and perspectives. Hence, the information collected will be greatly affected too.

FOCUS GROUPS: ADVANTAGES AND LIMITATIONS

As with other qualitative methods, focus groups have both advantages and limitations.

Advantages

- Focus groups allow a researcher to explore an in-depth knowledge of the participants quickly and at less cost than individual interviews. However, this does not mean that the method is a 'quick and cheap' approach, as commonly perceived (Morgan 1997; Morgan and Krueger 1993). To conduct focus groups takes as much time and money as other types of qualitative methods.

- Focus groups are excellent when a researcher needs to obtain in-depth knowledge on sensitive subject matters in order to provide an appropriate health service, to improve health care, or to develop health interventions that will be utilised by people in the community.

- Because of the flexible nature of focus groups, a researcher may discover some 'hidden' or 'unexpected' information that may be invaluable for the research project and have significant implications for developing health programs that are appropriate to the local people.

- The most visible strength of focus groups is their emphasis on interaction in the group in order to produce information. Participants compare and contrast their experiences and views. Morgan and Krueger (1993) argue that focus groups provide valuable insights into the complex behaviours and thoughts of people that are less accessible in other types of research methods.

- Since focus groups focus on interaction between the participants, they may help some people to discuss issues that they feel too uncomfortable or intimidated to talk about in an individual interview. This is particularly so when the topic is very sensitive (for example, issues related to sexuality, domestic violence or illicit drug use). When a person sees that someone else has similar experiences or views, they may feel more relaxed about talking.

- Group interaction can also encourage participants who might otherwise say little. Hearing about other people's experiences may help to stimulate them to contribute their point of view or to remind them of their own experiences which otherwise they would not have remembered. It also may help to 'break the ice' for shy participants.

- Focus groups reduce the chance of misunderstanding of research questions since participants can query anything during the discussion. They also help to correct any unintentional mistakes made by some members in the group through others challenging them.

- In focus groups the researcher and the participants are able to interact directly. The researcher may help with an immediate clarification, follow-up and probing of responses. This also allows direct observation of non-verbal responses among the participants, which may be valuable in the interpretation of the information gathered.

- Focus groups are invaluable when the researcher needs to gather information from some marginalised groups, such as illiterate communities, poor people from rural areas, prostitutes, drug users, children and minority groups, who may have difficulties in expressing their views via other forms of research methods such as a questionnaire, or who may have fears about expressing their own views. Indeed, the method assists in the empowerment process of these marginalised groups since the participants can become an active part of the research process (Kitzinger 1995).

• Focus group sessions are usually fun for the participants and the researcher. Fun assists the flow of lively discussion as well as building a sense of trust among the group members. Sometimes, the participants form friendships within the group and this helps to extend their social network.

Limitations

• Information gathered from focus groups can only represent the perspective of the participants. They can only indicate the range of views in a community, not their prevalence. They cannot be used, therefore, to statistically represent the wider community.

• Results from focus groups are meant to be in 'quality'. They are used to indicate some information that the researcher does not know about the participants. They are not meant to specify the 'quantity' of the knowledge. Statistical data should not therefore be generated from focus group results.

• Although focus groups can generate in-depth information, they cannot explore the complex beliefs and practices of an individual person, as can be obtained from an in-depth interview. This is mainly due to the nature of group interaction and time limitations. It is impossible to generate in-depth information from eight to ten people within one or two hours.

• Focus groups can examine participants' knowledge of, and attitudes on, certain issues. They cannot, however, investigate actual behaviours, as can be obtained from participant observation. People may say what they think, but that is not necessarily what they will do. In this case, information obtained from focus groups may not be accurate.

• Because of the nature of group talk, some participants may conform with the responses of other members in the group even though they may not agree. On the other hand, some may not wish to speak about their 'secret' in a group for fear of gossip being spread in the community, but may talk about it in private (see also MacDougall and Baum 1997).

• Focus groups are 'driven' by the researcher and they reflect the researcher's interests. This may have some biases on the intended outcomes since they may not reflect the participants' interests.

• Focus group sessions are directed and controlled by a moderator. As Morgan (1997, p. 14) points out, 'there is a very real concern that the moderator, in the name of maintaining the interview's focus, will influence the group's interactions'. An inexperienced or biased moderator may prevent the participants from expressing their true concerns about the issue. This has a major effect, therefore, on the information gathered from focus groups.

- Focus groups generate a large quantity of data. This may present some problems in particular areas, such as in cross-cultural focus group research. With this type of research, translation and back-translation are essential in the analysis process. The amount of data generated through focus groups may make this task difficult. Apart from errors that can easily occur with large data, it is also very time-consuming.

CONCLUSION

As illustrated throughout this chapter, focus groups are invaluable in obtaining in-depth information within a short period of time. They are not an easy option. Some focus groups can be complex and the data generated can be bulky. However, the method is straightforward (Kitzinger 1995). With some training and intuition, researchers can achieve good-quality focus groups.

In the past decade, focus groups have become popular and evidence points to their being a valuable method for qualitative data collection (Morgan 1997). Despite this, they are still under scrutiny as a 'soft' option by researchers outside qualitative disciplines (Stewart and Shamdasani 1990). It is true that, although focus groups have invaluable benefits and may offer many useful insights, they of course have some pitfalls, as do other research methods. We will end this chapter with the writing of Kitzinger (1994, p. 117), who describes the benefits of focus groups succinctly:

> We are none of us self-contained, isolated, static entities; we are part of complex and overlapping social, familial and collegiate networks. Our personal behaviour is not cut off from public discourses and our actions do not happen in a cultural vacuum whether that is negotiating safer sex, sharing needles, attending for a smear test or going 'queer bashing'. We learn about the 'meaning' of AIDS (or sex or health or food or cigarettes) through talking with and observing other people, through conversations at home or at work; and we act (or fail to act) on that knowledge in a social context. When researchers want to explore people's understandings, or to influence them, it makes sense to employ methods which actively encourage the examination of these social processes in action.

We also believe focus groups can provide a window into the richness and complexity of social life in general and health behaviours in particular.

Tutorial exercise

Gather a group of five people (for the sake of time, your acquaintances may be a good choice) and select a discussion topic relevant to public health. Research questions need to be developed to suit a 20-minute session. Act as moderator and assign someone else to take notes. What information do you obtain by the end of a 20-minute focus group discussion?

Further reading

Dawson, S., Manderson, L. and Tallo, V.L., 1993, *A Manual for the Use of Focus Groups*, International Nutrition Foundation for Developing Countries (INFDC), Boston.

Kitzinger, J., 1994, 'The Methodology of Focus Groups: The Importance of Interaction between Research Participants', *Sociology of Health and Illness*, vol. 16, no. 1, pp. 103–21.

Krueger, R., 1994, *Focus Groups: A Practical Guide for Applied Research*, 2nd edn, Sage, London.

Morgan, D.L. (ed.), 1993, *Successful Focus Groups: Advancing the State of the Art*, Sage, Newbury Park.

Morgan, D.L., 1997, *Focus Groups as Qualitative Research*, 2nd edn, Sage, Newbury Park.

Stewart, D.W. and Shamdasani, P.N., 1990, *Focus Groups: Theory and Practice*, Sage, Newbury Park.

5

Unobtrusive Methods

The fog had probably just cleared. The singular Sherlock Holmes had been reunited with his old friend, Dr. Watson ... and both walked to Watson's newly acquired office. The practice was located in a duplex of two physician's suites, both of which have been for sale. No doubt sucking on his calabash, Holmes summarily told Watson that he had made a wise choice in purchasing the practice that he did, rather than the one on the other side of the duplex. (Webb et al. 1966, p. 35)

INTRODUCTION

How could Sherlock Holmes tell that Watson had made a good decision in this instance? Well, he examined the steps of the property and found that they were more worn than the other one. Therefore, it indicated that the practice, which Watson had just purchased, was more popular than his competitor's. This is one of Sherlock Holmes' stories in his detective science. But what about in social science?

> In Managua, several motels were observed for a period of 7 hours during one week of investigation. Every couple was given a condom on payment before going into the room. The number of couples who entered the room and the time spent were recorded. After the couple had left, the room was carefully searched to see if the condom was there, if it contained semen. Actual rates of condom use were then calculated. (Gorter et al. 1993)

> In Sydney, the front-page coverage of medical and health stories in the Sydney Morning Herald was examined over the one-year period. In particular, features of the front-page stories including major topics, location, visual images, use of news actors and news sources, medical and health representation, language used in headlines and dominant and recurring discourses were analysed. (Lupton 1995)

These are just some examples of so-called 'unobtrusive' methods. The methods have been utilised for a long time, but they have not been very popular among researchers in the health area. As Kellehear (1993a), an exponent of unobtrusive methods, argues, this is mainly due to the fact that social science researchers have been occupied by more 'scientific' and 'rigorous' methods such as survey and other quantitative methods. Nevertheless, in recent years, we have seen increasing numbers of projects in health utilising unobtrusive methods and these will be discussed in this chapter.

The chapter begins with a definition of unobtrusive methods, followed by an analysis of their contribution to research, particularly health research, their history and their pros and cons. Some examples of health research utilising unobtrusive methods are also provided.

WHAT ARE UNOBTRUSIVE METHODS?

What are unobtrusive methods? Why are they termed as such? Essentially, unobtrusive methods are non-reactive research methods. The methods draw social and cultural meanings from existing sources, be they written records, audiovisual records, physical traces or human behaviours (Fetterman 1989; Kellehear 1993b).

According to Kellehear (1993b, p. 46), unobtrusive methods are so termed because they do not actively require the participation of others, whom researchers have referred to as 'subjects', 'respondents', 'participants', or 'informants'. The participants do not need to sacrifice their time to participate in research. Therefore, the 'social environment' of people is not disturbed.

In his *Research Methods in Anthropology*, Bernard (1995) points out that unobtrusive methods include all methods for studying human behaviour where informants do not know that they are being investigated. They include behaviour trace studies, archival research, content analysis, disguised observation, and naturalistic experiments.

There has been considerable debate about whether disguised or manipulative observation and naturalistic experiments should be classified under unobtrusive methods. Bernard includes them, but argues that they pose serious ethical problems. Berry (1979) and Kellehear (1993b) argue that manipulative experiments should not be included in unobtrusive methods. Kellehear (1993a, p. 4) points out that 'the method is ... socially as well as ethically intrusive' because people's 'activities have been disturbed by the researcher's activities'. Some manipulative experiments, such as fake collapses on trains to assess people's helpfulness (in Bochner's study 1979), may create a great deal of emotional turmoil and anxiety among people who participate without knowing.

In Kellehear's book on unobtrusive methods (1993a, p. 5), he argues that such methods include only the following: material culture; written records; observation; audiovisual records; and hardware techniques. This chapter follows

Kellehear's classificatory framework. Kellehear (1993c, p. 44) points out that unobtrusive methods are seen by many researchers as a qualitative method, but they are 'in fact, neither qualitative nor quantitative in any deterministic sense'. Nevertheless, since this book is about qualitative methods in health, we attempt to deal only with the 'ethnographic, inductive and thematic or interpretive' aspect of unobtrusive methods (for unobtrusive methods that deal with secondary analysis and meta-analysis of quantitative data, see Daly et al. 1997).

WHY USE UNOBTRUSIVE METHODS?

When people talk about doing qualitative research, most immediately think about talking with people either individually or in groups, or participating in other people activities. However, as Kellehear (1993a) argues, some research may not necessitate talking with people or participating in their routines when an answer to the research question may be found in existing literature and research. There are also some data that it may not be feasible to collect because of political sensitivity or simply because the informants no longer exist for researchers to interview. Furthermore, if the research questions deal with delicate situations or groups of people, such as people with HIV/AIDS or indigenous people, should the researcher intrude into these people's private lives when there is existing information that has not yet been examined (Daly et al. 1997)? Unobtrusive methods can offer answers to these situations. Further, because the data already exist, the research can be done relatively cheaply and quickly too.

Even when people tell you what they believe or do in the interview situation, do they tell you the truth? They may not do so because of some personal, social, cultural or political situations. Take the research on screwdrivers as an example (Carpenter 1977). When people were asked what they did with a screwdriver, most said they used it for turning screws. However, upon close examination of screwdrivers, Carpenter found several traces that indicated that they had been used as can or tin openers, chisels, stirrers, knives, and so on. Because of the limitations in talking to people, Kellehear (1993c, p. 48) argues that unobtrusive methods 'help restore meaning and context to confessions of belief, attitude and knowledge'. This is particularly so when unobtrusive methods are used with other qualitative methods.

Unobtrusive methods can be used to supplement other interactive methods of data collection, such as those of ethnography and in-depth interviews. As Fetterman (1989) points out, unobtrusive methods only require the researchers to keep their eyes and ears open. Anything that 'sticks out', such as burned-out buildings, graffiti, the smell of urine on the streets or a syringe in the schoolyard, may help researchers to estimate the relative wealth, poverty and well-being of the area (see also Chapter 8).

As a self-contained approach, unobtrusive methods can, as Kellehear (1993a, p. 48) also points out, 'supply surprising insights which challenge the information we have from other sources'. For example, Hahn's (1987) study of the medicalisation of childbirth from obstetric texts in the USA, and Koutroulis's (1990) study of sexism in gynaecological and obstetric texts used in medical schools in Australia, reveal many hidden realities that we may not have been able to extract from other types of qualitative methods. There are many research findings that provide some 'never-thought-before' information in the health area. These will be discussed in later sections.

HISTORY OF UNOBTRUSIVE METHODS

If we start to look closely, we find that unobtrusive methods have been employed for a long time. In detective science, fingerprints; footprints; traces of hair, buttons and clothes; the location such as a room, a park; objects such as a car, a chair; and so on have been examined to determine who has committed particular crimes (Kaye 1995). In the mainstream media, these procedures are commonly used in many detective series, such as 'Sherlock Holmes', 'Murder She Wrote', 'Miss Marple', 'Hetty Wainthropp Investigates', and many more. In anthropology and archaeology, as Bernard (1995) points out, unobtrusive methods have been used extensively, particularly in physical trace studies. One of the earliest and well-known research projects that employed unobtrusive methods was the 'Garbage Project', developed by archaeologist William Rathje at the University of Arizona in 1973 (Rathje 1979). Since that time, Rathje and his colleagues have studied the consumer behaviour patterns of Tucson, Arizona, by examining the rubbish from a representative sample of local residents. In order to prevent reactivity, people are not informed that their rubbish is being sorted and analysed. By looking through people's rubbish bins, researchers on the project have learned many interesting things about Americans' food consumption and waste. For example, squash is a popular baby food among Hispanic-Americans. About 35 per cent of food from chicken meat bought from restaurants is thrown away. Children generate as much plastic trash as adults do. Mexican-American households throw out less food than Anglo households do. With proper consideration, trace studies can be invaluable in cultural anthropology in order to generate useful information about human consumption (Bernard 1995).

In sociology, several well-known sociologists, such as Marx, Durkheim and Weber, spent most of their time in libraries (Kellehear 1993a; MacDonald and Tipton 1993). MacDonald and Tipton (1993, p. 188) point out that in his work Marx made use of government statistics and Civil Service reports referred to as 'Blue Books'. Durkheim's famous work *Suicide* was based on official statistics and on the unpublished reports on suicides which were held by the Ministry of Justice. Weber started his career in sociology by his studies of the Hamburg Stock Exchange and of the peasant problem in eastern Germany. These two studies were documentary studies and 'they led him to conclusions which he felt needed sociological explanations rather than economic ones'.

Unobtrusive methods in health, however, have not received as much attention as in other social science areas. Only in the last two decades have such methods been employed in the health area. Some of these studies will be dealt with in greater detail in the 'Unobtrusive methods in health: some examples' section.

UNOBTRUSIVE METHODS AS A METHOD

In this section we will outline some of the important issues to consider when employing unobtrusive methods, but this is not a step-by-step guide. There have been several well-known books providing detailed guides to unobtrusive methods that readers may consult further (see Sechrest 1979; Webb et al. 1966). Kellehear's book (1993a) is the most up-to-date and detailed description of these methods and we highly recommend it for researchers who wish to utilise unobtrusive methods in health research.

Here, we examine the main issues. First, where can researchers obtain information? Second, how do we make sense of the data obtained through unobtrusive methods?

Where can we obtain the data?

Everywhere you look, there is plenty of material that you can examine using unobtrusive methods. Have you ever walked in the cemetery and started to notice some common patterns or obvious strange-looking tombs, or looked to see who has been buried there and for how long? Have you ever followed writings about women's or men's health in magazines or newspapers? Have you ever considered how people express their feelings in the 'lost pet' notices? Have you ever observed interactions between mothers and infants in shopping centres? And have you ever compared the reactions of mothers and fathers to their children's behaviours, particularly when the children throw a tantrum in a toy shop? Simply, material can be easily obtained in most locations and situations. However, Kellehear (1993a) suggests five main ways of obtaining information when employing unobtrusive methods.

Material culture
Material culture includes physical objects (cutlery, syringes, medical equipment); physical traces (condoms in a rubbish bin, household garbage, graffiti,

erosion of floors); and settings (organisation of birthing rooms, clinics, hospitals). Through the study of these elements of material culture, many human behaviours can be revealed, as in Rathje's Garbage Project discussed earlier.

Graffiti can tell us many interesting things about a community. Sechrest and Flores (1969) conducted one interesting study that examined graffiti about homosexuality. They wanted to look at attitudes towards sexuality in the Philippines and in the USA, so they examined graffiti in men's public toilets in Manila and Chicago. What they found was that the percentage of graffiti that dealt with heterosexual themes was similar in the two cultures. However, there were more expressions of graffiti dealing with homosexuality in the Chicago setting than in Manila (42 per cent, compared with only 2 per cent). Sechrest and Flores argued that there was a clear difference in the level of concern with homosexuality between these two settings. There have been two subsequent studies of graffiti. One was by Blake (1981), who looked at graffiti in male toilets at the University of Hawaii in order to study inter-racial content. The other study was conducted by Bruner and Kelso (1980), who examined communication by people of the same sex through graffiti in toilets. The results of both studies were fascinating.

Settings can also be a good source of data for unobtrusive researchers. The way people organise their room, kitchen, house or workplace can offer insights into their social and cultural ideology. Miller (1988), for example, examined kitchens in public housing as a way to understand the 'social and biographical tastes and values' of people who live in the 'alien' environment of public housing. Particularly, he wanted to see who changed the kitchens and what the change (or absence of change) revealed about people's lives. Miller found that lonely, isolated or depressed people did not change their public housing kitchens. Single women displayed their personal belongings in their kitchens. Full intact families tended to make changes, by either altering or replacing their kitchens. In his conclusion, Miller suggests that kitchens are closely linked to people's patterns of socialising and sociability. The more people were able to socialise, the more they paid attention to their kitchens.

Maisano's study (1996) is another interesting unobtrusive research project. She looked at the ways in which birthing rooms in maternity hospitals and birth centres are organised. Are the rooms friendly or distant? What do the rooms offer to women in labour and to their families? From an examination of the layout of furniture, equipment, lighting and decorative objects, six key themes were apparent: space, time, privacy, choice, safety and homeliness. Maisano's observation showed that 'a standard code of aesthetics and value system is operative in Melbourne delivery and birth rooms. The western style of birthing practices is reflected in the birth settings' (p. 88). Therefore, women are placed as a homogeneous group. In her conclusion, Maisano argued that birth rooms are not only 'adjuncts to care' but they also have a role in communicating about birth managed by hospitals. Through this research, Maisano called for the alternative birth movement to establish birth settings that offer choices to women in childbirth.

The written record

Written records can be obtained in most libraries, archives and private collections. These include business archives and government records; published materials such as books, journals, magazines and newspapers; and personal documents such as life histories, diaries and letters. Nowadays, there are many unpublished theses available in most university libraries, which can be a valuable source of information.

Among written records, archival work is of value. Archival resources offer an invaluable source for studying cultural processes through time (a longitudinal study, in Kellehear's term (1993b)). As Bernard (1995) points out, the best-known study of cultural process using archival sources is Alfred Kroeber's study (1919) on long-term trends and cycles of behaviour. Kroeber studied women's fashions and his study became a classic in anthropology. Where were his data taken from? Archival records, of course.

Another important source of archive work that is invaluable to social science researchers is the Human Relation Area Files (HRAF): a 900 000-page data source of ethnographic studies collected by ethnographers on 350 cultural groups from all over the world (Bernard 1995; Kellehear 1993a). HRAF has turned the ethnographic studies into a data source for content analysis as well as cross-cultural tests of hypotheses (Bernard 1995). One good example of studies using the HRAF is that of Bart (1969). Bart wanted to find out why women in some cultures do not experience the negative effects of menopause experienced by most Western women. She used data from the HRAF to search for some possible explanations that might be associated with the lack of menopausal symptoms in many cultures. What she found was fascinating. The status of women within the society has a major influence on their experiences of menopause. Bart argued that the increased social status of women with ageing protects them from negative menopause experiences. This is commonly found in traditional societies where kinship retains its pre-eminent role in social organisation and economic life. From the data in the HRAF, Bart (1969, p. 14) came up with six themes or cultural characteristics that serve to protect middle-aged women: 'strong ties to family of origin and kin, extended family system, the residence patterns keeping one close to the family of orientation, strong mother–child relationship reciprocal in later life, institutionalised grandmother role, and institutionalised mother-in-law role'. A more recent study using the HRAF is that of Levinson (1978) who looked at cross-cultural research on family violence. Again, his study revealed many interesting aspects of so-called 'family violence' in different cultures.

Published material offers a great deal of data for examination. Most of it— for example, textbooks, government policy documents, journals, newspapers and magazines—is readily available in most libraries. Many social science researchers have used such library material as their primary data sources for their unobtrusive research. Koutroulis's interesting work on sexism in textbooks used by Australian medical students in obstetrics and gynaecology (1990) is just one example. In this case, several textbooks written by male medical academics were examined for their 'hidden' ideology of sexism.

Personal documents can also offer a great deal of information about people's health, sickness, life and suffering. Life history or story telling by people in their diaries and letters, or as folktales, can be illuminating. Plummer's *Telling Sexual Stories* (1995), for example, documents stories about sex, particularly 'personal experience narratives around the intimate', among rape survivors and lesbian and gay people. These people make sense of 'suffering, surviving and surpassing' through their stories. Plummer argues that personal documents such as 'sexual stories can be seen as issues to be investigated in their own right. They become topics to investigate, not merely resources to draw upon' (p. 5).

In some cultures, people's way of life is recorded in 'folktales'. Fetterman (1989, p. 70) asserts that folktales are important to both literate and non-literate societies since 'they crystallize an ethos or a way of being'. Most cultures use folktales to pass on their 'critical cultural values' from one generation to another. Although they draw on local physical surroundings and figures, the stories themselves are 'facades', because 'beneath the thin veneer is another layer of meaning'. They reveal underlying values that provide researchers with an understanding of the life of a people. In most literate societies, folktales are recorded so that they are not lost to younger generations. Therefore, they also are an available source of data that unobtrusive researchers may pursue.

The audiovisual record

The audiovisual record includes films, television programs, videos, images, music and photographs. Again, most of these materials are available in most libraries. Audiovisual records offer a great deal of information for investigation by unobtrusive researchers. As Kellehear (1993a, pp. 73–4) argues, audiovisual records such as images and music can be 'important clues' to the 'cultural world' of non-literate people, people 'whose communication emphasis is not strongly placed on speaking', such as young children and people who may not be able to express their perspectives in the language of the researchers (including non-English speaking background communities in Australia).

Consider the image in Figure 5.1. What can you see? What can you tell about the life of these people? This is an image of a Kiowa Indian birth in a teepee. The mother is grasping poles for support during labour. Who is around her? What does this tell you about the importance of social support at birth in

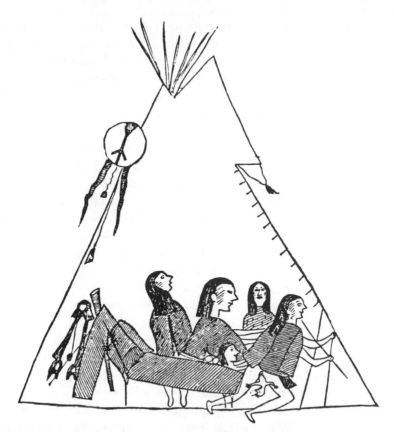

Figure 5.1   A Kiowa Indian birth in a teepee   *Source*: Englemann 1882

Kiowa Indian culture? What about the object hanging on the teepee or the one near the bed? What are their roles in childbirth? Might they say something about protecting the mother and her newborn from evil spirits or other bad influences? As you can see, an image can tell us many things about people's lives.

There is another type of audiovisual record, found not in libraries but in other important places. We are referring to inscriptions and drawings on the walls of a building or cave. This is one way that illiterate people recorded their way of life in the past. There are several such records that offer a valuable source of information about health and medicine in many countries. For example, the inscriptions and drawings of traditional medicines on the walls of Wat Pho temple in Bangkok, Thailand (van Esterik 1988), reveal the complexity and extent of traditional therapies in Thai people's lives in the past and present. The inscriptions and drawings were recorded over the past few centuries and they are still an important 'textbook' for traditional healers in Thailand.

Photographs can also be a data source for the study of cultural patterns. At a very basic level, family photographs can tell us many things about the family, such as who the firstborn child is (because he or she has more photographs than the rest of the siblings), and what the relationships are between siblings and parents, grandchildren and grandparents, and so on. Williamson (1986) records that her family described her as a young child who easily accepted her newborn sister. Yet, every photograph not in the family album showed her as jealous, anxious, suspicious and sulky towards her sister. Where is the truth?

At a more complicated level, there are many types of photographs that unobtrusive researchers may wish to examine. Take, for example, photographs of mental health hospitals, such as in the study of Dowdall and Golden (1989). They can record many things about the social and ideological assumptions of mental institutions. Dowdall and Golden were interested in these issues, so they examined over 300 photographs taken from the hospital office and staff donations, from printed sources such as medical journals and annual reports, and from major photographic collections in the local area and from antique bookshops. In addition, they analysed written documents of the times against which to compare their findings. What did they find? Interestingly, they found: a misrepresentation of sex ratios (more men than women); a projection of a rural image of the hospital, which was, in fact, situated in the city; and an overall impression of attendants and patients, not doctors. These findings revealed a more 'custodial and coercive' image than the written records. In this case, the photographs 'helped to deconstruct the public relations image portrayed in the written materials of the time' (Kellehear 1993a, p. 76).

Nowadays, video and television programs are available for unobtrusive researchers to pursue their research. Even some entertaining television series provide excellent opportunities to examine issues such as eating patterns, relationships between parents and children, and medical practices. Take any American drama series on medical professions. Do they tell us anything about medical dominance and gender roles in medicine? There has been some unobtrusive research using information from videos, films and television series. For example, Story and Faulkner (1990) were able to identify and analyse messages relating to food and the eating behaviour of American people by examining dramatic or situational comedies on television shown in prime time (8.00–11.00 pm). And what did they find? 'The prime time diet is inconsistent with dietary guidelines for healthy Americans' (p. 738). Other interesting studies include those of Sherman and Dominick (1986), who looked at sex and violence in music videos, and Denzin's (1991) study of dominant cultural ideas in films such as *Wall Street* and *Sex, Lies and Videotape*.

Simple observation
Simple observation can be carried out by systematically watching and recording people's behaviours, clothing, expressions and interaction in a particular location or several settings. In addition, physical signs and physical location can be

observed. Simple observation, as Kellehear (1993a) points out, can be done just about anywhere in public settings. It is therefore reasonably easy to conduct this type of unobtrusive research. However, in private locations, permission needs to be sought beforehand.

Observation of clothing is an interesting aspect of unobtrusive research technique. Palca (1981) argues that clothes can 'talk' and have meanings, and their meanings depend largely on the context or situation in which the clothes are worn. Williamson (1986), for example, suggests that 'leg warmers' worn by 'tall leggy' women in jeans or aerobic suits are symbols of the modern woman who has a career and who is still sexy and soft. And when Hmong people celebrate their important functions, such as Hmong New Year, what do they wear? They wear traditional costumes that are extremely colourful and decorated with silver. The costumes not only imply the solidarity of the Hmong people but also wealth and the care of family members. The wealthier the family, the more silver they use. More decorated and colourful costumes mean that the mothers and daughters spend a large amount of their time making them because they want their family members to look good on special days. And this implies family care.

Simple observation of people's behaviours also offers a great deal of information for unobtrusive researchers. Yule (1987), for example, argues that an observational study is very simple and can be done by anyone. In her own study she observed the interactions of eighty-five adult–child pairs for three minutes each. Within that period, she looked for facial expressions and other bodily movements. She found that adults were rude, asocial, intolerant, insensitive and aggressive towards their children. However, she concluded that these behaviours might be the extreme end of the spectrum of 'normal behaviour' of parents rather than child abuse.

More recently, Clark and Bowling (1990), Threlfall (1992), and Gorter and colleagues (1993) have conducted observational studies that attempt to understand human behaviours. Clark and Bowling's study (1990) is a particularly good example of the usefulness of observation techniques. The authors not only critically argue for the value of such methods, but also outline some practical methodological considerations (see also the later section in this chapter).

The use of hardware

Hardware allows simple observations to be detailed, to be available for later inter-rater analysis, and to be re-analysed in the future (Kellehear 1993a). The use of the camera is a good example. Threlfall (1992) photographed people who wore sunglasses, and their clothing, for his analysis of sun-protecting behaviours in Western Australia. From the pictures, he was able to make a link between clothes and the wearing of sunglasses.

Computers, and CD-ROMs, allow unobtrusive researchers to analyse existing literature. For example, Skolbekken (1995), in his study of a risk epidemic, obtained his data through searching the medical literature on MEDLINE databases. By using this type of unobtrusive method, he was able to find out how the epidemic arose.

How do we make sense of the data obtained?

There are many techniques that unobtrusive researchers can use to interpret patterns in their data. Kellehear (1993a, 1993b) proposes three principles of pattern recognition: content analysis, thematic analysis, and semiotic analysis. (For greater detail on these analyses, see Chapter 10.)

Content analysis is popular and frequently used in unobtrusive methods. Bernard (1995, p. 339) describes it as 'a blend of qualitative and quantitative, positivistic and interpretive methods'. Researchers start with their qualitative data (text), 'make hypotheses about what they think is "in there", do systematic coding and statistical analysis, and interpret the results in the light of historical or ethnographic information'. This type of analysis is, therefore, influenced by positivist theoretical tradition (see Chapter 1).

With the thematic type of analysis, themes of important messages inherent in the material are looked for. These messages emerge from the perspective of the material under examination. The emerging themes are then the categories of the analysis. In thematic analysis, frequency is not a major concern as it is in content analysis, but the 'position of the idea in the narrative' is more important (Daly et al. 1997, p. 135).

Semiotic analysis goes a step further. When employing this approach, researchers look for the 'hidden' agenda within the narrative material. In other words, this type of analysis attempts to reveal what is not said but may be hidden in the narrative material. Repressed and suppressed meanings may then become clear.

With thematic and semiotic analysis, hermeneutics and postmodernism traditions largely influence the interpretation of data. In some unobtrusive research projects we may also see the influence of feminism (see also Chapter 1).

UNOBTRUSIVE METHODS IN HEALTH: SOME EXAMPLES

In the last decade or so, we have seen more publications in health research utilising unobtrusive methods. In this section, we attempt to summarise several projects to illustrate the value of unobtrusive methods in health.

Within the medical text domain, Hahn (1987) examined relations between obstetricians and childbearing women as presented in the first seventeen editions of *Williams Obstetrics*, the central reference text of obstetrics and gynaecology in the USA that was originally developed by J. Whitridge. Williams was a powerful obstetrician in the early part of this century. Hahn's analysis was both thematic and semiotic in nature. In this study, Hahn attempted to examine the 'framework of concepts, premises, logic, and values' that underlie the obstetrical pedagogy. Examining the development of this text, Hahn argues, 'provides a window onto the profession of obstetrics, its work, its socialization, and the way it has conducted birth during this century' (p. 257). What he has found is as fascinating as that of Koutroulis. From the first edition in 1903 to the most recent one in 1985, this text has guided, and also reflected, the development of beliefs and practices in obstetrics in American medicine. The early editions reflect a strong belief that childbirth is an essentially pathological event. Women in childbirth are seen as patients who require extensive medical monitoring and intervention. Hahn found that, in the early editions that Williams himself wrote, women and childbearing are perceived as having four characteristics:

> First, the woman is conceived as 'the maternal organism' and 'the generative tract'—that is, the organ system is abstracted from the person so that the woman is no longer seen. Second, the course of childbirth is viewed as so danger-ridden as to be inherently pathological in need of pervasive medical attention and control ... Third, the parturient is ascribed an essentially passive role, while the physician assumes the central agency in delivery ... Finally, where childbearing women and their consociates are ascribed any agency, it is essentially as adversaries obstructing their own childbirths. (Hahn 1987, pp. 261–2)

Recent editions contain a view that indicates that childbirth is also considered as a social and psychological event. However, Hahn argues that this view has not really informed the beliefs and practices that characterise the text and hence obstetrics remains an essentially biological science in both its theory and practice. Hahn concludes that Williams aimed to achieve legitimate control of child-bearing by biomedical obstetrics and he did so via his influence on the obstetrics text used widely in obstetrical medicine. It is indeed a product of Williams' influence that 'in the divisions of labor, obstetrics continues to cast itself in the dominant role' (p. 279). As a result, childbirth continues to be medicalised by biomedical obstetrics.

That is how women and childbirth were portrayed in medical texts. What about women and premenstrual syndrome in the media? Chrisler and Levy (1990) looked at how premenstrual syndrome is constructed in magazine articles, by conducting a content analysis of magazines published in England between 1980 and 1987. Seventy-eight articles were identified and examined for their discussion of symptoms and treatments, the language and terms used in the articles and titles, and the types of issues covered in different types of magazines.

Chrisler and Levy found that most magazines tend to favour reporting premenstrual syndrome (PMS) as negative changes since they are more newsworthy and more dramatic. They tend to discuss the causes and treatment of PMS within the biological perspective, ignoring the social circumstances of young women. More importantly, the description of premenstrual syndrome is confusing. With so many different symptoms classified as negative, almost every woman can find some aspects of her experience in the list. Treatment recommendations are contradictory from one press to another. In short, the media coverage of PMS reinforces 'the stereotype of the maladjusted woman'. Chrisler and Levy (1990, p. 103) argued that 'these articles are not in the best interest of young women who may learn only what they read in the popular press and whose attitudes toward the menstrual cycle are being shaped as they read'.

In the area of child health, Gartner and Stone (1994) examined advice on breastfeeding in medical texts. They compared and contrasted published text-book material in Chinese and Western texts over the past 2000 years. The authors argued that breastfeeding was ideal for examination because it could be assumed that the physiology of lactation and breastfeeding had not changed over that period and its basic biology was similar in both cultures. Therefore, 'variations in the medical writings would be expected to reflect differing attitudes of both the medical establishment and of society as a whole in each culture' (p. 532). The authors used texts from library and archival sources in the Republic of China (Taiwan), the People's Republic of China, and in the USA. They employed a thematic analysis to examine the texts.

Gartner and Stone (1994) found that Chinese writings seem to approach breastfeeding from a more natural and supportive perspective. However, Western medical advice, both ancient and more recent, often implied the inadequacy of the mother to breastfeed her infant, particularly in the early weeks of life. One important aspect of Western medicine was its emphasis on the testing of mother's milk for its adequacy. The authors argued that this focus on testing might 'represent an early example of the reliance on laboratory diagnosis that has so heavily dominated western medicine in recent years' (p. 536). From the study, Gartner and Stone concluded that 'Western medicine seems more managerial with regard to breastfeeding than Chinese medicine, and has perhaps "medicalized" breastfeeding, a complaint often voiced even now in late 20th century America'. Nonetheless, both literatures show that, throughout the history of medicine, doctors have been concerned with 'promoting optimal breastfeeding and have understood the importance of human milk for the survival, growth, and development of the infant' (p. 536).

Unobtrusive research was used by Bammer and associates (1995) in their study of drug and alcohol. They examined heroin overdoses through an analysis of the report sheets completed by ambulance officers in the Australian Capital Territory (ACT) between August 1990 and July 1993. Using a content analysis, the cases were categorised into three groups: likely heroin overdoses, unlikely heroin overdoses, and possible heroin overdoses. Bammer and colleagues found that the number of overdoses dramatically increased in the second half of 1992 and the first half of 1993, but they could not identify the cause of this increase. In the 'likely' and 'possible' groups, most overdoses occurred to men under the age of 30 years, happened indoors and were treated on site. Frequently, there was not enough information in the records to explain why the overdoses happened. However, the available information indicated that, in half of the cases, users took heroin in combination with other drugs.

Another interesting study utilising unobtrusive research methods looked at injecting equipment in prisons. Seamark and Gaughwin (1994) examined injecting equipment found in three prisons in the Adelaide metropolitan area, between June 1991 and June 1992. Content analysis was used to classify the equipment according to four characteristics: the volume of the syringe; the type of syringe; physical appearance; and the presence of blood in the syringe barrel or in the needle cap. Syringes were categorised as new, little used, used, or very used, depending on the presence or absence of volume markings on the syringe barrel as well as the condition of the plunger. Fifty-eight syringes were examined. Their appearance suggested that most of them had been used more than once. This, the authors argued, suggested that syringe and needle-sharing might be taking place in prisons. One intriguing finding was that, even though the syringes were in poor condition, most did not contain visible blood. However, blood was visible in about one-third of the examined syringes. This suggested that most of the drug users cleaned their syringes and needles, but there were some that did not do so.

In the area of drug advertising, Kleinman and Cohen (1991) explored the 'decontextualization' of mental illness in psychiatric drug advertisements in the USA. They employed a semiotic approach to analyse the image of 'work' in drug advertisements appearing in the *American Journal of Psychiatry* between 1980 and 1988. From all advertisements that contained work and work-related themes such as domestic work, commuting and vacations, thirty-nine were selected for analysis that the authors believed most clearly drew on common-sense American images of work in their promotion of the drug product. Intriguingly, Kleinman and Cohen's unobtrusive study found that the advertisements tended to individualise mental illness. The treatment of the drugs also fails to consider the social realities that may be associated with mental illness. Take the following as examples (Kleinman and Cohen 1991, p. 869):

A young carpenter, clad in a flannel work shirt, holds a two-by-four and smiles at us. To his left is a quotation. He tells us: 'Everything seems to work better … *including me.*' Above the drug's logo a line reads 'It feels good to feel useful again'.

The patient pictured is a female radio disc jockey. She stares blankly at us, and does not look at the dial she turns with her right hand or the paper copy she holds with her left. 'She went into the hospital with a psychiatric emergency ... delusions, hallucinations, and other psychotic ... symptoms ...' But Thorazine *'brought her back to reality'*.

These two advertisements indicate that the mental health problem lies within the 'patient'. Hence, to be able to 'get back to reality', the focus is again on the individual person. Here is another fascinating ad (p. 872):

Her doctor helped her save a lot by prescribing Sinequan ... her family life.

This ad not only emphasises the benevolence of the physician and the traditional family role of the woman but also individualises the woman. These messages, as Kleinman and Cohen (1991, p. 872) argue, 'portray and reinforce a view of mental illness that localizes pathology within the individual patient. Economic and social contexts are assumed to be irrelevant, or are "givens" to which the afflicted patient must accommodate.'

In relation to work, an ad for the tranquiliser Tranxene pictured a young mother happily cutting a birthday cake for her three children. In this ad, the drug was advertised as 'effective, not overpowering', 'provides effective relief of anxiety symptoms' and hence allows the patient to 'function normally'. The drug helps not only mom but also 'the people who rely on ... [mom] every day'. This ad did not acknowledge anything about the dad because clearly the drug helped mom to manage her domestic work without having to rely on dad's assistance. Again, Kleinman and Cohen (1991, p. 870) argued that 'the message is clear: the original problem was with the mother, not the organization of domestic labor. From the point of view of the manufacturers of Tranxene, it makes no sense to suggest that there is something dysfunctional or anxiety-producing about the organization of the family.'

In conclusion, Kleinman and Cohen point out some of the dangers in the discrepancy between the world of the advertisements and the more complex nature of reality. First, the ads distort the debate over treatment options for mental illness, having more reliance on drugs than on other psychosocial therapies. Second, they reinforce and legitimise existing social relations and attitudes, such as sexism and alienating working conditions, that may contribute to mental illness. Last, most drug consumers are not aware of the ads and their impacts since the drug ads target physicians. Therefore, drug consumers do not have even the limited choices that household consumers have. The authors urged physicians to look carefully at the messages embedded in the ads before recommending drugs to their patients.

AIDS has become an alarming health problem worldwide. How AIDS has been constructed in society is interesting. This has led Herzlich and Pierret (1989) to examine the construction of AIDS as a social phenomenon in the French press. They analysed a total of 412 articles about AIDS published between January 1982 (the date of the first article) and June 1986 (the date of the Second International AIDS Conference) in six national French dailies. The newspapers were chosen on the basis that they have a national circulation, they provide regular coverage of medicine and they cover most of the political spectrum. In this study, the authors claimed that they did not intend to conduct a thematic analysis of the articles about AIDS, but 'rather to analyse how the French press started and abetted this process of social construction' (p. 1236). Therefore, the study utilises a form of semiotic analysis.

The study revealed how the AIDS social phenomenon was constructed during the period of study (1982–6). Herzlich and Pierret (1989, p. 1235) found that the media passed information about the new disease from the medical sphere into the public domain. As it did so, and at the same time emphasised 'the rapid extension and catastrophic proportions of this unforeseen "epidemic", AIDS became an issue around which social relations polarized'. The construction of AIDS as a social phenomenon involved the following processes: 'naming, comparing with past epidemics, popularizing medical knowledge and symbolic values, competing over claims to discoveries and patents, and talking about the other (homosexuals in particular)'. Through these processes, AIDS has entered the public sphere in France and, as the authors pointed out, it was the press that helped to make this disease into a social phenomenon.

Issues of smoking and tobacco have also attracted some unobtrusive researchers. The issue of tobacco use in popular films was examined by Hazan and colleagues in the USA (1994). In this study, two feature-length films on video, for each year from 1960 to 1990, were randomly selected from the twenty top films. The title, year of release, genre, target audience, rating (G, PG, PG13, R or X) and historical era of each film were recorded. The presence of tobacco events in each five-minute interval of film time was recorded. These events included implied or actual consumption of tobacco, the presence of ashtrays and matches, talking about tobacco, 'no smoking' signs, and logos of the tobacco product. The researchers invented twenty-five variables for coding the events, including the characteristics of the smokers (age, sex, role); the characteristics of the tobacco (product, brandnames and paraphernalia); and the characteristics of the particular scene (number of smokers, health message).

This study showed that films typically presented a smoker as a 'White, male, middle class, successful, and attractive' person. Hazan and others (1994, p. 999) argued that the picture of a typical smoker in popular films reinforced the tobacco advertising in the USA with 'youthful vigor, good health, good looks, and personal and professional acceptance'. Across the thirty years of films investigated, there was no significant decline in overall tobacco use. However, they found changes in tobacco presentation: smoking became less personal and more social. This, the researchers claimed, suggested that smoking had more 'populist appeal'. Interestingly, the study found that 'smoking was used as an anxiolytic, reinforcing its "healthful" properties as a stress reducer'. This finding was consistent with the efforts of the tobacco industry that aimed to promote tobacco use as an 'alternative intervention to improve mental health' (p. 999). The popular films studied also reflected real life situations in that they showed that those from better educated and higher socio-economic backgrounds smoked less over time. However, smoking was still presented as an acceptable behaviour because it always represented a majority behaviour in the films. The researchers concluded that 'films reinforce misleading images and overstate the normalcy of smoking, which may encourage children and teenagers, the major movie audience, to smoke' (p. 1000).

Whenever the government and the public try to reduce tobacco consumption in the community, the tobacco industry feels threatened. In response, the industry has published smokers' rights to protect their consumers. These publications were examined by Cardador and colleagues (1995). Fifty-eight issues of smokers' rights publications from 1987 to 1992 were randomly selected from 134 issues, from publication mailing lists and from tobacco control organisations around the USA. The publications were studied for their themes using the content analysis method. In particular, the researchers examined the number of publications per year, the number of sentences on different themes per year, and the number of sentences per theme per publication. The content was coded into four thematic categories: perceived threat; undermining the opposition; creating legitimacy; and political and social action.

Cardador and others found that the number of issues of smokers' rights publications increased dramatically from thirteen in 1987 to thirty in 1992. The number of sentences across all themes also increased over time. However, the largest number appeared in 1990, 1991 and 1992, and the highest average number of sentences across the years was on the theme of 'political and social action'.

As a result of their findings, Cardador and colleagues (1995, p. 1215) argue that smokers' rights publications are clearly designed to legitimise smoking and to make smokers more aware of, and active in, pro-smoking political activity. The themes in the publications were designed to 'move smokers toward social and political action by giving readers skills, strategies, and information to facilitate a behavioral change from nonparticipation to involvement in the smokers' rights movement'. Within the 'perceived threat' theme, for example, essential messages were that smokers were targets of 'discrimination and harassment', and that the tobacco control movement was 'a threat' to personal freedom. Indeed, the publications were used as a power tool for presenting smoking as a rights issue and hence encouraging smokers to protect their rights. Cardador and colleagues argue that the efforts of the tobacco industry were designed to 'maintain high cigarette profits both by mobilizing public opinion in their favor and by delaying shifts in societal perceptions and attitudes about the acceptability of smoking, environmental tobacco smoke, and attendant controls on tobacco use' (p. 1216).

In general public health, Lupton (1995) examined medical and public health stories on the front pages of the *Sydney Morning Herald*. A total of 311 issues, published between 1 April 1992 and 31 March 1993, was examined. An initial quantitative content analysis was conducted on all of the front-page news stories that featured a medical or public health issue or event. In addition, a qualitative discourse analysis of the language used in the headlines, main text and captions, and of the visual images such as photographs, cartoons and drawings accompanying the news stories, was carried out. Lupton argued that this was to 'go beyond the text' in order to 'discern the subtextual discourses evident in the news texts in the context of the wider socioeconomic and political settings in which they were expressed' (p. 502).

From the 311 front pages examined, 140 medical or public health stories were identified in 117 editions. Over one-third of all editions published at least one health or medical story on the front page, suggesting the newsworthiness of such topics, the major ones of which included health service delivery, tobacco and smoking, cancer, AIDS, environmental health, diet, drugs, swimming pool safety, contraception, sexual activity, work-related illness, alcohol, and obesity.

The discourse analysis yielded fascinating results. The language used in headlines was interesting. Lupton found that the recurrence of nouns and active verbs that refer to life and death, pain, distress, anger and panic not only reflected the subject matter, but also served to 'heighten their drama and sense of urgency'. Take, for example, headlines like 'The deadly virus that threatens Australia' or 'New clue to cancer's cause' (p. 506), which would quickly grab readers' attention.

Lupton (1995) also looked at news actors and news sources in the front-page news. Most stories cited news actors and news sources to give credibility to the details reported. Most of these actors and sources came from government, academe or research, and the medical profession. This, Lupton argued 'showed the power structure of Australian society and the tendency of elites to make the news, and therefore shape its meaning' (p. 506). What is more interesting is that where the gender of the news actors was identified, a gender imbalance was found: 72.8 per cent of news actors were male and only 27.2 per cent were female. Many stories contained only male news actors and sources and most news actors were government officials, politicians, spokespeople, academics, and members of the medical profession. Only stories about illnesses or diseases that predominantly affected women, or stories of 'victims' of diseases such as cancer, contained female news actors. Lupton argued that 'the impression conveyed is that of men as "experts", the active and knowledgeable participants and leaders in the medico-scientific domain, and women as the passive recipients of authoritative medical knowledge or the handmaidens of doctors' (p. 507). Lastly, Lupton found that the front-page news stories tended to find someone to blame for a health problem and to ignore socio-economic complexities.

Another interesting piece of unobtrusive research is Clark and Bowling's (1990) study of long-stay hospital and nursing home care in London. This study was part of a quantitative research project employing a randomised control trial and survey techniques. In selecting a simple observation method as their unobtrusive research tool, Clark and Bowling (1990, p. 1201) argued that:

> Observational methods are particularly appropriate when the study requires an examination of complex social relationships or intricate patterns of interaction. Institutions are ideal settings within which ... observation can take place in an unobtrusive manner. Observational methods are essential in evaluation studies of long stay care where the dynamics of the caring process and the content of everyday life are either unknown or difficult to measure using other techniques (e.g. survey methods) ... The rationale behind the use of observational techniques in sociological research is that the sociologist should become party to a set of social actions sufficiently to assess directly the social relationships and interactions involved.

With this theoretical framework in mind, Clark and Bowling began to observe the dynamics of everyday activities and the quality of interactions in a National Health Service (NHS) long-stay female geriatric ward and in two NHS nursing homes for the elderly within the same health district in London. Observations on the ward were supplemented by observation of the patients' club where less confused patients sometimes spent their time (an hour a day) in the basement of the hospital.

Clark and Bowling constructed the observation schedule to record data. The schedule consisted of a structured section involving logging activities, interactions and moods in fifteen-minute blocks. The log activities only included the recording of general activity, personal relationships and interaction between patients and staff. Additionally, a qualitative observational log was used to supplement the structured log. In this log, the observer recorded what she had observed over a fifteen-minute period. The observations were conducted at the part of the setting where most patients sat and activities were likely to occur, as well as at different times of the day, to ensure comparable periods in each setting.

Following Goffman's concept of the total institution, Clark and Bowling (1990, p. 1201) argued from the survey data that it appeared that 'block treatment' of patients in both long-stay hospital wards and smaller nursing homes was similarly evident. However, the observational study showed that only the ward setting conformed closely to this 'block treatment'. Staff in nursing homes was more likely to respond to the individual needs of the elderly. In addition, the observational study revealed that involvement in activities and interaction with others promoted positive feelings among the elderly. This led Clark and Bowling to question the validity of the 'disengagement theory' that sociologists tend to use to explain the position of old people in Western societies. In their conclusion, they point out the value of using multimethods in conducting any one piece of research (p. 1209):

> This study ... has shown how essential it is not to rely solely on interview material and assessments of mental and physical functioning, and to view quality of life more broadly than simply in terms of outcome. Whereas no differences in outcome were found between settings relying on the survey data, the observational data support the conclusion that a different quality of life was apparent between settings.

WHAT DETERMINES GOOD QUALITY UNOBTRUSIVE RESEARCH?

The quality of data gathered from unobtrusive research is a controversial issue in qualitative methodology. The issue of accuracy seems to be at the core of the controversy. How can you be sure that what you take as a set of data is accurate in the first place? How can you make sense of information that other researchers have collected and with which you have not had any first-hand involvement?

To answer these questions, Kellehear (1993a) argues that if researchers have doubts about the accuracy of the data collected, they need to combine unobtrusive methods with other qualitative methods. This is in line with the triangulation approach in, say, ethnography and focus groups. The combination of research methods allows researchers to validate their findings from unobtrusive methods. If they appear to confirm each other, then the data collected should be good quality data.

UNOBTRUSIVE METHODS: ADVANTAGES AND LIMITATIONS

As with other types of qualitative research methods, unobtrusive methods offer several advantages and contain some limitations.

Advantages

* Unobtrusive methods reflect people's behaviours more accurately than their reports of their behaviours. If a researcher wanted to know what people eat, it would be more accurate to look at their rubbish than to ask them what they eat. They are more likely to give answers that will please the researchers or to tell a story that may not be really true. Unobtrusive methods allow researchers to literally see people's behaviour for themselves. In trace studies such as an investigation of food consumption by examining people's rubbish,

Rittenbaugh and Harrison (1984) point out that, when the people were told that their rubbish was being monitored, the number of empty bottles of alcoholic drink was significantly fewer.

- Unobtrusive methods are non-reactive and non-disruptive. They are, therefore, typically safe for the researchers and the researched.
- Unobtrusive methods are repeatable by other researchers. This has the advantage of the possibility of crosschecking and re-examination for reliability and validity.
- Unobtrusive methods typically allow easier access to data sites since they do not require human contact, such as in other more obtrusive methods like individual interviews. However, researchers may still need to obtain permission to get access to the data, even if only as a matter of courtesy.
- Unobtrusive methods are inexpensive, mainly requiring time and a record book. They do not need funding for the development of a survey questionnaire, for equipment such as a tape recorder, or for the transcription necessary in individual interviews.
- Unobtrusive methods are ideal for longitudinal studies, which require the follow-up of activities for a long period of time. An examination of household rubbish, for example, can be traced for a few weeks instead of one; or the content in a newspaper can be examined for a period of one year.

Limitations

- Unobtrusive methods reduce the possibility of studying people from their own perspective, such as in the individual interview situation. What the researchers report from their observation may reflect their own perspective rather than that of the researched.
- The original records may be distorted or selective because of some biases of the persons who recorded them, whether due to hiding some information, to impress others, or due to their backgrounds. Therefore, the information analysed may not be accurate.
- Information from unobtrusive methods may be distorted because of 'intervening variables' (Kellehear 1993a, p. 7). In the Garbage Project, for example, Rathje (1984) did not initially take into account the recycling practices of some households. Only later was it realised that some families recycled their aluminum cans and others had compost heaps for making fertiliser for their vegetables. As a consequence, the earlier findings were distorted due to 'intervening variables'.
- Unobtrusive methods tend to rely on a single approach. For example, in Threlfall's (1992) study of the correlation between wearing sunglasses and type of clothing in Perth, he relied only on photographs of people. What he

observed on two Saturday mornings may not reflect real behaviours. If he had also used other methods to assess the issue, he may have come up with a different conclusion. For example, you cannot see whether people are wearing sunscreen in a photograph. You would have to ask them.

CONCLUSION

In this chapter we have outlined some major issues concerning unobtrusive methods in the social sciences, and particularly the importance of these research methods in the health sciences. As Kellehear (1993a, p. 161) succinctly puts it:

> Unobtrusive methods are able to make the silent past accessible to researchers of the present. The unobtrusive researcher is able to enter places, see people and events, and listen to voices that pollsters and interviewers are unable to hear, see or visit with their methods.

With this in mind, we hope that those who have embarked or wish to embark on research using unobtrusive methods may uncover new, interesting and important discoveries.

Tutorial exercise

Collect articles on health issues published in your local newspaper over a one-week period. Analyse these articles using content, thematic and semiotic analysis. What are the main ideas you receive from the media?

Further reading

Daly, J., Kellehear, A. and Gliksman, M., 1997, *The Public Health Researcher: A Methodological Approach*, Oxford University Press, Melbourne.

Kellehear, A., 1993, *The Unobtrusive Researcher: A Guide to Methods*, Allen & Unwin, Sydney.

Koutroulis, G., 1990, 'The Orifice Revisited: Women in Gynaecological Texts', *Community Health Studies*, vol. 14, no. 2, pp. 73–84.

Lupton, D., 1994, 'Femininity, Responsibility and the Technological Imperative: Discourse on Breast Cancer in the Australian Press', *International Journal of Health Services*, vol. 24, no. 1, pp. 73–89.

Sechrest, L. (ed.), 1979, *Unobtrusive Measurement Today*, Jossey-Bass, San Francisco.

Webb, E.L., Campbell, D.T., Schwartz, R.D. and Sechrest, L., 1966, *Unobtrusive Measures: Non-Reactive Research in the Social Sciences*, Rand McNally & Co., Chicago.

6

Narrative Analysis and Life History

Introduction

A man [sic] is always a teller of stories, he lives surrounded by his own stories and those of other people, he sees everything that happens to him in terms of those stories and he tries to live his life as if he were recounting it. (Sartre, quoted in Bruner 1987, p. 21)

One of the most powerful forms for expressing suffering and experiences related to suffering is the narrative. Patients' narratives give voice to suffering in a way that lies outside the domain of the biomedical voice. (Hyden 1997, p. 49)

When human beings make their lives meaningful they primarily do this by telling a story (Polkinghorne 1988). Narrative analysis examines these stories. As several recent reviews have noted, narrative analysis is an interdisciplinary approach covering a very wide range of topics, methodologies and techniques (Hyden 1997; Mishler 1995; Riessman 1993). This chapter focuses on some of the more common methods and techniques of narrative analysis that have been used in studies of health and illness.

Narrative analysis is distinguished from other qualitative research methodologies by its attention to the structure of narratives as a whole. Many qualitative methodologies fragment texts, or people, through the process of observation and analysis. Narrative analysis typically works with larger units of analysis, such as an interview as a whole, or a person's biography as a whole. An emphasis on narrative also allows a researcher to draw on studies of narrative in literary theory. This typically shifts the focus of a qualitative research project further away from positivistic methodologies and closer to hermeneutic or poststructuralist orientations.

WHY USE NARRATIVE ANALYSIS?

Narrative analysis is an approach to qualitative research that emphasises the narrative, or story-based, nature of human understanding. 'Narrative analysis takes as its object of investigation the story itself' (Riessman 1993, p. 1). Narrative thinking, or rationality, is very different to scientific thinking, or rationality (Bruner 1986). The goal of both is to establish a causal account (Robinson and Hawpe 1986). However, they do this in very different ways.

Scientific rationality is built out of logical, well-formed arguments that are designed to convince of truth through reference to repeatable scientifically constructed empirical tests. The aim is to produce general laws that can be applied to particular events to explain why things happen. These laws are usually abstract and context-free. There is no place for context-dependent flexibility or ambiguity in scientific rationality. Randomised control trials or epidemiological surveys are typically justified in this way.

In contrast, narrative rationality is formed through telling a good story that is designed to convince through its 'life-likeness', and that can be tested through ordinary interpersonal checking (Robinson and Hawpe 1986). Narratives focus on the details of the story and emphasise the context-dependent nature of the particular story told. Narratives change depending on who tells them and ambiguity is a central part of a good story. Narrative rationality convinces through gripping drama and believable history.

While logico-scientific rationality may be useful for understanding chemistry or biology, its usefulness is very limited in studies of meaning and human action. The consequence of this is perhaps most graphically illustrated in the development of psychological theory. In its quest to be scientific, psychology has almost completely forgotten to study people. 'Nearly all published psychological studies up to 1978 do not attempt to study a whole individual person, and of those that do, the whole person is not the point of the research, so much as an illustration of a point' (Polkinghorne 1988, p. 104). Psychology ignores the whole person because the person cannot be measured or categorised using scientific rationality. The self can only be studied as a whole when past, present and future are understood as integrated into a whole through a narrative.

The usefulness of a narrative approach is perhaps best illustrated through the responses obtained from interviews. Interviewers often expect categorical answers that fit with a scientific model of the person, but get narratives instead (Bruner 1990; Mishler 1986). For example, when Douglas (Ezzy 1996) was conducting his interviews with unemployed people as part of a study of job loss and mental health, one early interview significantly changed the way he thought about interviewing people:

Doug:	Tell me about how you felt about your work? Did you enjoy it? Did you get on well with people there?
Chris:	Well ... it's very difficult to give you a short answer about my working career and if you don't mind I think I'll give you a long answer.
Doug:	That's fine.
Chris:	I started as a representative, working from home ...

Douglas had been looking for a response along the lines of 'Work is enjoyable, but I didn't like one of the people involved'. That is to say, Douglas was thinking of people as made up of a set of characteristics or dimensions, along which various responses could be measured. Chris, for example, had low levels of work enjoyment but good relations with his work colleagues. However, he did not like thinking about himself in these terms, as bundles of variables. Instead, he preferred to tell a story that illustrated his experience. This difference between the responses expected by Douglas and Chris' preferred mode of response came to a head when Chris was asked:

Doug:	Can you give me ten words or phrases in response to the question 'Who am I?'?
Chris:	I've been down this track before and I don't like it.
Doug:	What do you mean?
Chris:	I've done this on various personality check-ups and so on. Well, the other day my wife and I went to Jenny and Alex's for New Year's Eve. I had a ball asking both of them their life story and went right through and it was fascinating as you would know. Afterwards my wife was making a comment about how I'm a terror for asking all these questions, but that people wake up to me and start throwing them back at me and asking questions and then I have a bit of trouble. I'm more of a question asker than answerer. So this is what's happening now. Who am I? What a ripper.

The response seemed strange. The Ten (or Twenty) Statements Test is a well-established technique utilised by a variety of researchers (Kuhn and McPartland 1954). Respondents are expected to give a list of words or phrases that summarise their self-concept. Why did Chris refuse? When asked to explain this refusal he first says that he does not like personality tests, and then he tells a story about how he sees himself more as a person who asks questions than one who answers them. Yet Chris provided many long responses to the questions he was asked in the interview. He certainly had no problem answering questions.

At the end of the interview Douglas realised why Chris had refused to answer the Ten Statements Test question as it was asked. Chris understood his life in stories. He easily answered questions that asked for a story, but struggled with categorical questions that treated him as an object to be measured. It is possible that Chris had had a previous bad experience with personality tests, which had made him cautious about questions such as the Ten Statements Test. However, the content of the interview suggests that the main reason he felt uncomfortable was that he had been asked these sorts of questions before, both by friends and more formally. Chris was an insurance salesman and perhaps he routinely asked, and assessed his clients by means of, categorical questions that rated them on various scales. Chris was self-aware enough to know that he did not think about himself in these terms. While most people happily provide a list of phrases or words in response to the Ten Statements Test, this list can only be interpreted within the context of the stories that they tell about these words or phrases. After the above response Douglas asked Chris a series of questions about his work, his family, his church involvement, and other aspects of his life. In response to each question Chris told a long story that illustrated how he felt about that aspect of his life. These stories were full of detail and typically made clear, for example, the relative importance of work and family.

This experience appears to be relatively common among qualitative interviewers (Mishler 1986). For example, Chase (1995, p. 4) reports that during her interviews, she 'dropped her sociological questions and began to ask for life stories ... when she realised that the general processes she sought to understand are embedded in women's lives'. Narrative analysis aims to understand the way in which general social processes are interpreted through their place in the narrative.

Heidegger (1962) argued that human beings do not understand themselves as detached beings, but through engaged activity. In the interview, Chris refused to discuss himself as an abstract entity or self-concept, or to place his experience on a scale of work satisfaction. Rather, he told a story about his life as an engaged activity. In everyday life, the question 'Who am I?' is not typically answered by describing the properties of a substance. When people are asked, 'Who are you?', they do not typically respond: 'I am a male. I am a father. I am an insurance salesman.' Rather, the self-concept is formed in a narrative. 'The everyday answer is given as a narration of the sort: "I was born in St. Louis, and then I went to school, which got me interested in these things" and so on' (Polkinghorne 1988, p. 152).

Most modernist psychology uses a root metaphor of a machine (Sarbin 1986), along with logico-scientific rationality. The world, and people, are thought of as machines, whose properties can be measured and whose behaviour can be predicted on the basis of causal models. Behaviourism and radical empiricism in psychology exemplify this approach. The attempt to classify people using the Ten Statements Test has elements of this mechanistic method. These models are not very useful when it comes to dealing with the contingent, complex and ongoing construction of everyday experience that is examined in qualitative research in general, and in studies of health and illness in particular.

The problem with the metaphor of the machine is that people do not understand themselves in this way. In contrast, the social psychological tradition of authors such as C.S. Pierce, William James and G.H. Mead uses a root metaphor of an historical event (Sarbin 1986). The world, and people, are like historical stories. If people are thought of as machines, there is little room for flexibility, for ambiguity, for multiple interpretations. In contrast, stories are often ambiguous and open-ended, and contain multiple interpretations. While the causal methodologies and mechanistic metaphors of physics and economics can offer a great deal, they cannot capture the richness and complexity of human lives, nor can they capture their historical depth. These can only be plumbed through a narrative methodology. Meanings are not objects but actions (Polkinghorne 1988).

The realist, positivist, or scientific psychologist, wants to avoid, or ignore, the influence of human creativity on the events described in a narrative. However, it is this creativity that interests the narrative analyst most: 'In the form a particular narrator gives to a history we read the more or less abiding concerns and constraints of the individual and his or her community' (Rosenwald and Ochberg 1992, p. 4).

To some extent, many qualitative research methodologies still reflect the influence of a scientific logical rationality that attempts to conceptualise people and experiences as objects that can be measured on variables. Narrative analysis embraces more fully the meaning dependent and ambiguous nature of human action:

> Unlike traditional qualitative methods, [narrative analysis] does not fragment the text into discrete content categories for coding purposes but, instead, identifies longer stretches of talk that take the form of a narrative—a discourse organized around time and consequential events in a world recreated by the narrator. (Riessman 1990a, p. 1195)

Why use narrative analysis? Because it provides a way of understanding human experience that is consistent with the way that people make sense of their own lives:

> Narrative is a scheme by means of which humans give meaning to their experiences of temporality and personal actions. Narrative meaning functions to give form to the understanding of a purpose to life and to bring everyday actions and events into episodic units. (Polkinghorne 1988, p. 11)

WHAT IS A NARRATIVE?

Narrative is defined in different ways, depending on the subject of study, how it is to be studied and the purpose of the study. Robinson and Hawpe (1986, p. 112) argue that 'there is no rigid recipe of what counts as a story'. Some definitions are so broad that they include nearly everything (Riessman 1993). Other definitions are quite limited, focusing on one aspect of narratives (Labov and Waletzky 1997).

Bal's definition (quoted in Toolan 1988, p. 9) contains the important elements: 'A *fabula* [story] is a series of logically and chronologically related events that are caused or experienced by actors.' Narratives require a narrator and they order events temporally in sequences, include references to the past as well as current understandings, and have a structure around a plot or theme that has a point or moral (Bertaux and Kohli 1984, p. 224).

Bruner (1990) suggests that stories have two main components, which must be grasped in order for the meaning of a narrative to be understood. First, a narrative has a configuring plot, an overall structure within which the constituent parts make sense. Second, the plot is constructed out of these parts, out of a succession of events, and the power of the story derives from understanding this sequence of events. Narratives join events together and display their significance for one another. Plot is the organising theme of a narrative. Plot weaves together the events into a single story.

Narratives can refer to either the process of making a story, to the cognitive scheme of the story, or to the result of the process—the written stories. Following Polkinghorne (1988), we use narratives to refer to both the process and the result. However, it is important that researchers make clear the particular definition, and referent, of 'narrative' that they are using.

NARRATIVELY ORIENTED INTERVIEWING

> A basic question drives the interpretive project in the human disciplines: how do men and women live and give meaning to their lives and capture these meanings in written, narrative and oral forms? (Denzin 1989b, p. 10)

Data for narrative analysis derives from two main sources. First, most qualitative research projects draw on oral interviews in which narratives are recorded. However, there are a variety of other sources of data that can be analysed using narrative methods, including autobiographies, written records, newspapers and other documents (see Chapter 5 on unobtrusive methods).

Chase (1995) points out that many interviews elicit reports about events that do not evaluate these events through placing them in a coherent narrative. In contrast, narratively oriented interviews elicit stories where the respondent takes responsibility for interpreting their experiences through contextualising them in a story: 'If we want to hear stories rather than reports then our task as interviewers is to invite others to tell their stories, to encourage them to take responsibility for the meaning of their talk' (Chase 1995, p. 3).

Bertaux and Kohli (1984, p. 224) suggest that a narratively oriented interview consists of two distinct parts. First, the interview contains 'a preferably extensive narration by the interviewee/narrator'. During this phase, the interviewer restricts their involvement to encouraging the continuation of the story. Second, the authors suggest a period when the interviewer actively engages with topics discussed in the narrative, seeking clarification and introducing additional issues that may have been implied or omitted. Interviewers who aim for narratives need to think carefully about how questions are constructed. Questions should be avoided that ask for abstract arguments or logical defences (Bertaux and Kohli 1984). For example, try to avoid questions such as: 'How did you arrive at that decision?' Rather, aim to elicit narrative detail: 'Tell me about the events leading up to that.'

Narratively oriented interviewing also involves a different way of listening. In Douglas' (Ezzy 1996) interview with Chris, reported above, it was only at the end of the interview that Douglas realised that the information being sought was being reported in a story. Even though the stories were given in response to questions at the beginning of the interview, Douglas had not 'heard' the response because he had been trying to categorise these responses as if they could be measured on a scale. When an interviewer listens for the story, the details that are heard, and the follow-up questions, are likely to be very different. Douglas felt like going back and starting the interview all over again once he understood that the stories were where the information was located.

TYPES OF NARRATIVE ANALYSIS

There is a wide variety of approaches to data analysis in narrative methodologies (Cortazzi 1993; Toolan 1988). As with other forms of qualitative data analysis, narrative analysis involves reducing the data and re-interpreting it in order to present an analysis of the material under consideration (see Chapter 10). This section will provide some examples of distinctive analytic strategies utilised in narratively oriented qualitative studies.

One of the most common ways of analysing narrative data in qualitative health-related research is in terms of plot structure (Frank 1995; Hyden 1997; Mattingly 1994). Such studies typically draw on studies of plot structure in literary theory and develop these to analyse the form of narratives in the particular empirical cases under examination. Gergen and Gergen (1988) provide a useful summary of three rudimentary plot types: stability, regressive and progressive. A stability narrative is 'a narrative that links events in such a way that the individual remains essentially unchanged with respect to evaluative position' (p. 24). Regressive and progressive narratives link events together so that events reflect, respectively, either a decline or an improvement in evaluations over time. Regressive and progressive narratives parallel the classic literary forms of tragic and romantic narratives. Combinations of these rudimentary types lead to more complex forms such as the romantic saga.

Apart from models of overall plot structure, Riessman (1993, p. 18) describes three other common types of analysis on narrative structures used by Labov, Burke, and Gee. Labov (Labov and Waletzky 1997) analyses narratives through identifying six elements of story structure, including the abstract, orientation, complicating action, evaluations, resolution, and coda. From a different perspective, Burke (1945) provides a dramatic analysis of grammatical resources: act, scene, agent, agency, purpose. Finally, Gee (1986) analyses the oral aspects of stories, such as pitch, pauses, and other features.

Narrative analysis is distinguished from other forms of qualitative data analysis by its attention to the structure of the narrative as a whole. Traditional thematic analysis typically fragments texts, coding small chunks and then collating them. Narrative analysis searches for larger units of discourse and codes their structure and thematic content. Riessman (1993, p. 44) reports that, when she began analysing her interviews, 'I found myself not wanting to fragment it into discrete thematic categories but to treat it instead as a unit of discourse' (see Chapter 10 for more detail on the methods of qualitative data analysis).

POLITICS, ETHICS AND NARRATIVE ANALYSIS

> The only life worth living is a well-examined one. But … if we can learn how people put their narratives together when they tell stories from life, considering as well how they might have proceeded, we might then have contributed something new to that great ideal. (Bruner 1987, p. 32)

Stories are not only historical, about what has happened, they are also about the possible, about what might happen. Narrative theory has recently become influential in various forms of psychotherapy (Wiersma 1992). Wiersma argues that one of the major consequences of psychotherapy is that it allows a person to reconstruct their history, or self-story, so that they can act with a sense of self-worth in the present and confidence for the future. Wiersma shows how, over several interviews, 'Karen' changed her story about her life, from an initial tragic story of exaggerated passivity as a wife and graduate student to a more complex appreciation of 'the bittersweet ambiguity of her life and of all lives' (p. 211):

But it is not just Karen's stories that are better. As story and action mutually elicited each other, her life became better … she felt better: happier; freer to exercise independence, autonomy, and agency; more knowledgeable, mature and self-confident; and more able to cope with her life.

To tell a story is to take a moral stance (Bruner 1990). Similarly, Ricoeur (1988, p. 249) argues that 'narratives are never ethically neutral and narrative identity is therefore always evaluative and normative in its claims'. Categorical and mechanistic models of the self typically separate out this moral dimension. However, a narrative conception of identity and experience is inextricably a moral conception of identity and experience (Taylor 1989). Telling a story about oneself involves telling a story about choice and action, which have integrally moral and ethical dimensions. Further, narratives have transformative potential beyond the level of individual experience. Narratives sit at the intersection of history, biography and society. As Bertaux and Kohli (1984, p. 230) observe, 'lives are totalities, even if broken ones. They develop simultaneously at several levels: the historical, the societal, the ethnosocial, the personal.'

Most research projects tend to separate the analysis of individual identity and the analysis of society. However, as Brown (1987, p. 58) has pointed out, a theory of narrative transcends this bifurcation through an examination of 'vocabularies of motives and the grammars of interest that are encoded in and realised through various forms of discourse'. This approach leads to an analysis more sensitive to the role of power in shaping the cultural repertoires and discourses that a person employs to make sense of their experience. For example, some feminist researchers have pointed to the androcentric hegemonic narratives that shape the lives of women, contrasting these to counter narratives that are both feminist and inspirational (Personal Narratives Group 1989).

From a public health perspective, narrative analysis can also be utilised to examine the political influences and implications of health practices. Lupton (1992), for example, advocates that public health practitioners employ discourse analysis, which is a form of narrative analysis that focuses on the sociocultural and political contexts in which narratives are formed. Lupton argues that discourse analysis is potentially important as a mode of public health research because 'it has the potential to lay bare the ideological dimension of such phenomena as lay health beliefs, the doctor–patient relationship, and the dissemination of health information in the entertainment mass media' (p. 145).

Finally, Denzin (1986, p. 17) reminds us that as qualitative researchers we should be responsible with our data, treating it with respect: 'It must be remembered that we do not own the lives and the stories we tell. They are lent to us, given provisionally, if they are given at all. They remain, always, and irrevocably the lives and stories of those who have told them to us.'

LIFE HISTORY AND NARRATIVE ANALYSIS

Life histories can be constructed from either primary or secondary data (Denzin 1970). Primary data derive directly from the person and include interviews, official reports, medical records and other similar documents. Secondary data indirectly provide information about a life history via the person's membership in a group about which there are official statistics, or a report on an organisation. According to Denzin, 'the life history presents the experiences and definitions held by one person, one group, or one organization as this person, group, or organization interprets those experiences' (pp. 220–1). This approach emphasises that life history is to be studied from the perspective of the person involved.

There are two main types of life history studies: 'life history as a topic', and 'life history as a means' (Helling 1988). On the one hand, some studies examine biography as a topic in and of itself. The aim is to describe the structure of events that make up a person's life history. On the other hand, many studies gather biographical information as 'a means of answering established sociological questions' (p. 214). In health social research, for example, a study might examine how previous illness experiences shape people's responses to cancer later in life.

The 'life history as a topic' is best illustrated by what Plummer (1983, p. 14) describes as 'the cornerstone of social science life document research', that is, 'the full length book account of one person's life in his or her own words'. The sociological classic of this genre is the 300-page story of Wladek Wisniewski, a Polish émigré to America, published as one entire volume of Thomas and Znaniecki's *The Polish Peasant in Europe and America* (1918–20). A more recent example is Bogdan's (1974) life history of Jane Fry. (Examples of 'life history as a means' are provided in the next section of this chapter.)

Chambron (1995, p. 127) observed that 'life history as method has not benefited much from existing tools of analysis'. This is a product of the narrative configuration of life stories. Methods that seek to avoid narrative rationality are not particularly useful in studying people's lives as wholes. The life story refers implicitly to a person's experience as a whole (Bertaux and Kohli 1984).

In qualitative research, life histories are typically elicited during long interviews. Interviews are not opportunities to discover pre-existing life stories (see Chapter 3). An autobiography is not simply a record of a life as it was lived (Bruner 1995). Rather, while events and stories predate the interview, the life story is recreated in the interview as part of a conversation with the interviewer. The structure and content of the life story is significantly shaped through the dialogue that occurs during the interview (Chambron 1995). According to this understanding, the aim of a life history interview is not to discover or reveal the correct events, or to uncover hidden memories. Rather, the interview involves the active construction of these events into a story (for more detail, see the discussion of hermeneutics in Chapter 1).

However, if a life history is actively constructed in an interview, this does not mean that it is completely fiction. There are limits on the types of story that can be told: socially constituted boundaries of possibility. Narratives of the self are not individual possessions, but the product of interaction (Gergen and Gergen 1988). As Denzin (1986, p. 17) puts it, 'lives are the expression of personal and social history, as well as relational webs of influence'. And 'the meaning of life-study inquiry lies in the discovery of the difference that sets the subject apart from others, yet joins her in the common epoch she shares with other ordinary people' (p. 16).

NARRATIVE ANALYSIS IN HEALTH: SOME EXAMPLES

In the interactionist tradition, life history analysis has focused on turning points that result in significantly restructured life projects (Denzin 1986). Illness is typically disruptive to people's life projects and may constitute a turning point. Narrative analysis is an incisive way of studying these turning points associated with illness experiences. 'Telling narratives is a major way that individuals make sense of disruptive events in their lives' (Riessman 1990a, p. 1199).

The place of narrative analysis in health research has had three distinct phases (Hyden 1997, p. 48). In the first, when biomedical definitions were taken for granted, narrative studies were used to examine patients' perspectives or behaviours, linked to terms such as 'illness-behaviour' or 'lay-perspective'. In the second phase, following on from the distinction between illness and disease, 'the possibility opened up for the study of the patient's speech ... as an integral and important part of the course of the illness' (p. 49). Finally, the transition from studies of clinical practice and illness experiences to studies focusing on the experience of suffering gave narrative an even more important place alongside biomedical accounts. The following three examples include a narrative conception of occupational therapists' clinical encounters, a broad study of the shape of illness narratives, and a public health-oriented study of the narratives of intravenous drug users.

A recent edition of the *American Journal of Occupational Therapy* was devoted to narrative research (Frank 1996; Larson and Franchiang 1996). Larson and Franchiang (1996, p. 247) argue that 'narrative and life history research are two approaches that can assist occupational therapists in better understanding the complexity and contexts of the client and his or her experience in the therapeutic process'. A 'better understanding' of the therapeutic process is important not only from the perspective of improved treatment for the patient, but also from the perspective of increasing pressure to provide cost-effective services.

On the basis of her research, Mattingly (1994, p. 811) argues that occupational therapists attempt to 'emplot' clinical encounters by enfolding them into larger developing narrative structures. Emplotment is the process by which individual events are pulled together into a narrative that gives them meaning, by placing them in the context of a larger narrative structure, or plot. This process of actively constructing life stories is crucial to the understanding of clinical and therapeutic interactions. Emphasising the central role of narrative emplotment to the clinical therapeutic encounters suggests a broader understanding of the experience of illness and healing:

> The central difficulty with the usual clinical depictions of patient sufferings is that in their abstractedness, the world of the patient is left out. This world is above all a practical and moral one in which patients have life projects and everyday concerns. (Mattingly 1994, p. 819)

Illness narratives do not simply report the events of an illness from the perspective of the patient. Illness narratives shape both the reality of the illness as it is experienced, and the responses of people to the illness.

In a more general light, Frank's (1995) discussion of *The Wounded Storyteller* places narrative reconstruction at the centre of the healing process for people experiencing a variety of different illnesses. Illness, suggests Frank, destroys people's self-understandings, particularly their assumptions about the future, making ill people a 'narrative wreck'. For this reason, he argues, ill people need to tell their stories 'in order to construct new maps and new perceptions of their relationships to the world' (p. 3). Frank's analysis of illness is distinctive because his use of narrative theory allows the ill person to be seen as a whole. Whereas an analysis using the Ten Statements Test may have segmented a person into various identities, narrative theory allows Frank to investigate the way that past experiences are related to present understandings that are in turn related to hopes for the future.

Frank (1995) identifies three types of illness narratives. First, the *restitution narrative* minimises the experience of illness, limiting the individual's responsibility to taking medicine and trying to get well. Illness is an interruption to be overcome. Parson's sick role theory is a clear restitution narrative: while a person can expect allowances due to their illness, this is only the case while they are trying to return themselves to normal functioning. Second, Frank identifies *chaos narratives* as the inverse of restitution narratives, where the person loses control and expects terrible things to keep happening without any order, meaning or purpose. The chaos narrative portrays the person as passive victim, in contrast to the agency of the restitution narrative. Finally, Frank (1995, p. 115) describes the *quest narrative*. In contrast to the restitution narrative, which treats illness simply as an interruption, quest narratives 'meet suffering head on; they accept illness and seek to use it. Illness is the occasion of a journey that becomes a quest.' Quest narratives typically involve a refiguring of the self-story with new emphases, often with the narrator as a hero or phoenix who reinvents himself or herself through suffering.

Finally, Hassin (1994) examines the public health implications of the narratives of female intravenous (IV) drug users in American society. Drawing on thirty-nine taped interviews along with additional informal interviews and participant observation, Hassin notes that there are two main images of female IV drug users in general American culture. First, they are viewed as unbridled dope fiends. Second, as the bearers of children they should be responsible citizens and 'clean up their act' for their children. At the heart of the tension between these images is the problem of agency. The 'dope fiend' image denies their agency, but the 'responsible citizen' image requires them to have agency. This problem has significant public health implications as most studies of AIDS focus on 'the problems and methods of educating IV drug users' (Hassin 1994, p. 392). These studies, and associated public health campaigns, assume agency. However, to understand how people choose to act 'responsibly', with agency, requires an analysis of identity construction and, particularly, an analysis of the narratives through which identity, agency and a sense of responsibility are attained.

All but one of the women Hassin approached were eager to tell their story. 'Yet, contrary to focusing on "the life," these stories were used by the speakers to negotiate and construct their identities for their audience and themselves' (p. 393). To illustrate this process, Hassin quotes extensively from an interview with 'Roberta'. Roberta uses the interview to redefine the stigmatising images of the junkie and HIV-positive person. She constructs her actions as moral, suggesting that her infection was the fault of a promiscuous previous husband, and that the withdrawal experience of her daughter was a consequence of Roberta being legitimately on methadone. These narrative strategies grant Roberta a level of dignity and acceptance that both reduces their suffering and allows Roberta to take an active role in actions that might reduce risky behaviour among the community.

Hassin argues that narrative analysis allows public health researchers to see the importance of the consequences of how IV drug users are portrayed. Images of IV drug users that deny them agency not only deny them dignity, and increase their suffering, but also make it more difficult for them to take responsibility for their actions and to participate in public health prevention campaigns. Further, 'the telling [of these stories] itself, within a supportive environment, sustains healthy behaviors allowing users to assume, with the legitimacy of moral acceptance, a positive identity within the society they live and accept as their own ideological base' (Hassin 1994, p. 398).

NARRATIVE ANALYSIS: ADVANTAGES AND LIMITATIONS

As with all other methods, narrative analysis has both advantages and limitations.

Advantages

- A narrative approach analyses interview data in a way that is consistent with how most people themselves make sense of their identity and their experiences. This methodology keeps the researcher close to the experience of their participants.
- Narrative analysis conceptualises stories as wholes, reducing the decontextualising and fragmenting effect of other qualitative methods.
- Narrative analysis explicitly incorporates moral and political dimensions into its framework.
- Narrative analysis addresses some of the problematic philosophical issues raised about the role of subjectivity in interviews and interpretative practice. This derives from the theoretical framework of hermeneutics that informs narrative analysis (see Chapter 1).

Limitations

- Some forms of narrative analysis cannot be easily codified and systematised because it focuses on the ambiguity of meaning and interpretation.
- Narrative analysis requires high investments of time and energy because of the focus on careful analysis of meanings and interpretations. This attention to detail may frustrate researchers with tight time lines or intolerance of complexity.
- As a consequence, 'narrative analysis is not useful for studies of large numbers of nameless, faceless subjects' (Riessman 1993, p. 69).

CONCLUSION

Research reports based on narrative analysis are more like history. They do not attempt to identify general laws that would enable prediction. However, they are also not typically oriented only towards the past. Rather, research reports based on a narrative methodology 'locate the decision points at which a different action could have produced a different ending' (Polkinghorne 1988, p. 171). The same idea is suggested by Ricoeur (1984, p. 52) when he argues that 'time becomes human to the extent that it is articulated through a narrative mode'. Past, present and possible futures are integrated in the plot of a narrative.

Narrative analysis explicitly incorporates the moral dimension, linked to antici-pated futures and the ability to choose how to act, into its conception of human experience. With this framework comes a more sophisticated understanding of suffering that is of major significance for studies of health and illness: 'Suffering is not defined solely by physical pain, nor even by mental pain, but by the reduction, even the destruction of the capacity for acting, of being-able-to-act, experienced as a violation of self-integrity' (Ricoeur 1992, p. 190).

Tutorial exercise

Select a health-related story from a recent edition of a local newspaper. The story could be about an individual, a disease, or a health-related organisation such as a hospital. Identify and summarise the plot of the story. Is it a tragedy or a story of heroism? What are the key events in the story? What does the story suggest about the future? Can you identify any ways in which the reporter has emphasised specific events to shape the story in a particular way? Is there another way that the story could be told? For example, if it is a tragic story, could it be told in such a way that it suggested a hopeful future? What would you need to know in order to know whether this alternative telling of the story might be plausible? Can you suggest why the media report chose to portray this particular health-related story in this particular way?

Further reading

Bruner, J., 1990, *Acts of Meaning*, Harvard University Press, Cambridge, Mass.

Cortazzi, M., 1993, *Narrative Analysis*, Falmer Press, London.

Denzin, N., 1989, *Interpretive Biography*, Sage, Newbury Park.

Frank, A., 1995, *The Wounded Storyteller*, University of Chicago Press, Chicago.

Hyden, L., 1997, 'Illness and Narrative', *Sociology of Health and Illness*, vol. 19, no. 1, pp. 48–69.

Lupton, D., 1992, 'Discourse Analysis: A New Methodology for Understanding Ideologies of Health and Illness', *Australian Journal of Public Health*, vol. 16, pp. 145–50.

Mattingly, C., 1994, 'The Concept of Therapeutic Emplotment', *Social Science and Medicine*, vol. 38, pp. 811–22.

Polkinghorne, D., 1988, *Narrative Knowing and the Human Sciences*, State University of New York Press, Albany.

Riessman, C., 1993, *Narrative Analysis*, Sage, Newbury Park.

Rosenwald, G. and Ochberg, R. (eds), 1992, *Storied Lives*, Yale University Press, New Haven.

7

Memory-Work

Introduction

The father is an amateur photographer. He works in his darkroom, developing films. The assembled family sits looking at the photos he has taken. 'You ought to watch your daughter, her tummy's too fat.' 'Oh, come on, she's only a child, it's puppy fat. It'll disappear of its own accord when she gets older.'

What passes through the mind of the child in the course of the conversation?—Perhaps:

> *There he goes again, finding fault with me: does she have to be so noisy, she disturbs him on Sundays when he's trying to sleep off Saturday excesses, what's more she's a girl, something he never wanted (so her mother says), and now to cap it all her tummy's too fat—after all, she is a girl',*

he has said. She doesn't care, of course. Her 'strength' is in her position at school—'strength' in the literal sense. She has a friend, too, who is clearly in awe of her. Both of them used to have long plaits, she cut hers off and her friend followed suit. Her friend is pretty and dainty. She tyrannizes her.

She enjoys the fights she often gets into with boys. They've made it into a game in which points are awarded for victories and defeats. Her points total places her in the top third. One day she managed to get one boy on the floor. She held his legs high against her chest so as to be able to kick his behind. He kicked out at her chest. She felt a sudden searing pain, like nothing she'd ever felt before. She kept going, emerged the victor once again, then went on her way and—burst out crying. It was over. She was turning into a girl. No longer would she be stronger than the boys, she was turning into a weakling, becoming girlish. No differences from all the stupid cry-babies, dirty fighters who scratched and bit and pulled your hair!

She began to pick fights with girls who annoyed her; one who couldn't speak German, whose skirts were too long—facts to which the boys had been indifferent. At some point in this period she must also have begun to look at herself more often in the mirror and to see that she was simply overweight. Above all, it was her stomach that was too fat. (Haug 1987, pp. 85–6)

This is a story about childhood experience in response to the body, written by a German woman involved in research examining the process of female sexualisation using a method called 'memory-work' (Haug 1987).

In this chapter, we will provide readers with a description of memory-work, its history, its method and its benefits and pitfalls. Several examples of research projects utilising memory-work will also be discussed.

WHAT IS MEMORY-WORK?

In its original form, Frigga Haug and her colleagues (1987) developed memory-work to discover the process of sexualisation in German culture. In their work, which appears in the book *Female Sexualization*, Haug and her colleagues write about a collective's attempts to analyse women's 'specialization' by writing stories of their own personal memories, 'stories within which socialization comes to appear as a process of sexualization of the female body' (p. 13). Memory-work, in Haug's perspective, is seen as a 'method for the unraveling of gender socialization'. Haug and her colleagues (1987, p. 36) write:

> Our research ... focused on individuals who, having submitted already to their own subordination, had no access to any alternative language, nor to any possible means of conceptualizing alternative action. And yet they shared one strength in common. Those who suffer in their subordination—however inarticulate that suffering may be—are many: potentially, they include all women. Thus our work began not only from the premise that the subject and object of research were one; our second premise was that research itself should be a collective process. It was as a collective that we recorded and analysed our personal memories.

The method involved selecting a theme related to the body, including legs, hair, stomach and height, and requiring the group members to write down their memories of past events that focus on this bodily area. The stories are then circulated among the group for discussion, reassessing and rewriting. The group looks for absences in the text, for contradictions, for 'clichéd formulations covering knots of emotion or painful detail' (p. 13). Collectively rewritten, the final text becomes 'a finely textured account of the process of production of the sexualized female body' (p. 13).

Memory-work is a new and distinctive qualitative research method in the social sciences. It is seen as a feminist research process in which memories are the raw data for analysis. However, memory-work is also influenced by other theoretical traditions, including phenomenology, symbolic interactionism, postmodernism and hermeneutics (see Chapter 1). In memory-work, memories are important and a legitimate source of knowledge. Memory-work accepts the notion that what a person remembers is 'a relevant trace in his or her construction of self' (Schratz-Hadwich 1995, p. 41). The significance of memories is that they are not just people's true records, 'but their active role in the construction of identity' (Schratz-Hadwich 1995, p. 41). Memories reflect the lived experiences of people, as Kippax (1990, p. 93) points out:

> Memory-work is based on an assumption that what is remembered is remembered because it is, in some way, problematic. The actions and episodes are remembered because they are significant, because they involve the unfamiliar or because they involve contradiction or conflict ... Because memories are more likely to point up contradiction, show up absences and gaps, as well as refuted connections, they are more likely to reveal the processes of construction.

The aim of memory-work as a social research method is 'liberation', as Haug (1987, p. 34) notes:

> However enchanted we may have been by ... fairytale heroes who ... release the spellbound from their chains we were ... determined to strip these dreams of their tempting character, and instead to rehearse the painful lesson that liberation is dependent upon liberation of the self. Our intervention is itself an act of liberation.

So what is the task of memory-work? Memory-work, in Haug and her colleagues' approach (1987), is to fill the gap between theory and everyday experience. Its task is to discover and reveal our earlier experiences in the light of our current understandings in such a way that the underlying processes can be uncovered (Kippax 1990). As Schratz-Hadwich (1995, p. 42) puts it, 'the key question for memory-work is not, who am I?, but, how did we get to be the way we are and how can we change?'.

> [Memory-work] is a method par excellence for exploring the processes of [the] construction of self and understanding of the ways in which emotions, motives, actions, choices, play their part in that construction. It gives an insight into the way we appropriate the social world and in so doing transform ourselves and it. (Kippax 1990, p. 94)

There are several key features of memory-work (Small 1997, abstract page):
- Memories are the raw data.
- The 'researcher' is equal to other members of the research group; each member is a 'co-researcher'.

- The subject and object of the research become one; the participant produces the data (memory) and subjects data to a progressive process of theorisation.
- There is a collective interpretation and theorisation of the memories; the social meaning is examined.
- The collective approach allows for the possibility of liberation.

If we compare memory-work with other qualitative methods presented in this volume, we may agree with Koutroulis (1996, p. 13), who argues that memory-work is similar to the philosophy and aim of participatory action research (PAR) in that it aims to empower people who engage in the research process: 'The liberatory aims of memory-work emulate aspects of Freire's "Pedagogy of the Oppressed", tying in with Freire's notion of conscientisation brought about by reflection, action and dialogue.' Considering the method itself, Koutroulis (1996, p. 42) points out that memory-work and participatory action research resemble each other in the following areas:

- The research is participatory and its ultimate aim is liberation.
- A collective of co-researchers searches for a problem and its related themes to research.
- An attempt is made to equalise power relationships between the researcher and the researched.
- The research process diminishes alienation and the individualisation of discontent.
- There is a reflexive quality to the research process.
- There is a recognition that reflection on the self and the alterations to consciousness which occur as part of the research process are reconstructive of the self. These understandings are likely to result in confrontation with some dominant cultural and social ideologies.
- It promises empowerment and liberation.

How is memory-work different from PAR? One central difference can be illustrated through the different understandings of empowerment. Memory-work as empowerment, in its original form developed by Haug and colleagues (1987) and that adapted by Crawford and others (1992), is questioned by some feminist researchers. Small (1997), for example, asks if these groups of feminist researchers really need empowerment since they already have considerable power in comparison with many other oppressed women. Small argues that women who need to be empowered are more likely to be those who lack education, are poor and illiterate. Since memory-work requires writing skills and the ability to link memories with theories, many women who really need empowerment will miss out. This is one pitfall of memory-work, as we see it, and this is the marked difference between participatory action research and memory-work. PAR aims to empower poor, illiterate and marginalised women and, because of the methods it employs (that do not require writing and theorising skills), the women have the chance to participate in the research process and this helps to empower them (see also Chapter 9).

WHY USE MEMORY-WORK?

Memory-work emerges from feminist ideology that sees women as oppressed and dominated by patriarchal ideology. Women's everyday experiences are marked by domination and power. Yet their experiences are absent from dominant social theories. In order to help women to see this, some feminists sought a new method that builds on women's subjective experiences in a way that might help them to see the social structures lying beneath their experiences (Schratz-Hadwich 1995). In memory-work, it is argued that, as individuals, women are suppressed and subordinated, but, collectively, they can be seen and their voices heard. Memory-work is seen as a feminist method (Haug 1992; Koutroulis 1993, 1996; Small 1997). However, as a feminist methodology, memory-work is rather distinctive and unique. As Haug (1987, p. 14) argues, 'no other feminist work has examined in such detail the means by which memory may be mobilized collectively to chart the progress of women through discourse, via their subjective experience of the body'.

Memory-work is seen as a way to raise the consciousness of the people involved, as Kippax (1990, p. 93) points out:

> The individual members of the memory-work groups, who each have produced one or more memories, together and collectively interpret and theorise the memories. New meanings and understandings are reached, but they are reached by the subjects themselves. They are reached by the memory-work group; there is a striving for a 'common' sense. The method thus has a political force and, in this way, has links with consciousness raising.

Memory-work is also seen as a way to bridge the gap between theoretical knowledge and the everyday experience of people. Haug and colleagues (1987) argue that, with the development of modern academic disciplines, scientific knowledge or theory has become alienated from everyday experience. They argued that in order to understand the ways in which we socialised ourselves into our societies a new methodology had to be developed. This method was memory-work.

HISTORY OF MEMORY-WORK

Frigga Haug is a German feminist and sociologist. She developed memory-work with a group of academic and professional women who took part in the student movement in the 1960s and who have been members of women's socialist groups. They had found themselves 'increasingly alienated from research, feeling that the process of creating research "products" left them disconnected from the research process, both as researchers and, even more, as research subjects' (Schratz-Hadwich 1995, p. 39). Haug and her colleagues were very concerned about the gap between theory and everyday experience, as well as about the individualistic approach of most research, which had undermined the capacity for collective action that they had learned from women's groups. Their experiences of research therefore reflected many of their other experiences as women in a patriarchal social world.

Because of these concerns, Haug and her colleagues (1987) searched for a method that might close the gap between the researchers and the researched and to make the research a collective process. They then set up a memory-work group to examine female sexualisation. In this work, they wrote stories about memories of different aspects of their bodies. In the process, they read their stories to each other, compared their experiences, discussed the stories and then wrote their analysis drawing on social theory. They 'developed complex ideas about how girls are socialized to be sexual beings alienated from their bodies' (Reinharz 1992, p. 223). The strength of the memory-work method developed by Haug is that, as Kippax (1990, p. 93) points out, 'it is integral to her theory of socialisation; her theory of how we become ourselves and the part we play in that construction'.

It is in this work that Haug and her colleagues challenge the implications of childhood memories for female sexualisation. An important theme emerging from the study is that of the relationship between class and sexuality:

> Two consequences flow, it seems to us, from the ordering of bodies in the ways described: the subjection of women to an actively slavish existence and, at the same time, their subjection to standard social relations. We are defined as social beings by our own social significance, our position in society and our general capacity for action: all three definitions are shot through with the questions of class and gender. In relations between the sexes, the subordination of women ensures the dominance of men, who can thus receive compensation for and validation of the general subordination of either sex. (Haug 1987, p. 277)

Up until now, very few researchers have adopted memory-work as a method. Since the writing of Haug and colleagues (1987), there have been only a few studies in Australia and in Germany that utilised memory-work. Schratz-Hadwich (1995) employed the method to help students develop an understanding of their own racism in an everyday and institutional setting in a course dealing with the difficulties of living together in culturally diverse groups. In Australia, the first memory-work research project was done by Crawford and her colleagues (1992) in Sydney in their study of emotion and gender. Following this, Kippax and associates (1990) used memory-work to look at heterosexual negotiation in a group of women in Sydney. Since then, there have been a few other memory-work research projects. In the tourism area, Small (1997) and Hohnen (1996) utilised the method to look at women's tourist experiences. In the educational area, Fitzclarence (1991) used memory-work as a way to help student teachers understand the nature of authority in the process of dealing with the difficult transition between the roles of student and teacher. In the health area, Farrar (1994) and Mitchell (1991) made use of the method to explore the experience of menopause among older women. Lastly, Davies (1990), and most recently Koutroulis (1996), employed it to examine women's construction of menstruation. Some of this research will be discussed later in the chapter (see the 'Memory-work in health: some examples' section).

MEMORY-WORK AS A METHOD

Memory-work has several components and steps. These are discussed in the following sections.

The theme and the 'trigger'

What theme should a memory-work group focus on? This is the task of the group to decide. The memory-work process commences with the selection of a theme or topic among the co-researchers. Once this is agreed, then the 'triggers' need to be invented. In the study of emotion by Crawford and her colleagues (1992), their triggers include, for example, 'saying you are sorry', 'crying', 'danger', and 'holidays'. Kippax (1990) argues that the trigger is largely dependent on the topic under investigation. However, the choice is very important as some triggers do not provide 'the expected'. As Kippax and her colleagues (1988) point out, the trigger of 'saying you are sorry' did not prompt the members to write memories that reflect guilt or shame. Instead, they wrote memories that reveal anger and a sense of injustice. The trigger 'secrets', however, also produce reflection on guilt and shame more.

An obvious trigger is not always helpful. Obvious triggers 'produced obvious and somewhat over-rehearsed responses. The memories were rounded and smooth, they lacked any sense of contradiction; their meanings in general were glib' (Crawford et al. 1992, p. 45). Kippax and her colleagues (1990) observed in their study of women's sexuality that triggers such as 'first love' and 'loss of virginity' produced memories of events that represent sex and love in their clearest and least problematic form. However, with triggers such as 'initiating', 'touching', and 'penetration', they produced more 'subtle and informative descriptions of sexual episodes' than the first two triggers.

The writing

Haug and her colleagues insist that memories must be written down. They argue that writing is important, since 'writing is a transgression of boundaries, an exploration of new territory. It involves making public the events of our lives, wriggling free of the constraints of purely private and individual experiences' (Haug 1987, p. 36).

Writing has several advantages (Crawford et al. 1992). First, writing provides the memory-work group with a discipline to adhere to. Second, writing avoids some aspects of self-presentation that tend to emerge in a talking situation. When we speak, there is a tendency to justify and interpret the events as we present ourselves to others. Third, writing provides a permanent record that can be used in the future. Last, writing makes our everyday experiences more interesting and important. Writing is, therefore, particularly important for women because women 'see writing as an impossibility, since [they believe] there is nothing to write about. The things we experience seem unimportant and uninteresting; they are banal' (Haug 1987, p. 38). Haug and her colleagues believe strongly that writing is a weapon that women use to defend themselves from being seen and controlled through the eyes of others (particularly through male eyes).

However, the writing in memory-work must be in the third person. Haug (1987) argues that, unless we have some ways to distance ourselves from our past experiences, writing may be impossible. Distancing ourselves can be done by writing about our experiences in the third person, as if these events do not represent ourselves. 'By translating our own experiences into the third person, we were able to be more attentive to ourselves. Thus the gaze we cast today on ourselves of yesterday becomes the gaze cast by one stranger on another' (Haug 1987, p. 46). Similarly, Crawford and others (1992, p. 47) argue that:

> Writing in the third person enables the subject to have a 'bird's eye view' of the scene, to picture the detail. The subject reflects on herself/himself from the outside—from the point of view of the observer, and so is encouraged to describe rather than warrant.

Another important point about writing in memory-work is to avoid biography and autobiography (Haug 1987). Biography tends to bring coherence, 'the coherence of the reinterpretation of past events as antecedents of what follows. That is, of what we "know" to be the consequences' (Kippax 1990, p. 95). Coherence hides resistance. And so it works against the method. As Haug (1987, p. 41) argues, memory-work is a method in which the analysis 'has to be seen as a field of conflict between dominant cultural values and oppositional attempts to wrest cultural meaning and pleasure from life'.

The researcher and the researched

Haug (1987) insists that participants are 'co-researchers', that is, the researched become co-researchers. This process helps to eliminate the hierarchy of 'experiment and subject' that exists in most other research methods.

She suggests that in any piece of research, if people's subjective experiences are to be pieced together, it is necessary that the objects of research become the co-researchers. In their work on emotion, Crawford and her co-researchers (1992, p. 43) started their project by forming themselves into a memory-work group: 'We were our own subjects; the distinctions between researcher and "subject" disappeared.'

Before the commencement of memory-work, a group of co-researchers must be formed. Crawford and others (1992) point out that this can be done in two ways: by creating a group with several researchers as full members, or one with one or more of the researchers as facilitator. How do we choose the co-researchers or co-workers? Crawford and others (1992, p. 44) prefer to have a group of members who share some criterion that 'we regarded as relevant'. In their work, they set up memory-work groups of 'older women', 'young women', and 'young men'. They also point out that a group of close friends is as effective as a group of strangers. Whatever group is to be selected, the main issue to be considered for success is 'mutual trust', since the group has to work together for a long period of time.

Collective nature

Memory-work is carried out by a 'collective' of co-researchers. Haug (1987) argues that the collective process is essential if women are to be liberated and if the memory-work project is to be achieved. She contends that, with a collective approach, the co-researchers can complement each other, can decide on the themes of common importance, and can share the workload. The collective approach is particularly important in choosing the theme, if we wish to 'guarantee that it is generalizable' (p. 56). As well, the collective approach is essential in the analysis process when the co-researchers compare memories, make comments and fill the gaps. As Haug maintains, 'in attempting to produce compatible accounts, we were at the same time demanding explanations, searching for an understanding of our own actions' (p. 56). This can only be done through a collective approach.

As Schratz-Hadwich (1995, p. 44) points out, memory-work does not reflect 'the insights, predilections or obsessions' of just one researcher; all co-researchers are involved in the research process. A memory-work group is usually a self-selected group of people who wish to work together and who have some sympathy for the ideas that inform the method. A small group of four or five members gathers together to work on a particular theme of memory-work. The group usually meets once a week over a lengthy period of time, mostly about two or three months, but sometimes longer (as in Crawford and colleagues' study of emotion and gender).

MEMORY-WORK: THE PROCESS

In summary, memory-work has three important phases (Crawford et al. 1992; Kippax 1990). It should be noted, however, that the phases are 'recursive: they feed into and off each other' (Crawford et al. 1992, p. 1). In practice, the three are not easily separated.

Phase one: the collection of written memories

In this phase, once a theme or topic has been collectively agreed, the memories are written according to a set of rules. Following Haug (1987), Crawford and her colleagues (1992, p. 45) suggest five steps in writing memories:
- Write a memory, usually about one to several pages,
- of a particular episode, action or event,
- in the third person,
- in as much detail as is possible, even some trivial detail,
- without interpretation, explanation or biography.

However, in Crawford and others' work, they add a sixth step:
- Write one of the earliest memories. This will help to reveal the processes of construction of self more clearly than writing about a recent event.

Crawford and others point out that the writing process needs at least a week's gestation. Some memories can be easily written since there are some triggers to help, but at other times people may need some time to recall their memories. Therefore, one week is recommended.

Phase two: the analysis of memories

In this phase, the memory of each member is read and discussed. The text of memories is exchanged and analysed by the group members. Schratz-Hadwich (1995) points out that by analysing each other's memories, each member is involved in the research process. Each one acts as both a subject and object in the research. All members thus become co-researchers. This phase aims to reveal the common understandings contained in memories. What is important at this stage is not why someone's father did such things but why fathers do these things. The aim of the analysis is to 'uncover the social meanings embodied by the actions described in the written accounts and to uncover the processes whereby the meanings—both then and now—are arrived at' (Crawford et al. 1992, p. 49).

Following Crawford and her colleagues (1992, p. 49), the processes in phase two are as follows:
- Each memory-work group member expresses views and ideas about each memory in turn.

- Similarities and differences, the continuous elements of memories and the elements that do not fit in, are explored.
- Clichés, generalisations, contradictions, cultural imperatives, and metaphors are identified.
- Theories, popular conceptions, sayings and images about the topic are discussed.
- What is not written in the memories, but what might be expected to be written, is examined.
- The memories are rewritten.

In the analysis of memories, each co-researcher expresses his or her views and ideas about a particular memory with which the group has chosen to start. The task is to search for the author's motives and other meanings that 'lie between the lines' of the memory. In the analysis, the memory is treated as a text, not a testimony. Therefore, a question like 'What did you mean when you wrote … ?' is to be avoided (Schratz-Hadwich 1995, p. 48). At this stage, similarities and differences between the memories are examined for 'continuous elements' among the memories, as well as those that do not seem to fit.

The final task in phase two is to rewrite each person's original memory. In the rewriting process, each member must pay attention to the questions raised by the co-researchers in the analysis process. Schratz-Hadwich points out that, 'by modifying the texts, the authors engage in a reflective process, which brings to light new "data" from their memory. These memories might have been suppressed and may suggest starting points for the reinterpretation of the construction of self' (p. 49).

Phase three: theorising of memories

In phase three, the rewritten memories are discussed again. At this stage, the original and the revised memories are compared, contrasted and examined further. Common themes that emerged from the memories are discussed in view of new understandings. Additionally, at this stage, if there are other memory-work groups involved, the results are discussed and exchanged across the groups. Schratz-Hadwich (1995, p. 49) argues that 'this process of collective theorising is a powerful feature of memory-work and often involves relating to other theoretical positions and other kinds of research'.

MEMORY-WORK IN HEALTH: SOME EXAMPLES

This method is still in its infancy in the health area. There have been only a handful of research projects that employed memory-work as a method. Some of these are discussed in this section.

Crawford and her colleagues (1992) were the first group of academic women who adopted memory-work in the Australian context. Their group consisted of five women who were academics at one Australian university. Their project stemmed from feelings of isolation in the academic world. In order to fight this isolation, they took on memory-work developed by Frigga Haug. Their memory-work project was focused, however, on emotion and gender. They examined several triggers: 'saying sorry and being sorry', 'happiness', and 'fear and danger'. The group met and worked together over a long period of time and they eventually produced *Emotion and Gender: Constructing Meaning from Memory* (Crawford et al. 1992).

Crawford and her colleagues (1992, p. 185) state that memory-work enabled them to trace the way they constructed themselves through specific experiences in their world. In this study they identified several obvious themes of gender. The main themes included: responsibility, autonomy and agency. Social responsibility stood out as a strong theme. From a very young age, people learned that they were held responsible for the well-being of others. The sense of responsibility also extended to difficult and dangerous situations. If they got themselves into trouble or danger, it was their own fault for which they must take full responsibility. Autonomy was another core theme that emerged from this study. Children, girls or boys, wanted to be responsible for themselves as part of forming their sense of autonomy. In doing so, children tried to behave like adults and to be taken seriously by them. Sometimes this was successful. But other times, people pushed the boundaries too far so that the attempts were met with reprimands and shame. Girls and boys achieved autonomy by breaking adult rules. They both expected punishment. However, at the same time, boys believed that such rule-breaking was expected of them and that they were not responsible for anyone but themselves. Crawford and her colleagues (1992, p. 187) suggest that 'both boys and girls experience subordination of themselves as children, but boys experience subordination secure in the knowledge that it will be transformed collectively into male dominance'.

Another recurring theme that Crawford and her colleagues discovered was that of the 'inside/outside' pattern of events. Some memories happened inside, particularly inside the home. Others memories occurred outside. The inside/outside dichotomy was loaded with symbolic meaning. They were intrigued by 'the rich sensuous detail associated with the warmth and security' of inside, in contrast to 'the harsh and exciting coldness' of outside. In other words, in people's construction as children, inside was safe. However, Crawford and her colleagues draw attention to the contradiction between people's memories and the reality that inside was not necessarily safe for women and young girls. Most crimes of violence, such as domestic violence, rape and murder, occur inside the home.

Lastly, Crawford and her colleagues identified the theme of support and isolation. Many of the memories as girls were of situations where they were alone and without support. Women's struggles were not witnessed and hence their experiences were unspoken. This was not true with the boys' memories, however.

Crawford and others (1992) argued that their memory-work project revealed that emotion was often gendered and power played a significant role in the construction of emotions. However, power often appeared in the form of powerlessness in memories. This powerlessness was a central issue for women, particularly the issue of women as victims. In order to give women power, women's emotions needed to be shared and a collective effort needed to be secured.

Kippax and others (1990) examined heterosexual negotiation, which would form the focus for behavioural change, using memory-work as a method. Memory-work, in this study, provided a way to examine how sexuality was produced and reproduced through the reflection and reconstruction of past experiences of a group of young women in Sydney. Memories were analysed by looking for gaps, clichés and metaphors in order to search for the common understandings and taken-for-granted assumptions, that set the boundaries within which encounters occurred. The women in this study met once a week for several months. Their memories were written in response to cues such as 'come up and see my etchings', 'saying no', 'saying no when you want to say yes', 'touching', 'initiating a sexual episode or encounter', and 'being picked up'.

Kippax and others (1990) point out that the memories obtained in this study could be understood in terms of three discourses: the male sex drive, the have/hold discourse, and the permissive discourse. They could also be understood in relation to three permissible figures for women: virgin, wife–mother, or whore. In tying their data to these theories, the researchers identified three themes in the representation of the feminine: women as objects of desire, women as committed and faithful partners, and women as seductive. Kippax and her colleagues (1990) argue that, if women were positioned as objects of desire, they were not in a position to negotiate sex. What was interesting was that women who were faithful partners were not really in a position to negotiate sex either. 'The characteristics of virgin, intact, untouched, pristine, pure, or wife/mother, nurture, faithful, committed, selfless, acquiescent, are not the characteristics of the skillful negotiator' (p. 541). However, women who were seductive, who had the characteristics of 'lover, desiring, passionate, seductive, inventive', were the skilful negotiators of safe sex.

The study also demonstrated that some common understandings underlying sexual encounters render negotiation not only impossible but also largely unintelligible:

> Negotiation is rendered intelligible when men and women acknowledge women's sexual desire and women are empowered to give voice to that desire. Women say 'I do/don't want to', not 'I can't'; women return the gaze; initiate sexual encounters; in short, women become active subjects of desire. Sexual experience empowers. (Kippax et al. 1990, p. 541)

The findings of this research suggested that 'the much touted monogamy solution' to the problem of AIDS was not a feasible solution for all women. Even the use of condoms would only be likely if women had a stronger voice.

Mitchell (1991) explored the possibility of nurses using memory-work as a primary health care strategy. In this project, a group of older women in Adelaide were invited to explore memories relating to their health and illness, in order to search for the ways in which these had been formulated. Mitchell argued that older women themselves had the right to speak out about how their health needs could be met, and that their health experiences needed to be listened to. Through the collective process of memory-work, 'menopause', a medicalised aspect of older women's health, was identified as one of the main focuses of the study. Mitchell's study aimed not only to assist the women to be more aware of the significance of the health and illness events in their lives, but also to provide an opportunity for empowerment so that they could make the positive changes they wanted.

In this study, the group of older women agreed to write memories relating to their health. Collectively, they identified a series of themes that were important indicators of the health of older women in general. They then wrote a specific memory relating to that theme. The women agreed to recall and write their earliest memory relating to menopause during a one-week period. The written memories became part of the data in the study. At the next meeting, the women shared their memories and discussed and analysed them. The group meetings were tape-recorded and a written journal relating to the experience of the memory-work group was also kept. These were later used as part of the analysis.

The women's memories varied markedly, but they reflected the 'mystery, myths, misinformation' and medicalisation of menopause. Two women wrote about positive experiences, 'reflecting on it as a time of new found freedom and relief associated with being past childbearing age'. Menopause, however, was a traumatic experience for three of the women. What was intriguing was that two memories reflected the notion that if women were busy and got on with their life, they would not think about menopause, which was a product of patriarchal thinking. This reflection was hotly discussed in the memory-work group, particularly among women who had had traumatic menopause experiences.

Mitchell (1991) pointed out that the processes of memory-work provided the women with the opportunity to see and to understand how their health patterns had been socially constructed. More importantly, the sharing of the memories had therapeutic value as the women examined significant events in their lives. One woman wrote that 'writing about past experiences helps one to clarify ones thought and thereby get some order in ones thinking, thus enabling one even if sad to experience some quieting of the mind' (p. 51). And another one said that 'thinking things through and writing about them helps to unravel the tight knots that unhappy events leave' (p. 51). There were several positive personal benefits for participating in the memory-work. However, of significance was the increased level of self-awareness that each woman experienced. This was empowerment. Additionally, validation of one's experience by other members enhanced this process and provided the support strategies that were essential when 'old wounds' were opened up. This might not have been possible if the memories had not been written and shared.

The most recent research employing memory-work is that of Koutroulis (1996), who examined the construction of menstruation via women's memories. This study focused on the embodied experience of menstruation. Through memories, the meanings women gave to menstruation were examined. Additionally, the taken-for-granted rules and social practices about the management of menstruation and how women negotiated the rules were also examined.

A group of women, including Koutroulis herself, wrote their memories about significant menstruation experiences; eight memories in total were written. 'Written memories are the principal data and provide the basis for analysis. They are the catalyst, the prompt, the inspirer of other stories that are as much about menstruation as they are about what it means to be a woman, in this society' (Koutroulis 1996, p. 6). Exploring women's memories about menstruation offered a means to tap into wider social issues. The memories were then discussed and analysed, using feminist theories as a framework. The group met once a month for a period of several months.

The women's memories together revealed a wide but connected range of themes. The memories were connected by the core concept of 'secrecy' and by themes such as 'dirt, power and emotions'. Koutroulis argued that the meanings of concepts ('clean' and 'dirty') were socially constructed and transcended class, ethnicity, gender and age. The meanings of menstruation in a patriarchal society like Australia, reflected in her memory-work, revealed that menstruation was dirty and this was a detrimental way for women and men to think about women's bodies. Koutroulis and colleagues found that the way in which women themselves described and experienced menstruation, and the way in which they were treated by others because of menstruation, was often socially mediated.

For Koutroulis (1996), the findings of her study indicated that menstruation was an embodiment of human relationships. Mother–daughter relationships and male views of menstruation contributed to the way in which women's own meanings of menstruation were constructed. Women responded to menstruation in contradictory forms because it was a hidden but powerful event in their lives. There were many rules that women were expected to observe. Some women complied with these rules, but others asserted themselves autonomously by ignoring or breaking them. Koutroulis's study challenged homogeneous conceptualisations of the menstrual experience and highlighted that women do not have uniform views about menstruation.

CAN MEMORY-WORK DATA BE GENERALISED?

In traditional qualitative research, generalisation is not a major concern since it is believed that the examination of subjective experience in depth is more important than numbers. This too holds true for memory-work. However, Frigga Haug (1987, p. 44) believes that what is generated from memory-work can be generalisable:

> We live according to a whole series of imperatives: social pressures, natural limitations, the imperative of economic survival, the given conditions of history and culture. Human beings produce their lives collectively. It is within the domain of collective production that individual experience becomes possible. If therefore a given experience is possible, it is also subject to universalization. What we perceive as 'personal' ways of adapting to the social are also potentially generalizable modes of appropriation.

Haug further argues that using our own experiences, both positive and negative, as the basis for our investigation opens up the possibility of examining the experiences of others in detail. We can compare our experiences with others. We can enjoy each other's experiences. We can develop new possibilities for our actions. These ultimately lead to the ability to generalise our experiences.

THE DETERMINANTS OF SUCCESSFUL MEMORY-WORK

Not all memory-work groups will work well and succeed. What determines a group's success? Schratz-Hadwich (1995, p. 60) argues that 'what determines success is in part the development of the group as a group. Memory-work requires both a serious intent and a degree of conviviality.' Memory-work works well when the group is a real group: the members have shared values and interests, they enjoy each other's company and they are willing to work together for a long period of time. Most important of all is the trust between them. Without this trust, the memory-work may not succeed.

MEMORY-WORK: ADVANTAGES AND LIMITATIONS

Memory-work has its pros and cons, as with other research methods. In this section, we attempt to outline some of these advantages and limitations.

Advantages

- The basic material of memory-work is memories, and memories are not difficult to access. Hence, the data gathered through memory-work can be easily obtained.

- Memory-work allows people to examine and connect their individual experiences with social structures. It enables individual persons to realise that what is happening in their everyday life and what has been taken for granted as non-significant in their daily routine is located within social structures. This helps people to deflect undeserved blame, thus empowering them.
- Existing theories often do not take into account the personal experiences of people involved. In memory-work, however, theories are built on personal experiences. Memory-work provides a way of looking at the social world from a personal point of view. It constitutes a theory, not just a method (Schratz-Hadwich 1995). And as Koutroulis (1996, p. 332) argues, the contribution of memory-work to the 'experience–theory' link 'makes this method accessible to many ways of thinking and knowledge'.
- However, memory-work also provides a collective understanding of the matter of concern. The collective nature of memory-work 'serves to emphasise the common socializing influences and practices in our society as they affect people and are appropriated and transformed by them' (Kippax et al. 1990, p. 534).
- Since memory-work is a collective approach, researchers do not work alone. This helps to reduce the social isolation that most researchers experience, not only in terms of the research methodology but also in the theorising process of their findings. Hence, memory-work can be seen as 'a form of mental health healing' (Mitchell 1991, p. 52).
- Additionally, because of its collective nature, memory-work avoids the hierarchy of researcher and researched and breaks down the dominance of an 'expert'. Since all members are involved in the process, everyone is equal in terms of power relationships.
- The method is flexible enough to allow its adaptation to suit the particular nature of most research topics. This can be seen clearly from the several examples cited in this chapter. Memory-work has been adopted in research ranging from tourism and education to health.

Limitations

- Memory-work in its original form (as proposed by Haug 1987) is limited in its application. The method works well when each 'co-researcher' has an equal investment in the research. However, what happens when each member does not have equal interest or time to spend on the project, or when there is an unequal relationship among the members? As Small (1997, p. 16) argues, 'the implications ... are problematic. If memory-work is, as claimed, highly political, concerned with changing women at both the individual and social level, then in its purest form, it is only groups such as academics who can be changed. Perhaps these groups are not those most in need of empowerment.' If this is the case, the method may not be feasible for conducting a research project with women who are in less powerful positions than the researcher (Small 1997).

- The method requires that the co-researchers are able to write. Therefore, memory-work excludes those who are illiterate or who feel threatened by the writing process. And these groups of people may be the ones who need empowerment most.

- Memories cannot warrant people's actions or events. Memories offer descriptions of actions and events but cannot provide detailed analysis of the reasons for actions and events.

- The ideology of 'co-researchers' may not be always practical. In some studies, there may be a need to have a claim of ownership by a particular researcher (such as in the case of a doctoral thesis; see Koutroulis 1996 and Small 1997). In this case, a breakdown of the power relationship between the researcher and the participants as co-researchers, as the method strongly advocates, may not be feasible.

- The process requires members to meet for a long period of time, in some cases for several months. Each meeting also requires intensive discussions over long hours. This may not be practical for some groups of people, such as those with young children, older people, or those who have many commitments.

- Successful memory-work is built on mutual trust between members, where each one enjoys working together with the group. Some memory-work groups may not go well if these features cannot be achieved.

CONCLUSION

In the conclusion to her book *Female Sexualization*, Frigga Haug succinctly suggests:

> We aim to develop ways of living collectively, and thus to escape individual isolation. *Our aim is to change the world lovingly.* (Haug 1987, p. 282, our emphasis)

Our hope is that, through this research method, the world of many women and men who are oppressed may be improved.

Tutorial exercise

Conduct memory-work with a group of your friends (three or four), choosing one particular memory, such as the illness of a family member during summer holidays, the first experience of menstruation, emotional turmoil in the family. Note all the essential requirements of the method described in this chapter.

Further reading

Crawford, J., Kippax, S., Onyx, J., Gault, U. and Benton, P., 1992, *Emotion and Gender: Constructing Meaning from Memory*, Sage, London.

Haug, F. (ed.), 1987, *Female Sexualization*, Verso, London.

Koutroulis, G., 1993, 'Memory Work: A Critique', in B.S. Turner, L. Eckermann, D. Colquhoun and P. Crotty (eds), *Annual Review of Health Social Sciences: Methodological Issues in Health Research*, vol. 3, pp. 76–96.

Schratz-Hadwich, B., 1995, 'Collective Memory-Work: The Self as a Re/Source for Re/Search', in M. Schratz and R. Walker (eds), *Research as Social Change: New Opportunities for Qualitative Research*, Routledge, London.

Small, J., 1997, *Memory-Work: A Feminist Social Constructionist Method for Researching Tourist Behaviour*, Working Paper No. 7, School of Management, University of Technology, Sydney.

8

Ethnography

Introduction

Upon arriving in the field, I did everything I could to understand !Kung life: I learned language, went on gathering expeditions ... ate bush foods ... lived in grass huts in !Kung villages, and sat around their fires listening to discussions, arguments, and stories. I gained an invaluable perspective, participating and watching ... (Shostak 1981, p. 5)

During the first month or so [the ethnographer] proceeds slowly ... He walks warily and attempts to learn as quickly as possible ... important forms of native etiquette and taboos. . . [He] often experiences anxieties in a strange situation ... and [is] overwhelmed by the difficulties of really getting 'inside' an alien culture and of learning ... other strange language ... (Powdermaker 1968, p. 419)

Walking closer to the synagogue, I saw a room filled with some forty teenage boys ... And what would I do once inside? Pray with them? Perhaps. Participation in prayer would require feigning familiarity with the ... rituals of the prayer service. I decide to begin the research on the following day. (Shaffir 1991, p. 74)

I, as an anthropologist, had to involve myself ... to develop an adequate explanation of what was being observed ... I conducted [the] entry and participation phases of the research well; too well ... [However] the final phase of research, the ... writing [of] an ethnography for the eyes of outsiders, was nothing short of betrayal. (Wolf 1991, p. 223)

These excerpts give us an indication of the research methods of some well-known ethnographers. There are several important points to note: learning about 'other' people's lives and cultures; going to live in the community; learning the language; difficulties in undertaking many tasks in ethnography; and so on. These important issues in ethnography are the focus of this chapter. We also provide a brief discussion of the history of ethnography, some examples of its use in health research, as well as listing the advantages and disadvantages of the method. It must be noted that this chapter takes a cultural anthropological perspective more than a social one since it has been used by cultural anthropologists for many decades and continues to be an important approach today.

WHAT IS ETHNOGRAPHY?

Ethnography is a culture-studying-culture. It consists of a body of knowledge that includes research techniques, ethnographic theory, and hundreds of cultural descriptions. It seeks to build a systematic understanding of all human cultures from the perspective of those who have learned them. Ethnography is based on the following assumption: *knowledge of all cultures is valuable.* (Spradley 1979, p. 9, emphasis added)

Put simply, ethnography is the art and science of describing a group or culture. The description may be that of a small tribal group in some exotic land or a classroom in a university. The essential core of ethnography is, as Spradley (1979, p. 3) argues, 'to understand another way of life from the native point of view'. Malinowski (1922, p. 25) said this succinctly when he wrote that the goal of ethnography is to 'grasp the native's point of view, his relation to life, to realize his vision of his world'. In this sense, ethnography is heavily influenced by the ethnographic theoretical tradition. However, the method is also influenced by other theories, including phenomenology, symbolic interactionism, hermeneutics and feminism, depending on the topics and informants chosen in the study (see also Chapter 1).

What we have just said is perhaps what Atkinson and Hammersley (1994, p. 248) refer to as 'a philosophical paradigm to which one makes a total commitment'. In their writing, Atkinson and Hammersley (1994, p. 248) argue that ethnography is a form of social research that has several key features:
* a strong focus on exploring the nature of particular social phenomena;
* a tendency to work primarily with unstructured data;
* examination of a small number of people, perhaps just one in detail; and
* analysis of data which involves explicit interpretation of the meanings and functions of human actions. And descriptions and explanations of the events take priority.

Although, traditionally, ethnography is undertaken in a cultural group of a village or small town of a 'primitive' or 'non-literate' or 'underdeveloped' society, it can also be applied in health care research in contemporary societies. Many research settings can be considered as 'a cultural group'. Nursing homes, maternity wards, labour wards, ultrasound clinics, IVF clinics, intensive care units, and so on can be treated as legitimate cultural groups. Patients who suffer from, say, diabetes, women who have experienced a caesarean birth, people with weight problems, women who suffer domestic violence—each group is a cultural group that has a lot to offer ethnography. Therefore, ethnographic research has been widely conducted in Western societies like Australia, the USA and Canada (see the later section on 'Ethnography in health: some examples').

ETHNOGRAPHY FOR WHAT?

Many people may ask this question. Why can't we use other types of research methods that may be cheaper, quicker and able to include more people in the study? It is true that some methods are cheaper, obtain information more quickly and include larger numbers of respondents. However, will they help you to deeply understand people and hence offer ways in which people can be helped appropriately? Maybe not! In arguing about the above question, Spradley (1979) asserts that ethnography is not only for understanding the human being, but also for serving the needs of humankind. He particularly insists on the synchronisation of these two uses of ethnographic research. According to Spradley (1979, pp. 10–16), ethnography is invaluable in many ways:

* It helps to understand human behaviours. Therefore, it helps to understand complex societies where cultural diversity is great.
* It offers an excellent strategy for discovering grounded theory in social science.
* It helps to discover human needs. And therefore, it helps to find ways for meeting these needs.

Spradley's argument for ethnography applies as well in multicultural societies like Australia, the USA and the United Kingdom where there are a large number of immigrants who have come from diverse social and cultural backgrounds. Ethnography helps us to understand the behaviours and needs of the immigrants and this, in turn, helps to fulfil their needs. This can be seen clearly in the case of a woman from Pranee's ethnographic study among the Hmong community in Melbourne. Through ethnography, she discovered a Hmong woman who had suffered from soul loss due to a caesarean operation in a maternity hospital. Further, as a consequence of her ethnographic approach, Pranee understood that the solution involved bringing the woman back to the hospital and having a soul calling ceremony performed for her. This ceremony was performed and, as a consequence of being able to observe her cultural practices, the woman has been well since then (see Rice et al. 1994 for further details).

There has been some acknowledgment of the importance of ethnography in health care settings. Schmoll (1987, p. 1895), for example, argues that ethnography is 'well suited for the systematic study of clinical behaviors and their many inherent variables'. In Schmoll's case, ethnography is particularly useful for studying physical therapy in clinical settings. Similarly, Stein (1991) demonstrates that the ethnographic approach can be employed in health practitioner education and clinical work. Stein (1991, p. 8) argues that, in trying to reveal:

> the complex texture and weave of clinical thought and action, [ethnography] offers a more complete understanding of clinical decision making than is conveyed by such formal cultural and biomedical doctrines as medical science, professionalism, objectivity, rationality, efficiency, the sanctity of the doctor–patient relationship, and the best interests of the patient.

Savage (1995, p. 16) has also pointed out that 'ethnography, with its emphasis on the holistic description and understanding of a local world' is also valuable in examining the interaction between nurses and their patients.

Ethnography has been applied in order to develop questionnaires for use in a large-scale survey research. Coreil and others (1989), for example, employed an ethnographic approach to identify maternal knowledge of vaccines as an important variable in immunisation use in Haiti. The findings were then used to develop a set of questions for use in a case-control study, which compared users with non-users of childhood immunisations. Coreil and colleagues argued that the qualitative findings were useful in identifying factors that predisposed children to be incompletely immunised. From their study, Coreil and others concluded that 'epidemiological studies can benefit from the insights provided by qualitative data, particularly in the exploratory phases of research' (p. S37).

HISTORY OF ETHNOGRAPHY

Ethnography originated as a method in cultural anthropology (Atkinson and Hammersley 1994; Fielding 1993). Cultural anthropologists have been using ethnography as a major tool to understand people from different cultural and social settings. Morse (1992, p. 142), for example, argues that 'the foundations of ethnography lie in anthropology where the essence of good ethnography is understanding cultural rules, norms, and values'. Bronislaw Malinowski applied ethnography in his work among the Trobriand islanders in Melanesia (see, for example, *Argonauts of the Western Pacific*, 1922). Many other cultural anthropologists have followed his example.

Traditionally, ethnography has been associated with Western interest in the culture of non-Western societies. Most early Western ethnographers would travel significant distances to learn from people whose social lives and cultures are distinctive to them. And many ethnographers still continue this tradition. However, in recent times, more ethnographers conduct their fieldwork in their own cultures (Atkinson and Hammersley 1994). As Cole (1977) points out, many Western anthropologists and sociologists apply the ethnographic method to the investigation of their own societies. And this has been a central feature of twentieth-century social science.

It is only in recent decades that ethnography has become a popular method in social science and health research, along with other types of qualitative work (Hammersley and Atkinson 1995). This is partly due to dissatisfaction with the information collected by quantitative methods, which do not tell the whole story of the health behaviours of those whom the researcher wishes to understand (Rice 1996b). Ethnography provides in-depth understanding about people's behaviours, and this in turn offers greater ways to find some solutions to improve their health. Ethnography is particularly appropriate and popular among medical anthropologists and medical sociologists, who study health beliefs, attitudes, practices and patterns in different social and cultural settings. In the past decades, we have seen several such studies conducted in different parts of the world, both in Western and non-Western societies. Some of these will be discussed later in the chapter (see the 'Ethnography in health: some examples' section).

THE ETHNOGRAPHER

What does the ethnographer do? *He writes.* (Geertz 1973, p. 19, emphasis added)

A social science researcher who writes ethnography or studies ethnography is called an 'ethnographer'. The ethnographer writes the ethnography from all the data collected: from people's daily lives to their specific rituals. In order to write up this data correctly and clearly, they have first to make sense of it all. One important quality of a good ethnographer is the ability to keep an 'open mind' about the studied group or culture. Fetterman (1989, p. 11) argues that, since the ethnographer is 'interested in understanding and describing a social and cultural scene from the emic (an insider's) perspective, he or she is both storyteller and scientist; the closer the reader of an ethnography comes to understanding the native's point of view, the better the story and the better the science'.

However, this does not mean that the ethnographer enters the field with an 'empty head'. Most ethnographers start their fieldwork with a problem, a theory for their conceptual framework, people they will talk with or learn from, methods for data collection, techniques and tools for data analysis, and what they intend to do with the data.

One notable difference between an ethnographer and a researcher using other methods is that, rather than 'studying' people, the ethnographer attempts to 'learn from the people'. Thomas's (1958, p. 43) fascinating account of her fieldwork describes how, after travelling for miles across the Kalahari Desert with her family and other researchers, the group came to the homes of the families in the middle of the desert:

> And then a young woman who appeared to be in her early twenties came out of the house. Presently she smiled, pressed her hand to her chest, and said: 'Tsetchwe'. It was her name. 'Elizabeth', I said, pointing to myself. 'Nisabe', she answered, pronouncing after me and inclining her head graciously. She looked me over carefully without really staring, which to Bushmen is rude. Then, having surely suspected that I was a woman, she put her hand on my breast gravely, and, finding that I was, she gravely touched her own breast. Many bushmen do this; to them all Europeans look alike. 'Tsau si' (woman), she said. Then after a moment's pause, Tsetchwe began to teach me a few words, the names of a few objects around us, grass, rock, bean shell, so that we could have a conversation later.

'Tsetchwe began to teach me' is the essence of ethnography (Spradley 1979, p. 4). Ethnographers seek to 'learn' and to be taught by people, not to 'study' them as they are usually treated in other types of social science research:

> Ethnographers adopt a particular stance toward people with whom they work. By word and by action, in subtle ways and direct statements, they say, 'I want to understand the world from your point of view. I want to know what you know in the way you know it. I want to understand the meaning of your experience, to walk in your shoes, to feels things as you feel them, to explain things as you explain them. Will you become my teacher and help me understand?' This frame of reference is a radical departure from treating people as either subjects, respondents, or actors. (Spradley 1979, p. 34)

It has been argued that the gender of the ethnographer plays an important role in ethnographic studies (Bell 1993). Not only does it have an influence on the conduct of fieldwork to collect information, but also in the representation of the cultures one intends to learn from (see *Gendered Fields: Women, Men and Ethnography*, edited by Bell and others 1993, and also *Self, Sex, and Gender in Cross-Cultural Fieldwork*, edited by Whitehead and Conaway 1986, for good detail about gender in ethnography).

ETHNOGRAPHY AS A METHOD

In practical terms, ethnography usually refers to forms of social science research having a substantial number of essential features, as Hammersley and Atkinson (1995, p. 1) state:

> We see the term as referring primarily to a particular method or set of methods. In its most characteristic form it involves the ethnographer participating, overtly or covertly, in people's daily lives for an extended period of time, watching what happens, listening to what is said, asking questions—in fact, collecting whatever data are available to throw light on the issues that are the focus of the research.

This is why Denzin (1978, p. 183) refers to ethnography as 'a curious blending of methodological techniques'. There are several ways in which the ethnographer can obtain information and these are discussed below.

Fieldwork

The ethnographer strides into a social or cultural situation in order to explore the world of the people they intend to learn from and this begins with fieldwork. Hence, sometimes the term 'fieldworker' is used instead of 'ethnographer' (Fetterman 1989; Shaffir and Stebbins 1991).

Ethnographic fieldwork involves 'the disciplined study of what the world is like to people who have learned to see, hear, speak, think, and act in ways that are different' (Spradley 1979, p. 3). In doing ethnographic fieldwork, there are two important elements, as Emerson and others (1995, p. 1) state:

> First, the ethnographer enters into a social setting and gets to know the people involved in it; usually, the setting is not previously known in an intimate way. The ethnographer participates in the daily routines of this setting, develops ongoing relations with the people in it, and observes all the while what is going on. Indeed, the term 'participant-observation' is often used to characterize this basic research approach. But, second, the ethnographer writes down in regular, systematic approach what she observes and learns while participating in the daily rounds of life of others ... These two interconnected activities comprise the core of ethnographic research: Firsthand participation in some initially unfamiliar social world and the production of a written account of that world by drawing upon such participation.

These two interconnected activities will be dealt with separately in the next section.

Fetterman (1989) points out that fieldwork is the basic and most important part of any ethnographic study. Typically, the ethnographer learns the local language before starting fieldwork (Fielding 1993). The ethnographer then spends six months to two years or longer in the field. Most stay in the field for over a year (Bernard 1995). Some ethnographers may spend about a year on their initial fieldwork and then return for further fieldwork, while others stay in the field until they have to leave. Although a typical period of fieldwork in ethnography takes about one year or longer, Bernard (1995) points out that it can be done in a shorter period of time. This is particularly so if the ethnographer does not need to learn a new language and is well prepared. However, he also points out that the amount of time spent in the field makes a lot of difference in what the ethnographer may find. The longer the fieldwork period, the more likely it is that the ethnographer will learn about sensitive issues and obtain information about social change that is not possible in a short period.

Gaining entry

> Heroic literature is replete with tales in which the hero must pass a series of tests and questions before he is permitted to gain the prize. A similar experience, though less ritualized and unaccompanied by operatic music, awaits the sociologist in the hospital. (Mauksch 1970, p. 188)

Ethnographic fieldwork rarely commences as soon as the ethnographer moves into the area they have chosen as a study site. To begin with, the ethnographer has to seek permission from the 'gatekeeper' (Fielding 1993, p. 159), such as a government body, institution or community leaders, to conduct research. Obtaining a permit in most circumstances is just a matter of formality. However, in some cases, it can be difficult or even impossible to gain access to the research site (Howard 1996). To conduct a study in Thailand, for example, an ethnographer must seek a permit from the National Institute of Research, which enables entry to the research site with few difficulties. Where the ethnographer wishes to carry out research in a hospital, senior hospital staff must typically be contacted, but there are also other medical professions from whom the researcher may need to seek permission (see Danziger 1979, for example). At the community level, the community leaders must be approached. When Pranee conducted her ethnographic study of Hmong women in Melbourne, she had to seek permission from Hmong community leaders. Through her bicultural researcher, she asked if she could be present at one of the fortnightly meetings at which community members discussed community concerns. She was allowed to attend and she explained to the meeting what she wished to do in her study and who would be involved in it. Before agreeing to her request, the leaders asked her to assure them that the process and the results of the project would not harm their community. Once permission was granted, Pranee was able to enter the Hmong community in Melbourne.

Gaining access to the community will not guarantee the success or smooth operation of the research. Good rapport with the community and informants is essential (Danziger 1979). The ethnographer must be sincere and reassuring about the purpose of the study. In some cases, however, convincing people that the ethnographer is not a threat can be difficult (see, for example, the incident described by Gini Scott 1983 when other members of a black magic group in the USA discovered her position as covert observer). When Pranee conducted her study among Cambodian refugees in Melbourne, one man accused her of being a spy from the social security department, checking on Cambodian people. Although the accusation did not come from her informants, this could have been a threat to her study if the community had agreed with the man. Fortunately, Pranee had been in the community for some time and many people knew that she would not cause harm to them (see Rice 1996c for more detail about gaining entry into some ethnic communities in Melbourne; see also Chapters 3 and 8 in this volume).

Participant observation

> The concept of participant observation ... signifies the relation which the human observer of human beings cannot escape—having to participate in some fashion in the experience and action of those he observes. (Herbert Blumer 1969, p. vi)

Ethnography relies substantially on participant observation (Atkinson and Hammersley 1994). While ethnographers are in the field, they are required to become close to the everyday experience and activities of the people they wish to learn from. They must commit themselves to being as close as possible to the people. This can be achieved through participant observation. Fetterman (1989) argues that this technique is essential for effective fieldwork. According to Goffman (1989, p. 125), participant observation involves:

> subjecting yourself, your own body and your own personality, and your own situation, to the set of contingencies that play upon a set of individuals, so that you can physically and ecologically penetrate their circle of response to their social situation, or their work situation, or their ethnic situation.

To achieve this, ethnographers 'immerse' themselves in the culture. Immersion in ethnographic research is about being with other people; it is about learning about how people respond to situations, how they organise their lives; it is about learning what is meaningful in their lives. Through this immersion, the ethnographers themselves experience events in the same way as the local people. They then are able to see things from the people's perspectives and hence to have a deeper understanding of the people they are learning from. The term 'participant observation' suggests that, as Boyle (1991, p. 277) puts it:

the researcher is directly involved in the informant's life, observing and talking with people as he or she learns their view of reality. The end result is that participant observation allows the researcher to take a particular slice of behaviour and interpret it by putting it into context.

In conducting participant observation as fully as possible in the community under study, ethnographers learn how to live in the community, how to behave as a member of that community, and to experience events and meanings in the same way as the members of the community. Because of this full involvement, some ethnographers end up 'going native' (that is, they are drawn completely into the informants' lives, perhaps marrying a local person and staying in the field for most of their lives), but most 'maintain some distance and objectivity' (Bernard 1995, p. 137; see also Denzin 1978 for an excellent discussion on participant observation).

In participant observation, ethnographers may find themselves not only doing things with their informants, but also doing things for them. When Pranee was conducting her fieldwork in the Hmong community in Melbourne, she participated in many activities that Hmong women usually do. She sat in the kitchen with the women while chatting with them. She tried to do needlework (with difficulty), as most Hmong women and girls must know how to do. She took her daughter to see a magic man when her daughter was accidentally burnt by hot water. She walked with a medicine woman to learn what herbs cure what illness. She also took a Hmong woman to hospital for her soul calling ceremony. She was with the woman when the shaman was conducting a shamanic ritual to cure her illness, and she picked green herbs from a backyard garden to cook a chicken for a soul calling ceremony. The list could easily go on.

Participating in the local culture may sometimes entail a unique experience for the ethnographer (see Box 8.1). When Pranee participated in a *hu plig* (soul calling) ceremony for a newborn infant in one Hmong family, she was invited to sit at the table with the men (see also the 'Fieldnotes' section below). It is usual in Hmong culture for the men to sit at the table, while the women are in the kitchen or other parts of the house, but not sitting at the table with the men. Therefore, it was rather unusual to have Pranee at the table. She was told that, because she was known within the Hmong community and because she was highly educated, her status was therefore equal to men. As a consequence, she could legitimately sit at the table with them.

Pranee's experience (as related in Box 8.1) is not unusual. Many ethnographers have to confront many things which are not part of their own culture, and perhaps not part of their personal life, when they participate in a culture that they are trying to learn about and understand. However, this experience proved to be an extremely useful learning exercise for Pranee in the course of her

Box 8.1 The experience of participant observation

Before the eating started, the family members and junior men (younger men who did not sit at the table) said thank you to the senior members who had helped them in general and in the *hu plig* ceremony and asked the senior members to accept their thanks. They then bowed low on the floor three times. The senior members stood up and said they accepted the thanks and let the party begin. The alcohol tray was handed out to a man at the top of the table. He poured beer into two glasses (in full) and then handed them to the man next to him. The man drank the two glasses of beer continuously (so quick to me). I asked the man next to me why he had to drink two glasses at one time. 'There are always a pair in Hmong culture, like marriage which needs a pair of woman and a man, father and mother and so on', he said. The man who had drunk the beer then poured two more glasses of beer and handed them to the next person. I by now started to realise what was going to happen to me. I would have to drink two glasses of beer at once like the other men at the table. Oh dear! I started to panic since I cannot have alcohol. Every time I touch alcohol I become unconscious. 'What do I do?' I kept wondering. I decided to ask the man whom I had been talking with about the solution. I explained to him that I understood that this was the Hmong tradition and I indeed respected it, but I could not drink any kind of alcohol. He looked at me with funny eyes, and then he smiled and said, 'I will do my best to help you out'.

Then it was my turn. The beer was passed to me. I looked desperately at the man at the top of the table who was in charge of this drinking round. The man next to me whispered to me that I should seek permission from the in-charge man. I stood up and told him about my problem. Everyone laughed. The man in charge stood up and said that he accepted my problem and he knew that as a woman I should not drink alcohol anyhow. He then poured two glasses of Coke and passed them to me. What a relief! I thanked everyone at the table and then drank the Coke as quickly as I could.

Source: Rice fieldnotes

ethnographic study. And this is a common experience for most ethnographers who immerse themselves in a culture (see Styles 1979, for example, for an illuminating case example of his experience in learning about gay baths).

Although most ethnographic studies employ overt participant observation, covert participant observation can also be used. However, this has been criticised because of its ethical implications (Fielding 1993). Covert participant observation may be useful in areas involving sensitive issues, when the ethnographer cannot reveal herself in the research setting or perhaps when revealing her true identity might jeopardise the process of the research. In addition, covert participation helps to verify the results from interactive approaches, since people may not do as they say in the interview (see, for example, Naruemon 1988; Rosenhan 1992).

Fieldnotes

> The production of fieldnotes is the observer's raison d'être: if you do not record what happens you might as well not be in the setting. (Fielding 1993, p. 161)

The second part of doing fieldwork in ethnography is to document what is experienced. This is done through fieldnotes. According to Emerson and colleagues (1995, p. 4), 'fieldnotes are accounts describing experiences and observations the researcher has made while participating in an intense and involved manner'. What the ethnographer sees and experiences is 'put into words'. However, fieldnotes contain not only descriptions of what the ethnographer has seen and experienced, but also her perceptions and interpretations of the events. Consider the fieldnotes from Pranee's ethnographic study of reproductive health among Hmong women in Melbourne (Box 8.2).

Box 8.2 An example of fieldnotes

26 February 1995, Sunday morning
Hu plig ceremony for Xee and Lee's son. Missed the *hu plig* ceremony conducted early in the morning because Neng forgot to inform me about the time. What a pity! Never mind, there will be another one soon and I will not miss it again.

When I got there Hua, Lee's brother whom I have met and talked with many times, invited me to sit at the table near where the junior men were sitting, opposite the senior ones. I asked Hua if I should be with the women in the kitchen instead of at the table with the men. Hua said 'You are my guest and we know you. Also you are very educated, so you should be with us here'. Was I honoured as men in the community? This reminded me of what Pat Symonds has said in her thesis; very similar indeed. I thought perhaps I was honoured because I know the family quite well and have helped them on several occasions, and since I have been in the community for quite sometime, most people know me.

There was a great welcome for me at the party. Everyone tried their best to communicate with me in Thai and Lao as well as English. The man who was sitting next to me was very articulate and well spoken both in Thai and English.

I have not seen him before. Later, Blia told me that he is one of the well-established Hmong men in Melbourne because he has more education than most
Hmong men here.

Hu plig ceremony started. Cotton threads were given out to all men in the
room, as well as to me. People started to tie the cotton on the baby's wrist
(note—left side only, Why left side only, will ask Neng and Grandma Va later), as
well as on the mother and father's wrists. While tying the cotton thread, people
blessed for good future, wealth and good health. A tray was held by the father
and people put banknotes in the tray before tying the cotton thread. What was
the money for? When it was my turn I did what others did. I have intended to
help the family with the ceremony, so I put in a $50 banknote for the parents. I
should not have done that because it was more than anyone else had put in.
Would I offend those older men? But I hoped not. I kept wondering throughout
the ceremony. I had to ask Neng about this too.

Note: Names used in the fieldnotes are pseudonyms only.

Fieldnotes contain not only a passive account of the facts of an event, but
also the active processes of sense-making, of the ethnographer's feelings and
interpretations of what they see and experience during the participant observation. This will guide them to enquire further, hence obtaining more in-depth
understanding of the community group. Fielding (1993, p. 162) believes that
the researcher's personal feelings and impressions should be recorded in the
fieldnotes. Van Maanen (1988, p. ix) has asserted that ethnography is 'the peculiar practice of representing the social reality of others through the analysis of
one's own experience in the world of these others'. This 'peculiar practice' can
only be achieved when ethnographers deeply immerse themselves in the culture
they are studying. And, as Emerson and others (1995, p. 10) argue, 'it is exactly
this deep immersion—and the sense of place that such immersion assumes and
strengthens—that enables the ethnographer to inscribe detailed, context-sensi-
tive, and locally informed fieldnotes'.

Most ethnographers write up their fieldnotes as soon as they can. It may not
be possible to write while observing, so it is necessary to record the observation
as soon as the opportunity arises. Spradley (1970), for example, ran into a toilet
to record his fieldnotes after he had talked with drunks and this made the men
think that he had a problem with his bladder. Powdermaker (1966) sat in her
car for hours after interviews to write up her fieldnotes. This is also Pranee's way
of recording her notes. Most often she had to travel to different Melbourne
suburbs to participate and interview women. Afterwards, she sat in her car writing the fieldnotes to capture vivid information, before driving home.

Key informants

In social science research, the people who provide information to the researcher are often known as 'subjects' or 'respondents'. However, in ethnography, people whom the ethnographer learns from are called 'informants'. An informant has several characteristics (Spradley 1979, p. 25):

* is a native speaker;
* speaks in his or her own language or dialect when giving out information (note that the language of an informant can also be the language of the ethnographer);
* provides a model for the ethnographer to imitate; and
* is a source of information; in other words, an informant is a teacher of the ethnographer.

Ethnographers work with their informants to produce an accurate description of the culture. So, how are informants chosen? In general, ethnographers commence their fieldwork by talking to ordinary people, virtually with anyone they meet and wherever they can 'slip a foot in the door' (Fetterman 1989, p. 43). They build on their information from the informants' common experience. Through a series of interviews and participation, these ordinary people become well-informed informants. In addition, through general conversation, it will become clear that some people are more articulate and can provide much more information than others. These people then become the 'key informants'. By working closely with them, the ethnographer is able to provide a rich description of the culture. When Pranee conducted her study with Hmong women, she started off by interviewing anyone who could give their time. Gradually, she found several key informants with whom she spent more time. This is a common strategy in doing ethnographic study.

Bernard (1995, p. 165) points out that an important question that positivist scientists ask about ethnography is: 'Can a few informants really be capable of providing adequate information about a culture?' According to Bernard, the answer is yes. However, it depends on two things. First, the ethnographer must choose good informants with whom the ethnographer can easily talk, who understand the information the ethnographer needs, and who are willing to supply it. And, second, the ethnographer must ask them things they know about and know better than others. The ethnographer must choose informants for their 'competence', not for their representativeness.

Ethnography utilises several qualitative research methods in collecting information from informants. Most popular is the in-depth interview (see Chapter 3 for details of this method). However, in many ethnographic studies, we also have seen a combination of qualitative methods. These include focus group interviews, life history, and rapid assessment (see Chapters 4 and 6 for the first two methods; see Manderson and Aaby 1992, and Scrimshaw and Hurtado 1987, for rapid assessment). Some ethnographers also incorporate questionnaires in their studies when they need to gather information from a large group of respondents or to generalise their qualitative findings (see, for example, Chirawatkul 1993; Davis 1997; Inhorn 1994; Khanna 1997; Rao 1997; Whittaker 1994). The combination of research methods is used as a triangulation; that is, the results of each method are used to test the validity of information gathered.

Most of these methods are interactive and involve dealing with people. However, there are other non-interactive methods from which the ethnographer may obtain good information to supplement their interactive methods. They are known as 'unobtrusive methods' (see also Chapter 5) and include outcroppings, written information, and folktales (Fetterman 1989, p. 44). Outcropping is 'something that sticks out', which can be graffiti on a wall, the smell of urine on back streets, or syringes scattered in a park. The presence of these outcroppings assists the ethnographer to estimate the relative social situations of an area. Folktales are also useful in providing additional non-interactive information in ethnographic study with 'non-literate' societies, in which cultural values and lessons are transmitted through folktales. Folktales therefore reflect a society's way of life; 'stories provide ethnographers with an insight into the secular and the sacred, the intellectual and the emotional life of a people' (Fetterman 1989, p. 47). Other information, such as medical records, minutes from meetings, photographs, or anything that has been recorded about the cultural group, can be examined and used to supplement the ethnographer's material.

The 'story behind the story' (Stein 1991) gleaned by means of these unobtrusive methods, combined with other interactive methods, can help ethnographers to better understand the people they are studying.

ETHNOGRAPHY IN HEALTH: SOME EXAMPLES

In the last two decades there have been an increasing number of research projects in health that utilise ethnography as a method. It is difficult to discuss these studies in great detail because of space limitations. We will first provide some brief references to recent ethnographic research, which readers may pursue further if they wish. However, we also include detailed discussions of some ethnographic studies in order to provide a full picture of the method and information emerging from them.

Domestic violence, such as wife-beating, is a health-threatening factor facing many women in the world, particularly in poor countries. Despite this widespread threat to women's health, it has rarely been systematically studied. One reason for this lack of research is the sensitive nature of the subject, which makes it rather difficult to obtain good responses from orthodox quantitative surveys. Rao (1997) employed ethnography that included in-depth interviews, participant observation and focus group interviews to obtain sensitive information about the incidence and determinants of wife-beating from women in three villages of Karnataka State in southern India. The ethnographic results revealed that wife-beating was more prevalent when dowries were seen as inadequate, when husbands were alcoholic and when the reason for the abuse was seen as legitimate by the community. However, Rao wished to extend his results to a wider community. He used information gained from the ethnography to construct questionnaires and was able to elicit responses from 170 women. The questionnaire results allowed him to generalise the main themes of his qualitative findings. In addition, he found that women who had been sterilised or had fewer male children were more likely to be abused by their husbands and their families. Rao argued that the methodology employed in his study aimed 'to be informed by the richness, warmth and contextual nature of in-depth interviews, while benefiting from the ability to make generalisable statistical statements about the nature of social scientific interactions' (p. 1170).

Some ethnographic research has looked at the health of mothers and their infants. Zeitlyn and Rowshan (1997), for example, examined breastfeeding and the impact of reproductive technology on the health of women and their unborn children. Another interesting study examining infant health is that of Khanna (1997). Khanna examined the ethical and social implications of the introduction of reproductive technologies in many societies since the 1970s. While the ethical debate around the use of these technologies focuses in Western societies on abortion rights, parenthood rights, and the economic exploitation of infertility, in India the central concern is on sex-selective abortion following antenatal sex determination. This issue is a public health concern because, in India between 1978 and 1983, nearly 78,000 female foetuses were aborted after being detected via antenatal technologies. Since sex determination and the subsequent abortion of female foetuses has been controversial in India, health care providers, women and family members wish to keep it secret. As a result, previous studies have underreported the incidence of antenatal sex determination and sex-selective abortion.

To remedy this, and to understand the lives of Jat women in Shahargaon, in north India, Khanna (1997) adopted ethnography as her method. She conducted participant observation in the village as well as making repeated visits to sex-determination clinics. Khanna also conducted in-depth interviews with family members in order to understand the intrafamilial dynamics in the process leading to antenatal sex determination and sex-selective abortion. Through these methods she was able to crosscheck information on antenatal sex determination and sex-selective abortion.

Because of the preference for sons in the patriarchal ideology of India and because of the impact of urbanisation on family size and composition, reproductive technologies offered Jat women a means of knowing the sex of their unborn child. If the foetus was detected as female, the women would choose abortion. And because the women believed that it was more likely to detect the sex when they were three months pregnant, they delayed sex determination until the beginning of the second trimester. Abortion was not seen as posing any health risk, so there was little concern over the effect of late and repeated abortion on the women's health. Many of the women obeyed the decisions made by their husbands and family members and were willing to risk their health and lives for sons. However, Khanna pointed out that there were some women who resisted this ideology by refusing to have the test and to abort their female foetuses. These women inevitably met with retaliation from their husbands and families. They, and their unwanted daughters, had to bear the consequent physical and emotional abuse.

Khanna also found that most clinics did not keep records of the women, and test results were provided verbally. Also, women were not informed about the risks associated with late and repeated abortion. This had major consequences for the health of many Jat women.

Recently, ethnography has been applied in an attempt to understand health beliefs and attitudes towards HIV/AIDS (for example, Furin 1997; Waterston 1997; Whitehead 1997). Furin (1997) looked at the use of alternative therapies by gay men with AIDS in West Hollywood, California. During a two-year ethnographic study, eighty-nine different therapies for HIV and AIDS treatment were discovered. Furin found that most men in the study used some kind of alternative treatment. Interestingly, most of them also used Western medicine at the same time.

One question emerging from earlier AIDS studies is: why do people with AIDS, and gay men with AIDS in particular, turn to alternative therapies at such high rates? It has been argued that perhaps it is because there is no cure for AIDS (O'Connor 1995). This reason was confirmed in Furin's research. However, Furin also found that a majority of the men in her study turned to alternative therapies because they were dissatisfied with biomedical treatment. What is interesting is that this study found that the high rates of alternative therapies use among gay men were the result of the AIDS activism movement, which has formed in several gay communities throughout the USA in response to the epidemic. Furin (1997, p. 502) argued that the 'extensive therapeutic domain is tied to organized AIDS activism'. AIDS activism has allowed gay men to 'reclaim the technical sphere'; that is, it has allowed some gay men to 'become their own doctors', as one participant said:

> With this disease, you have to do it for yourself. You have to be 'your own doctor' ... You can't count on somebody ... especially when it doesn't matter as much to them and ... so many people don't even bother to learn about it ... You really have to become your own doctor. (Furin 1997, p. 502)

In public health in general, Winch and others (1994) set out to promote the use of mosquito nets to prevent malaria in Tanzania. Menegoni (1996) identified perceptions of tuberculosis and the choices of treatment in Highland Chiapas in Mexico, and Vecchiato (1997) examined the sociocultural aspects of tuberculosis control in Ethiopia. Whiteford (1997) examined the ethnoecology of dengue fever in the Dominican Republic.

There have been several ethnographic studies in the area of drug use. Grund and colleagues (1991) looked at needle-sharing among injecting drug users in The Netherlands. Moore (1993) conducted an ethnographic research project with the members of a social network of young users of recreational/illicit drugs in Perth, and Hassin (1994) examined the impact of AIDS on the social identity of intravenous drug users in the USA.

ETHNOGRAPHY: ADVANTAGES AND LIMITATIONS

As with other methods, ethnography has both advantages and pitfalls.

Advantages

- Ethnography requires the researcher to spend time in the field, talking with people and participating in their lives. Hence, it provides a deep and rich understanding of people in a way that is impossible in other qualitative methods.
- This deeper understanding helps prevent any ethnocentrism on the part of the researcher, encouraging the adoption of a cultural relativism, that is, seeing the world from the people's own perspective. As well, it prevents a false interpretation of the community studied as might be easily done in other methods that cannot elicit in-depth understanding of a people.
- Information obtained from an ethnographic study helps to formulate sensible questions in the native language for further quantitative research. Too often, questionnaires are formulated from the researcher's perspective and so do not make sense to the local people, or are culturally inappropriate. Ethnography can help to overcome this problem (see, for example, Coreil et al. 1989 for the use of the results of ethnography to construct questionnaires in an epidemiological study of immunisation in Haiti).
- Ethnographic research is not only concerned with understanding the world of people under study, but also with applying its findings to bring about change. This is particularly valuable in the health area, where information gathered from ethnographic research can be applied in order to change health practices (see Rice et al. 1994 as an example).

Limitations

*   Ethnography requires the researcher to see the world from the informants' perspective, which may be in marked contrast to the researcher's worldview. This can make some researchers feel uncomfortable about the information obtained or about continuing their ethnographic study.
*   Ethnography requires the researcher to spend a.long period of time in field-work. This may not be feasible for those who have limited time and budget. In addition, some ethnographers may experience emotional and physical health problems.
*   The most difficult part of ethnography is gaining entry into the cultural group or community. In most circumstances the researcher can find ways to overcome this, but, sometimes, it is impossible to gain access. As a result, the research proposal may have to be changed and the project may not be able to be completed as planned.
*   Information collected by means of ethnography from a relatively small number of people from one setting cannot be generalised to the wider population.

CONCLUSION

Ethnography has a long history in learning about what it is to be human. Cultural anthropologists have engaged in the ethnographic method in order to understand people, their cultures, their meanings and their ways of life. Medical anthropologists have used this method to understand health and illness among people in many parts of the world. In public health research, too, it can be an invaluable tool to understand, for example, why many mothers reject immunisation of their young children, why many women do not turn up for their Pap smear test, and why HIV/AIDS has penetrated women's lives and more and more women are facing this life-threatening disease. As Daly and others (1997, p. 157) point out 'ethnography is the classic method for studying a social or cultural niche about which we know very little'. We have to admit that health is a complex issue involving many facets of a person's life. This, coupled with different notions of culture, means that we often 'know very little' about people's health and illness. For us, ethnography is the way in which a researcher may come to have an incisive and deep understanding about the people with whom they intend to work.

Tutorial exercise

Imagine yourself as an ethnographer who wishes to understand why many women from Asian backgrounds do not want to have a Pap smear test. How would you go about finding this out? Set up a plan, using ethnography as a method, and incorporate the essential components discussed in this chapter.

Further reading

Atkinson, P. and Hammersley, M., 1994, 'Ethnography and Participant Observation', in N.K. Denzin and Y.S. Lincoln (eds), *Handbook of Qualitative Research*, Sage, Thousand Oaks.

Denzin, N.K., 1978, *The Research Act: A Theoretical Introduction to Sociological Methods*, 2nd edn, Aldine, Chicago.

Emerson, R.M., Fretz, R.I. and Shaw, L.L., 1995, *Writing Ethnographic Fieldnotes*, University of Chicago Press, Chicago.

Fetterman, D., 1989, *Ethnography: Step by Step*, Sage, Newbury Park.

Hammersley, M. and Atkinson, P., 1995, *Ethnography: Principles in Practice*, Routledge, London.

Powdermaker, H., 1968, 'Fieldwork', in D.L. Sills (ed.), *International Encyclopaedia of the Social Sciences*, vol. 5, Macmillan, New York, pp. 418–24.

Shaffir, W.B., 1991, 'Managing a Convincing Self-Presentation', in W.B. Shaffir and R.A. Stebbins (eds), *Experiencing Fieldwork*, Sage, Newbury Park, pp. 72–81.

Shaffir, W.B. and Stebbins, R.A., 1991, *Experiencing Fieldwork: An Inside View of Qualitative Research*, Sage, Newbury Park.

Shostak, M., 1981, *Nisa: The Life and Words of a !Kung Woman*, Vintage Books, New York.

Spradley, J.P., 1979, *The Ethnographic Interview*, Holt, Rinehart & Winston, New York.

Wolf, D.R., 1991, 'High-Risk Methodology: Reflections on Leaving an Outlaw Society', in W.B. Shaffir and R.A. Stebbins (eds), *Experiencing Fieldwork*, Sage, Newbury Park, pp. 211-23.

9

Participatory Action Research

Consciousness of the oppressed

Do you know who Lakshmi and who Swaraswati is?
Adivasi: Yes.
Who is Lakshmi?
Adivasi: Rice; clothes; hut.
And Swaraswati?
Adivasi: Sawkar's knowledge.
If you could have only one of them, what is your preference?
Adivasi: Swaraswati.
Why?
Adivasi: If everyone has knowledge, then no one can cheat others. Then
only can we have true equality. *(Rahman 1993, p. 74, emphasis ours)*

INTRODUCTION

While qualitative research in health has received much attention in the past few decades, participatory action research (PAR) as a concept and its practices have not received much attention in professional journals. In the last few years, however, we have seen some more publications examining the role of PAR in health and welfare areas in several underdeveloped countries, mainly Africa and India, as well as in Britain and Australia (see an excellent collection of papers in *Participatory Research in Health*, edited by Korrie de Koning and Marion Martin, 1996). In this chapter, we aim to provide readers with an overview of PAR, its history, its development and theory, its use in health research, and its advantages and pitfalls. What follows is our attempt to put together several facets of so-called PAR. The chapter relies heavily on the book edited by de Koning and Martin, as their work provides the clearest and most detailed accounts of PAR currently available.

WHAT IS PARTICIPATORY ACTION RESEARCH?

To pinpoint exactly the meaning of PAR is not straightforward. Reason (1994, p. 328) points out that 'there are several different communities of PAR practitioners who represent their work in different ways'. PAR means different things to different people, as de Koning and Martin (1996, p. 3) argue: 'For some, PR means involving field-level health workers in the research in order to sensitize them to the needs of the community; for others it means research which is an integrated part of a process towards empowerment and emancipation.' In principle, PAR aims to examine the political structures that disempower marginalised, deprived and oppressed groups of people and to find ways in which these structures can be changed. As such, PAR aims to create new forms of knowledge through a creative synthesis of the different understandings and experiences of those who take part. Since knowledge is created from the point of view of marginalised, deprived and oppressed groups of people and classes, it aims to transform 'social realities' (de Koning and Martin 1996, p. 14). Martin (1996, p. 82) argues that PAR is based on a 'strong commitment to social justice and a vision of a better world'. Fals-Borda and Rahman (1991) place PAR within the political aspects of knowledge production and the long tradition of liberationist movements (Reason 1994, p. 328). There are three important tasks of PAR commitments:

- The primary task of PAR is the 'enlightenment and awakening of common peoples' (Fals-Borda and Rahman 1991, p. vi). Within PAR, researchers are more concerned about the production and ownership of knowledge among powerless and 'oppressed' people. The so-called 'scientific methods' of data collection commonly practised among orthodox researchers are of less concern.

- Second, in the PAR tradition, the knowledge and lived experience of 'oppressed' people are valued. Therefore, as Reason (1994, p. 328) points out, the PAR strategy 'has a double standard objective. One aim is to produce knowledge and action directly useful to a group of people—through research, adult education, and sociopolitical action. The second aim is to empower people at a second and deeper level through the process of constructing and using their own knowledge.'

- Lastly, PAR researchers must have a genuine commitment towards 'oppressed' people. The researchers must authentically work in collaboration with the local people in order to improve their lives.

In practice, the key concepts and activities of PAR are interrelated and include participation, education and collective action (Martin 1996, p. 82). PAR aims to be a learning experience for the participants. Its focus is the interests of the participants. It requires active and informed participation by the community in establishing the directions of the research. Hence, community groups are seen as 'active subjects' of the research as opposed to 'passive objects having research done on them', as they are often considered in an orthodox research method. They take an active role from the beginning of the project and, through this active participation, they gain new knowledge and skills and hence increased self-confidence. This process is believed to empower the local community and assist them to change their lived situation. Cornwall (1996, p. 94) takes a similar standpoint, arguing that PAR has its focus on the process of research, not the product. Cornwall argues that actively engaging in a process of learning helps the local people to realise what they know, and that their knowledge is valuable. This in turn empowers them to be able to more effectively take control of their situations.

PAR represents an approach to the learning process in which research, reflection and action are continuing. Both the local people and the researcher play equal parts and the local people are involved in the process from the start. As Maguire (1987) points out, PAR is an approach in which the 'oppressed' and ordinary people join hands to take collective action for social change. As such, PAR aims to 'transform power structures and relationships and empower oppressed people' (George 1996, p. 119).

However, de Koning and Martin (1996, p. 3) point out that, in recent years, different interpretations of participatory action research have been emerging:
- the researcher and research community design the research together;
- the community helps in data collection after the researcher has designed the study; or
- the community works closely with the assistance of a non-governmental organisation (NGO).

Each interpretation has a different commitment and outcomes (see de Koning and Martin 1996 for more detail).

WHY USE PARTICIPATORY ACTION RESEARCH?

Conventional qualitative research aims to gain knowledge from the point of view of the local people. Participatory action research, however, steps beyond the collecting of information about the needs and lives of local people. Rather, it focuses on 'the process' of knowledge production and this emphasis is beneficial to the people involved in PAR research in many ways, as de Koning and Martin (1996, p. 4) argue:
- It assists those who are marginalised and deprived to 'gain self-confidence and pride in being able to provide a useful contribution to community life'.
- It allows 'respect and empathy in professional groups for the insights and knowledge people have and the problems they face'.

- It 'helps to avoid mistakes and to develop programmes that take into account the specific situation and conditions which will influence the outcome of programmes'. It also helps to explain why many health interventions and programs are only partly successful or not at all.

PARTICIPATORY ACTION RESEARCH AND ACTION RESEARCH

It is perhaps here that we need to clarify the concepts of 'participatory action research' and 'action research'. For 'PAR', some writers may only use the term 'participatory research', but others insist on using 'participatory action research'. Some PAR writers, such as McTaggart (1993), see the term as a convergence of two approaches: participatory research and action research. McTaggart points out that participatory research has its origin in community development approaches in underdeveloped countries, whereas action research was developed from Kurt Lewin's work (1946) and has been applied in education and management research in developed countries such as the USA, Britain and Australia (Hart and Bond 1995; Kemmis and McTaggart 1988). Action research argues for acting as a basis of learning and knowing. Ritchie (1996, p. 207) argues that the theoretical basis of both approaches in social science is similar. Both focus on 'emancipation, collaboration and empowerment'. However, the practice of each approach is different. She argues that, at least in Australia, action research has been undertaken by and with people who have considerable power and control, such as teachers and managers. But participatory research has been developed with 'disempowered' people. To Ritchie (1996, p. 207) the major difference between these two approaches lies in the description of the relationship between the researcher and other participants:

> In action research … the instigator is most likely to be one of their own kind, with shared values and similar use of language. In participatory research, the instigator may be from a different sub-culture if that person is better resourced and more highly educated than the other participants.

HISTORY OF PARTICIPATORY ACTION RESEARCH

PAR was originally developed in countries in Latin America, Africa and Asia. The common ground for the development of this approach was concern about marked inequalities in the distribution of resources and power between those who are privileged and dominant, and those who are marginalised and oppressed. It was, and still is, believed that, in order to fight oppression and to alleviate poverty, the feeling of helplessness associated with oppression must be addressed. More importantly, the need to link research with empowering education and action was strongly emphasised by pioneers in PAR, including Fals-Borda and Rahman (1991), Fernandes and Tandon (1981), and Hall (1981).

In his recent writing, Tandon (1996) argues that there are six significant trends that contributed to the evolution of the concept and practice of PAR:

- the debate about the sociology of knowledge and its implications for the formulation of knowing throughout human civilisation;
- the reformulation of adult education where the phrase 'participatory research' was first proposed';
- the alternative pedagogy as a basis for linking PAR as an educational process within the framework of popular education, developed by Paolo Freire;
- the contribution of 'action research', which argues for acting as a basis of learning and knowing, proposed by Kurt Lewin;
- the emergence and contribution of phenomenologists, who promote experience as a basis of knowing; and
- the promotion of participation as a central concept in the development process.

In more recent times, there have been other significant trends contributing to the development of this method. Among these is the development of feminist perspectives that have strengthened the work of PAR within the contemporary context (Tandon 1996).

Since its original establishment, many researchers have adopted PAR in different settings (for example, Cohen et al. 1992; Greenwood et al. 1993; Whyte 1991). Whyte et al. (1991), for example, applied PAR in a study of cost reduction and job preservation in the Xerox Corporation in New York and in the exploration of problems and to devise new organisational strategies in the Mondragon cooperative complex in the Basque country of Spain. In *Participatory Action Research*, Whyte (1991) covers many PAR practitioners who apply the approach in industrial and agricultural settings. Toulmin and Gustavsen (1996) discuss many issues concerning the application of PAR in industrial organisation and management that originated in an action research program in Sweden, known as the LOM program.

Among the pioneers in PAR, Hall (1981) was the first to argue for its use in the development of health programs. The emphasis on community participation in primary health care (PHC) has prompted many researchers and health professionals to adopt PAR in health areas (see, for example, Laurell et al. 1992; Nichter 1984; Schoepf 1993; Seeley et al. 1992).

THEORETICAL PERSPECTIVES

Participatory action research has its theoretical framework in 'linking the process of knowing to learning and action' (de Koning and Martin 1996, p. 5).

Paolo Freire, a Brazilian educator, had a significant influence on this process. In his writing of the *Pedagogy of the Oppressed*, Freire (1972) argues that 'linking knowing and learning through an ongoing cycle of action and reflection, leads to the development of a critical awareness about the world participants live in' (cited from de Koning and Martin 1996, p. 6). In criticising general practices in education, Freire argues that most educational activities do not challenge inequalities in the learners. Most keep the learners passive and uncritical. They fail to help people to question the situation they are forced to live in. De Koning and Martin (1996, p. 6) provide a good example of the application of Freire's theory in health. They argue that a conventional approach in health education that employs a didactic approach to teach people about hygiene and nutrition has failed to enable people to, for example, critically examine the reasons for there not being enough water and food and then to identify means in which 'political, social and personal action can change this situation'. Not surprisingly, we have seen many health education programs fail to reach target groups and achieve their goals.

Recently, we have seen the emergence of the feminist movement in the debate and development of PAR (de Koning and Martin 1996; Maguire 1987, 1996; Martin 1996; Tandon 1996; Thompson 1991). Feminist researchers and action groups in many countries have questioned the terminology, of the 'poor', the 'marginalised' and the 'oppressed', used in PAR. Although the method aims to empower the 'poor', the 'marginalised' or the 'oppressed' to take control over their lives, who are the 'poor', the 'marginalised' and the 'oppressed'? De Koning and Martin (1996) argue that there is a danger in the use of categories like these since they imply that these 'poor', 'marginalised' or 'oppressed' people are homogeneous. Feminist critiques contain three points of concern:

- Who is given a voice in a PAR project? That is, who are included as participants, and whose ideas are represented in the results? In the past, most of these projects represented mainly the voices of men. Women were largely excluded from the research (Maguire 1996).
- The use of categories like the 'poor', the 'marginalised' or the 'oppressed' by Paolo Freire raises questions about the development of theory in practice. As a male, in his early writing, Freire failed to address differences between and among groups of 'oppressed' people. (In his later writing, however, Freire acknowledges the critique of his work by feminist writers; see McLaren and Leonard 1993 for more detail.) De Koning and Martin (1996, p. 13) point out that Freire's examples include bosses oppressing workers and men oppressing other men. However, as Weiler (1991) argues, he did not look at situations where men who are oppressed in the workplace come home and start to oppress their wives or daughters.
- The meaning of being a woman differs depending on place, situation and time. Ethnicity, class and age also influence the experience of being a

woman. The use of 'women' as a unified group is therefore problematic, and feminist researchers, particularly in underdeveloped countries, have also challenged this.

With the development of feminist theory we have seen several PAR projects addressing the issue of 'differences' between men and women in the empowering process. Among the writers, Maguire is prominent. In her writing about PAR from a feminist perspective, Maguire (1996, p. 28) states that:

> Feminisms are about attempting to bring together, out of the margins, many voices and visions of a more just, loving, non-violent world. In that sense, feminism/s and PR share emancipatory, transformative intentions. Yet in practice and theory, PR has often ignored the gender factor in oppression.

Maguire argues that feminist perspectives have shifted the question of how PAR might be 'man-centred', as has been used in the past, to 'human-centred', which will include 'women' on the agenda of research.

In more recent times, Freire, Lewin and feminist theories are utilised in PAR projects. This is a good sign since it helps to strengthen this research approach in both developed and underdeveloped societies where there are inequalities in class, ethnicity and gender.

PARTICIPATORY ACTION RESEARCH AS A METHOD

How do we conduct participatory action research? If we scan through publications relating to PAR, we may find the ideology of the approach rather than a description of what actually happens (Reason 1994). Participatory action research is not a method per se but, rather, a methodology. Tandon (1988) argues that PAR is a methodology for an alternative system of knowledge production. It is based on the people's role in setting the agendas, participating in obtaining data and analysis, and controlling the use of the outcomes. If we examine the methodology of PAR from theoretical traditions (see Chapter 1), it can be seen that it is influenced by phenomenology and hermeneutics as well as feminism, as discussed above.

In the PAR approach, we may find a combination of quantitative and qualitative methods. However, in keeping with its philosophy, which emphasises the production of knowledge and empowerment, most PAR research employs qualitative research methods. A wide range of such methods is used. Most frequently utilised are in-depth interviews, focus group interviews, life history, and participant observation. George (1996), for example, employed several qualitative methods in a PAR project on the meaning of sexuality among poor women in Bombay. The project initially began with focus group discussions. However, later on it was realised that the women had a vast amount of knowledge and experience to offer, which was difficult to generate from group discussions. Life history was then undertaken as a first step. Through this method, the researcher was able to elicit many painful experiences in the women's lives, such as the extramarital relationships of their husbands, the social trauma of infertility and domestic violence, and the difficulty in seeking treatment for a sexually transmitted disease. After the life history was conducted, in-depth interviews followed for some women to clarify their narratives and to allow them to discuss their personal experience of their sexual lives. Focus group discussions followed the life histories to allow the women to share their experiences. George stated that it was easier for the researcher to raise some sensitive issues concerning sexuality in the focus groups following the life history interviews because the women felt more relaxed about talking once they knew that other women had had such experiences and had talked about it. Similarly, Mavalankar and colleagues (1996) used a combination of focus group discussions, in-depth interviews and participant observation with women of reproductive age, in trying to explore their perceptions and reasons for using or not using public health services such as immunisation, family planning, and antenatal and birthing care in north Gujarat, India.

In rural participatory action research, emerging in the last decade, rapid appraisal assessment methods were also used in conjunction with small-scale qualitative methods. These allow an in-depth understanding of people to be developed in a relatively short period. They help to identify the needs and priorities of the local people, place issues in the context of people's lives and assist in the development of programs and provision of services (see, for example, Annett and Rifkin 1988; Bentley et al. 1988; Scrimshaw and Hurtado 1987; Vlassoff and Tanner 1992).

Some innovative methods used within the participatory rural appraisal approach, including seasonal calendars (Welbourn 1992), body mapping (Cornwall 1996), and modelling (Marindo-Ranganai 1996), have been increasingly employed in PAR too. Marindo-Ranganai provides an account of an interesting PAR project in Zimbabwe, which attempted to obtain demographic data on fertility, population size and mortality in order to create a community-based information system. Through participatory modelling, area maps were drawn and quantitative data on birth and deaths among children within the communities were collected, despite the fact that most participants, particularly women, were illiterate.

PAR researchers also use community meetings and different types of community events, such as theatre, storytelling, puppets, song, drawing, and painting, as a means of gathering data among illiterate people. Preston-Whyte and Dalrymple (1996) and Dalrymple and Preston-Whyte (1992), for example, describe the use of drama as a method in a PAR project concerning AIDS education programs in black secondary schools in KwaZulu, South Africa.

Some PAR projects begin with an intervention that has the formal objective of developing health care or adult literacy. Through this intervention, the process of participation and dialogue flow and further developments follow. In their review of projects undertaken by Australian NGOs in various countries, Manderson and Mark (1997) provide two case studies of women's health and development projects in China and Indonesia. In China, village women attended pig and poultry husbandry courses to obtain new skills and thus to later generate income. The acquisition of new skills and the ability to raise income helped to empower the women, and hence enhanced their status. Later, they decided to provide basic health services for their communities in poor and underserviced areas using money that they had raised. As a result, the 'barefoot doctors' program was initiated and implemented.

In Indonesia, a literacy training project was established in response to the needs of illiterate members of a small traders group who ran a savings and loans scheme. As more than 70 per cent of the members were illiterate, the scheme did not function well. However, after gaining functional literacy, many of the women felt empowered and gained self-confidence. Three months later, the women identified access to clean water as crucial for their community. Because of their active involvement in the project, the women increased their capacity to work effectively and improved their personal status. This was reflected in the enhancement of their position at home, their improved understanding of legal documents, and their ability to manage household budgets and the savings and loans scheme. The project also reduced the pressure on divorced or widowed women to remarry. Many men were attracted by the project activities and later joined the program.

Many of these so-called 'unorthodox' methods employed in PAR are essential if the researchers wish to give local people the chance to participate fully. Salazar (1991) argues that it is necessary for 'oppressed' people to be able to find a way to tell their stories and this may help them to break 'a culture of silence' resulting from centuries of oppression.

Some 'orthodox' quantitative methods, such as survey techniques, are utilised in some PAR projects (see, for example, de Roux 1991; Gaventa and Horton 1981; Rahman 1991; Tandon and Brown 1981). However, Reason (1994, p. 329) argues that the results from these techniques need to be understood from the point of view of the community in order to promote the production of knowledge and empowerment.

PARTICIPATORY ACTION RESEARCH IN HEALTH: SOME EXAMPLES

Participatory action research is increasingly recognised as an important research tool in the health field. De Koning and Martin (1996, p. 1) argue that there are several reasons for the growing popularity of this method:

- It has become evident that there is a gap between the perceptions and attitudes towards health and illness held by health care professionals and lay people. Too often, the biomedical framework of illness and disease is in marked contrast to the understanding embedded in a local cultural setting.

*   There are many factors—cultural, historical, socio-economic and political— that are not easily measured in biomedical terms but which can have an impact on efforts to improve people's health. Therefore, when one attempts to measure health outcomes, one simply cannot ignore these factors and assume that 'the world outside the laboratory is the same as inside' (Lammerink and Wolffers 1994, p. 7).

Tandon (1996, p. 23) argues that PAR has become more popular in the health area because of its philosophical approach, which places an emphasis on the local people as a central point of concern both in the definition of health and the location of responsibility in maintaining and improving health. Tandon argues that the rise of medical knowledge, specialisation, technology and commercialisation has resulted in a narrow definition of health, one that focuses only on the disease model. This has made doctors and other medical experts the dominant group, with a 'legitimate right' to control people's lives and health. Since, in the PAR process, people are empowered to take control of their own lives and hence their health, its application in the health area is extremely useful for local people themselves.

It is perhaps here that we need to acknowledge the implications of the development of PAR for health care. Tandon (1996, pp. 24–5) argues that there are several points to address:

*   There is a need to redefine the concept of health. Health needs to be redefined as part of life and as a dimension of lifestyle since it cannot be separated from human life and lifestyle. Therefore, before one starts the endeavour to improve the health of people, one must address the issue of living situation and prerequisites of life. This is a fundamental way to improve the health of many 'oppressed' people.
*   It is essential to incorporate traditional health practices and healing systems into the health care system. Many of these traditions have been eroded and destroyed with the expansion of modern medicine, but in the last decade there has been a trend to bring them back. One powerful example among the many traditional practices and healing methods is the return of breast-feeding in many societies.
*   There is a need to 'demystify' modern knowledge and medical technology so that local people are not threatened or confused by the rise of modern science, and hence they may have a chance to take responsibility for their own health.
*   There is a need for local people to have the right to know about their health status; the causes, nature and treatment of their ill-health; and the resources available to improve their health. If this information need is met, the people will have more control over their lives.

- There is a need to recognise and accept the current state of knowledge and skills, regarding the health and health care of the local people, among health researchers and service providers. New knowledge and skills can only be learned if they build on existing knowledge and skills.
- There is a need to question the political economy of knowledge, science and education in medicine. Tandon (1996, p. 25) argues that a fundamental issue in health care is: 'Whose interests do health sciences, research in health care, knowledge about health care and health practices serve? Who has control over health, health care, health science, health research?' Tandon argues that, if in the end research in health care and practice only serves the interests of the medical professions and their associates, 'it will serve to perpetuate the current system of inequality and injustice related to health and health care'. The PAR approach addresses this tendency and provides some basis for redressing inequality and injustice.

There have been several PAR projects in health conducted in different parts of the world, mostly in underdeveloped countries, in the last few decades. In Thailand, as in many other underdeveloped countries, there have been several such health projects, aimed at empowering people. Yimyam and Suwanwong (1995), for example, showed that there are still many nutrition problems among infants in rural areas in Thailand. This prompted them to conduct a PAR project to determine the factors influencing supplementary feeding among mothers in a rural area in Chiang Mai and to find ways in which the nutritional status of the infants might be enhanced. Through the participation of the women in the project, several obstacles affecting supplementary feeding were identified, including inappropriate timing of the introduction of supplementary food, and the inappropriate quality and quantity of this food. The underlying obstacles, however, were those of cultural and traditional beliefs concerning infant feeding, problems with breastfeeding, economic pressure to seek paid employment, the commercialisation of infant food, maternal work, and maternal knowledge. Several culturally appropriate strategies for supplementary feeding promotion were developed to assist the mothers. The strategies were particularly useful for the mothers involved in the PAR project and included: obtaining ingredients available in the community or those that were in season; and using utensils available within the household for food preparation, such as a mortar and pestle, instead of a food processor, for those who could not afford to buy one.

We also have seen PAR projects in some developed countries. Dockery (1996), for example, has shown us that it is possible to apply the method even within non-participatory health care systems. He used the National Health Service (NHS) in the United Kingdom as a case in point. The NHS is one of the largest bureaucracies in Europe (Dockery 1996, p. 168). As a bureaucracy, it is hierarchical by nature and in practice. This has implications for any attempt to make structural changes, which is a fundamental aim of PAR in its purest form. What Dockery tried to say was that it was a difficult task to change structures and practices in a non-participatory and hierarchical organisation like the NHS. However, he proposed that PAR researchers needed to purposefully look for any opportunity within the research process where participation could be facilitated and to attempt to push it towards the ideal aim of PAR.

Ritchie's recent work in Australia (1996) is participatory action research. Ritchie attempted to enhance the health of workers in the work setting. Through her long association with health promotion programs in the workplace, she became aware that a conventional model of health promotion did not address the real health needs of the workers; rather, it reflected the decisions of the executives. Ritchie applied the PAR approach in trying to promote the health of semi-skilled blast-furnace operators and steelworkers and to enable these men to be able to take more control over their health. During the period of her research (over eighteen months), the men worked through the cyclical process of raising problems, debating the issues of concern and finding solutions.

> The range of issues dealt with was considerable. Overcoming the health impacts of shiftwork generated enormous interest in investigating alternative rostering schedules; concerns about company policies in relation to the wearing of protective gear led to the formal appointment of a sub-committee to investigate all heat-resistant clothing; a stop-smoking group asked for assistance from a consultant psychologist and gained permission for this to proceed; alternatives were explored to put more physical exercise into the day of technical assistants who spent all the shift in front of computer screens; an innovative hearing-conservation scheme was set up to promote positive rather than punitive ways of using noise-protective gear; the list went on and on. (Ritchie 1996, p. 213)

The work of Ritchie stresses the value for these working class men of actively participating in finding solutions to issues of concern. Many workers were empowered and made a particular effort to improve not only their own health but also that of other workers.

A more recent PAR project, conducted with Australian Aboriginal health workers, is that of Hecker (1997). Hecker employed PAR to examine the factors that affected the empowerment of these workers within the context of an Aboriginal-controlled primary health care service in South Australia. She argued that the method was particularly appropriate for conducting research with Aboriginal health workers, who historically have had very little control over the research process, because 'it enabled relatively unempowered groups to undertake research into their own situations' (p. 785).

Hecker found that there were three main issues that affected the empowerment of Aboriginal health workers: the low standard of training, the lack of skills in English literacy and numeracy, and the lack of active participation in planning and decision making within the health service. She concluded that the health workers were in a difficult position. While they had to play their role in the 'key delivery of primary health care', they had inadequate necessary training or English skills to fulfil and support their role. The lack of training and English skills, in turn, reduced their ability to take on more responsibility and control within health teams. This, Hecker argued, 'has created their low level of confidence and provides them with little incentive to develop consistent work patterns' (p. 787).

Hecker argued that her project was different from other research undertaken with Aboriginal health workers in remote areas for two reasons. First, PAR enabled the health workers to actively participate as co-researchers. Hecker argued that, when the 'researched' become the researcher and are given a genuine opportunity to set the agenda for the research, the process can develop initiative, strengthen decision making and hence increase 'self-reliance' (p. 788). Second, the project brought about action and positive changes for the health workers during the research process. These two aspects led to the process of empowerment among the health workers in remote areas. As a consequence, they have a greater chance of taking more responsibility in solving their problems and in achieving greater influence within the Australian health system.

In recent years, we have seen more research in women's health utilising PAR as an approach to empower women and to improve their health as well as that of their families and communities. Khanna (1996), for example, described an interesting PAR project on a women's health program in the Panchmahals District of Gujarat in western India. There were three parts to the program: maternal and child health; action research on traditional medicines; and training for gynaecology through the self-help approach. Khanna (1996) pointed out that PAR was built into the women's health program in three ways:

- The local women had raised concerns—with SARTHI (Social Action for Rural and Tribal Inhabitants of India), an independent entity that works closely with women in development projects in the district—about their general poor health, gynaecological problems and living conditions, as well as their low status within a society that had disempowered them. With the involvement of SARTHI and the women's participation, woman-centred holistic health care at the primary level was set up. An essential part of this initial work was to provide a chance for the women to share their stories, to talk about their experiences of childbirth and menstruation. Hence, they had a chance to realise how their bodies had been subordinated by men. It also helped them to abandon their sense of shame about their bodies, and so to revalue and claim for their own valuable selves.
- Activities involving traditional remedies for women's health were carried out. These included workshops with traditional healers; village meetings with elders; participatory field exercises with schoolchildren; and field visits with local women into the forests to identify herbal medicines traditionally used

for common health and gynaecological problems. These activities and their processes were empowering since they made the women realise the wealth of their knowledge of traditional medicines. The result of these PAR activities was that the women consciously propagated medicinal plants and revitalised the system of traditional medicine for their primary health care needs.

- Self-help workshops for training in gynaecology in a social and gender-sensitive way were also instituted. Regular three-day workshops were carried out over a year to learn about the basics of gynaecology by examining the participants' own bodies. The group also dealt with their own health problems with traditional medicines and other non-drug therapies. Because of the knowledge and skills gained from the PAR approach, many of the women have become 'barefoot gynaecologists' who travel to help other women in the area.

All of these areas of the PAR project have proved to be invaluable for a poor and marginalised group of women in Panchmahals. Khanna (1996, p. 66) pointed out that firstly, the process involved in PAR had the effect of transforming all participants in that their ways of seeing reality, and the responses they chose to deal with reality, were changed dramatically. Secondly, the women became aware of the gender imbalance that affected their lives and the society. As a consequence, PAR resulted in 'the politicalisation' of the women. This politicalisation process had helped many of them to initiate action to change their lives.

QUALITY OF PARTICIPATION: WHAT DETERMINES THIS?

How do we know if a PAR project contains a good quality of participation? De Koning and Martin (1996, p. 3) point out that quality can be assessed by examining the research process:
- Does community participation happen at all stages of the research?
- Which groups in the community represent which parts of the process?

Good quality participation occurs when the community participates in all stages of the research process. However, this may not be feasible as both the researchers and the community members may have different priorities and needs. For example, community members may have to work to maintain their daily income or care for their dependants; the research may not really focus on the needs of the community; or the researchers may want control over the research process (de Koning and Martin 1996; Pratt and Loizos 1992). Good quality participation also occurs when the same group from the community participates in all parts of the research process from the start. If the researchers can organise their PAR in this way, a process of learning and empowerment within the involved community group will result.

One of the unique qualities of PAR is that the research project should serve the shared interests of both the researchers and the researched community.

In achieving this, a complex negotiation process is usually needed and most often it involves a shift of power between the researcher and the community. Research conducted by Martin (1996) with a well-women group in the United Kingdom is a case in point. Martin points out that she had to negotiate with the women in the group during the period of the PAR. In the early stages of the project, the research aims were negotiated between her and the well-women group representatives, hence power was well balanced. However, the power balance changed dramatically in the later stages, particularly in the selection and design of the method and in the analysis and writing up of the report, where the major responsibility was given to her as a researcher. This was mainly due to the belief among the women that she had all the necessary skills to conduct research and that they did not have the time to take on additional tasks. In addition, the women had a 'mystique' idea about doing research and they did not feel confident enough to be totally involved in these stages. Had Martin not insisted on the full participation of the women, the consequence might have been that, instead of empowering them, the process might have disempowered them. Shared interests between researcher and community are therefore essential in conducting a good quality PAR.

PARTICIPATORY ACTION RESEARCH: ADVANTAGES AND LIMITATIONS

Like other qualitative research methods, the participatory action research method has its advantages and disadvantages.

Advantages

* As an alternative method to orthodox research, which is determined by dominant groups, PAR aims to produce knowledge from the point of view of marginalised, deprived and oppressed groups and classes. The emphasis is on transforming social realities so that the lives of such people are improved.
* PAR attempts to combine research, education and action in one endeavour. The isolation of orthodox research from these three aspects has been criticised strongly by PAR researchers (Hall 1993; Maguire 1996). Through the combination of the three perspectives, local people can use the method to create knowledge and take action for 'emancipatory and transformative structural and personal change' (Maguire 1996, p. 32).
* PAR attempts to link theory and practice, or knowing and doing. It therefore has the potential to transform social reality.
* PAR provides a way for people whose voices have been 'oppressed' or ignored to speak about their problems. They discover how their lives can be improved from their own perspective, not according to the researcher.
* PAR emphasises a balanced relationship in power between the different groups involved. Not only are health care workers or researchers seen as

powerful because they have more knowledge, but local women and men are also powerful because of their local knowledge. The method helps to merge these two perspectives of knowledge so that it strengthens local people's confidence and empowers them.

- The activities involved in PAR are largely expressive. They enrich the enquiry as well as provide a means through which ordinary people may experience and validate the data being used (Reason 1994).
- PAR can be applied in any part of the world. Although its original use was in underdeveloped countries, it is also a valuable approach in many developed countries where there are gaps between the rich and the poor, the privileged and the oppressed, the powerful and the powerless.

Limitations

- In PAR, open-ended questions are often used to elicit information relevant to local people. This means that they have the freedom to answer as they wish. Since local knowledge is a 'complex social construct' (Tolley and Bentley 1996, p. 53), researchers need to crosscheck their data by using a mix of methods and talking with a wide range of people. This is known as 'triangulation' in qualitative methods (Denzin 1978). This is not so much a limitation as a potential complexity.
- The issue of ownership of data or knowledge is important. In PAR, ownership of the process and the outcome is shared between the researcher and the local people (Tolley and Bentley 1996). What happens to the data when the researchers need to publish findings as required by their institutions? Because the data gained from PAR are shared, how can they be published? This needs to be negotiated between the researchers and the communities at an early stage in the development of the project. The local people need to be clear about this issue from the start.
- There may be problems associated with the different expectations of the PAR researchers and of the funding bodies or academic institutions. PAR cannot be undertaken in a short period of time, like survey methods. Involving local people in every stage of research consumes tremendous amounts of time, so PAR projects often take longer than a year. This may not be practical if funding bodies do not wish to fund a long-term project or have an unrealistic expectation about its timeline. This also may make an ongoing process problematic. The long process of projects may create a sense of lack of fulfilment or lack of accomplishment among PAR researchers.
- PAR practitioners are often accused of not being 'scientific' in their approach. Hence, they may have difficulties in attracting research funds and, to a lesser extent, in publishing their work in professional journals that emphasise the 'scientific' approach or conventional research methods.

- PAR researchers who come from an academic background may not be able to be involved in a project until the end of the process because of time and funding constraints. This may jeopardise the project in that it may not achieve its goal. However, this can be overcome by involving NGOs and government agencies from the beginning of the project. When the researcher has to retreat, these people can step in to complete the project (see, for example, Dockery 1996; Mavalankar et al. 1996).
- PAR requires an authentic attitude of mutuality and openness and a commitment to learning on the part of all people involved, particularly the researchers. This may present difficulties if some people have other political agendas that prevent them from meeting these requirements. This can be overcome by emphasising the importance of such requirements during the training process.
- One problem in implementing PAR in health research is that training in health science emphasises a biomedical model of health. This may make it more difficult for health workers to attempt PAR projects since this model does not correspond well with local notions of health and illness. The hierarchical nature of work may also place some strains on the workers, which may result in the same feelings of powerlessness and helplessness that 'oppressed' groups have. Training that aims at empowering PAR health practitioners is essential in this regard.
- PAR philosophy emphasises the role of 'participation and self-direction in development' of 'oppressed' people. Yet 'PAR projects may not occur without the initiative of someone with time, skill, and commitment, someone who will almost inevitably be a member of a privileged and educated group' (Reason 1994, p. 334). The method may therefore not have the results expected.
- There is a wide range of skills required for participatory research. These skills are very different from those of conventional research. They include, for example, 'personal skills of self-awareness and self-reflexiveness, facilitative skills in interpersonal and group settings, political skills, intellectual skills, and data management skills' (Reason 1994, p. 335). Some researchers who attempt to use the PAR approach may find that these skills are beyond their limited resources of time, money and energy. However, with 'authentic commitment' and patience, these can be overcome.

CONCLUSION

Participatory action research, in our sense, is research that is participatory and that unites with action. As we have illustrated, the method is of value in health research. Inequality is a common phenomenon in most societies, and this affects people's health and well-being. PAR is an approach that we believe can help to empower those who are 'oppressed' and hence reduce social inequalities. It allows people to acquire new knowledge and skills through their participation in the research, thereby empowering them and enabling them to take control over their health and lives. PAR prevents 'oppressed' people from becoming passive objects who have research 'done on them', as in conventional research methods, because they are able to have equal power in controlling the research. Through this empowerment and emancipation, we believe that injustices in health care, including health education and research, can be reduced. As Tandon (1996, p. 25) argues, 'it is only when the issues of control over health and the political economy of research in health sciences are addressed, both in our practice and in our theory, that we will be able to make health a truly human endeavour, and not one that is limited to experts, scientists, laboratories and medicines'. We too believe in this endeavour.

Tutorial exercise

Design a participatory action research project on an Aboriginal health issue (focusing on one of the following: breastfeeding, alcohol, or diabetes) in one community only. Write down the key components of the research plan, applying the main points discussed in this chapter in the research process. Make sure that the plan is realistic and feasible.

Further reading

de Koning, K. and Martin, M. (eds), 1996, *Participatory Research in Health: Issues and Experiences*, Zed Books, London.

Fals-Borda, O. and Rahman, M.A. (eds), 1991, *Action and Knowledge: Breaking the Monopoly with Participatory Action Research*, Apex Press, New York.

Fernandes, W. and Tandon, R., 1981, *Participatory Research and Evaluation: Experiments in Research as a Process of Liberation*, Indian Social Institute, New Delhi.

Freire, P., 1972, *Pedagogy of the Oppressed* (trans. M.B. Ramos), Penguin, Harmondsworth.

McTaggart, R., 1993, 'Dilemmas in Cross-Cultural Action Research', in D. Colquhoun and A. Kellehear (eds), *Health Research in Practice: Political, Ethical and Methodological Issues*, Chapman & Hall, London.

Rahman, M.D.A., 1993, *People's Self-Development: Perspectives on Participatory Action Research—A Journey through Experience*, Zed Books, London.

Reason, P., 1994, 'Three Approaches to Participative Inquiry', in N.K. Denzin and Y.S. Lincoln (eds), *Handbook of Qualitative Research*, Sage, Thousand Oaks.

10

Qualitative Data Analysis

There are many ways to move from the field to the text, many way to inscribe and describe experience. (Denzin 1994, p. 511)

Interpretation is an art that cannot be formalised. (Denzin 1994, p. 512)

INTRODUCTION

Qualitative research can be described as a strategy of 'calculated chaos' (Lofland and Lofland 1971, p. 69). Researchers intentionally immerse themselves in interviews and participant observation, and then in reading, and rereading, the data. The aim is to discover, to understand, through immersion in the data. The initial experience of immersion may result in a chaotic confusion as a consequence of the complexity of the data and of exploring multiple possible interpretations. However, out of this immersion emerges new perspectives, new linkages, new understandings and theories.

The phrase 'calculated chaos' is suggestive of two central, and potentially conflicting, processes that operate in qualitative research. First, qualitative research is calculated. There are established procedures, techniques and methods for conducting qualitative research and for analysing qualitative data. There are many different traditions that prescribe procedures and techniques for qualitative data, or, as Denzin (1994, p. 511) puts it, 'there are many ways to move from the field to the text'. Those reviewed in this chapter include content analysis, grounded theory, different types of coding, computer-assisted data analysis, and semiotic and poststructuralist approaches to data analysis. These established techniques have been demonstrated to be effective ways of producing useful results. They are part of the tradition of qualitative research.

However, qualitative data analysis is also chaotic. Qualitative research is often criticised for being too exploratory, and too unclear about its aims. However, it is not always clear what the specific nature of a problem is at the beginning of a research project. Further, when meanings and interpretations are the focus of a project, it is somewhat presumptuous to assume to know the interpretations that Aboriginal people, for example, give to hospitals before you have asked them. Qualitative research courts this uncertainty and lack of clarity. Qualitative research also provides a certain respect for intuitive 'hunches' (Strauss and Corbin 1990). For example, a theoretically informed hunch led Charmaz (1991) to explore the link between chronic illness, self-concept, and the experience of time. However much grant applications may claim otherwise, good qualitative research allows chaos. If the problem could be precisely defined, if the meanings of the participants were known completely beforehand, if it were clear that a theory would explain a particular experience, if the benefits of the research could be demonstrated with certainty, qualitative research would be irrelevant.

RESEARCH DESIGN AND DATA ANALYSIS

Qualitative data analysis should begin at the beginning of the study. It should be part of the research design, part of the literature review, part of the theory formation, part of the data collection, part of the data ordering, filing and reading, and part of the writing. From this perspective, the first step in qualitative data analysis involves conducting a literature review and developing a theoretical orientation and the method of data collection can all have significant implications for how data analysis is conducted.

For example, the extent to which theory is developed inductively or deductively will have a major impact on the method of data analysis (Kellehear 1993a). Deductively derived theories are built up, or deduced, from pre-existing theory. Deductively produced theories are then typically tested against the data. For example, it may be hypothesised that men are less likely to talk about their bodies than women, and a content analysis of interviews with chronically ill people could be conducted to test this. In contrast, inductively derived theory is developed from the empirical data, with limited reference to pre-existing theory. For example, a careful reading of a set of interviews with chronically ill people may discover that men are more likely to think of their bodies as machines, to be fixed, whereas women have a closer relationship to their bodies (Gergen and Gergen 1993).

However, most qualitative research involves a combination of inductive and deductive theorising. A new theoretical approach is derived deductively and then compared with, or tested against, inductively derived theory. The complexity of this process is most obvious in semiotic or poststructuralist data analysis techniques. They explicitly recognise the role of prior theory in framing both the content of the data and how it is analysed. However, as discussed below, grounded theory also involves a complex mixture of inductive and deductive modes of analysis.

THE FIRST STEPS: IDENTIFYING UNITS OF ANALYSIS

As in sampling (see Chapter 2), one of the first steps in qualitative data analysis is identification of the units of analysis. Lofland and Lofland (1971, p. 71) describe a unit of analysis as 'a tool to use in scrutinising your data log'. The unit may be meanings, practices, encounters, narrative structures, organisations, or lifestyles. The unit of analysis will usually be decided upon through examining previous research on the topic, the theory to be used, and the uses for which the research is designed. For example, one study of unemployment may focus on job-loss episodes as the unit of analysis, whereas another may concentrate on unemployed people's encounters with government officials as the unit of analysis. Once the units have been identified, the researcher begins to ask questions about them as they appear in their data. This is the beginning of coding and is described in detail below.

Content analysis, thematic analysis, grounded theory, and semiotic analysis all require a careful identification of the units of analysis. While some researchers may have a clear idea of their units of analysis, in exploratory studies the research may explore a number of different units concurrently, refining the analysis later in the project.

CONTENT ANALYSIS

Content analysis has been differentiated from thematic analysis (also referred to as grounded theory) on the basis that content analysis involves the identification of codes prior to searching for these in the data, and that thematic analysis involves the inductive identification of codes from the data. We provide a short description of content analysis, which leads into a more detailed discussion of thematic analysis and grounded theory.

As Berg (1989, p. 106) puts it, content analysis requires 'explicit rules called criteria of selection, which must be formally established before the actual analysis of data'. The principles of content analysis can be summarised following Kellehear (1993a):

• Develop categories prior to searching for them in the data.
• Select the sample to be categorised.
• Count, or systematically record, the number of times the categories occur.

For example, Hill and Radiner (1996) conducted a content analysis of the health and nutrition messages of food advertisements in Australian women's magazines. They sampled seventy-two different magazines published in 1992 and sorted advertisements into two basic categories: those that advertised core food groups, including the five main food groups, and those that advertised non-core foods such as alcohol, cocoa products, and supplements. They also differentiated between 'mature women's magazines' and 'young women's magazines'.

Hill and Radiner found that, in mature women's magazines, 47 per cent of advertisements were for core foods, and all five of the core food groups were noted. However, in young women's magazines, only 12 per cent of advertisements were for core foods, and only three of the five food groups were mentioned. The most common advertisements in young women's magazines were for non-core foods such as alcohol, and cocoa products.

Content analysis is often an initial step that leads into another type of qualitative data analysis. For example, Gergen and Gergen (1993) conducted a content analysis of twenty autobiographies from the US best-seller list, looking for descriptions of the body. They found that in childhood years men rarely mention the body, except to note its usefulness. However, women's stories are more embodied with numerous references to the body during their childhood. In adulthood, men again rarely mention their bodies, and when they do, they describe them as servants to their career. In contrast, women mention their bodies many more times, and women's sense of identity is more closely tied to their physical condition. This then leads Gergen and Gergen into a discussion of the relationship between the results of this content analysis and the way that discussions of the body fit into the narrative form of autobiography.

Some researchers use the term 'content analysis' differently. Altheide (1987), for example, uses 'ethnographic content analysis' to refer to the inductive methods of thematic analysis or grounded theory. We prefer to reserve the term 'content analysis' to refer to data analysis that involves the identification of categories prior to coding.

GROUNDED THEORY OR THEMATIC ANALYSIS

One of the more influential research methodologies utilised in qualitative health research is grounded theory (Glaser and Strauss 1968; Strauss and Corbin 1990). In the next two sections we review two aspects of this theory: first, the role of pre-existing theory in the development of grounded theory—this is important because many textbooks provide conflicting and confusing advice on this issue—and, second, the techniques of grounded theory, focusing on forms of coding and journalling.

The main difference between grounded theory and thematic analysis is that grounded theory includes theoretical sampling (see Chapter 2), whereas thematic analysis does not. The techniques used for analysing data in thematic analysis and grounded theory are broadly similar, and we discuss them together.

The theory of grounded theory

Grounded theory is consistent with the provisional and inductive approach of much qualitative research. In contrast to deductively derived propositions, grounded theory argues that theory can be built up through careful observation of the social world:

A grounded theory is one that is inductively derived from the study of the phenomenon it represents. That is, it is discovered, developed, and provisionally verified through systematic data collection and analysis of data pertaining to that phenomenon. (Strauss and Corbin 1990, p. 23)

According to the methods of grounded theory, concepts, categories and themes are identified and developed while the research is being conducted. Concepts are the basic units of analysis. These are then grouped and related to form more abstract categories. Relationships between categories are then identified to develop what Glaser and Strauss (1968) refer to as 'formal theory'. Glaser and Strauss' (1968) original work on grounded theory explicitly rejects the 'logico-deductive' method of theory building and verification. More recently, Strauss and Corbin (1990, p. 50) have also argued that 'it makes no sense to start with received theories or variables (categories)'. This rejection is consistent with the method's emphasis on the inductive nature of theory building. However, on closer examination, the concern of Strauss and his associates is not to reject logico-deductive theory completely. Rather, grounded theorists object to the typical way in which deductively derived theory is brought into relationship with the data:

> It makes no sense to start with received theories or variables (categories) *because* these are likely to inhibit or impede the development of new theoretical formulations, unless of course your purpose is to open these up and to find new meanings in them. (Strauss and Corbin 1990, p. 50, emphasis added)

That is to say, their objection is not to the use of pre-existing theory per se, but to the way in which it might influence the research process: 'it would hinder progress and stifle creativity' (Strauss and Corbin 1990, p. 53). Gerson (1991) demonstrates that grounded theory does make use of pre-existing theory, suggesting that the apparent antipathy to pre-existing theory was a consequence of a 'absurdly restricted and inadequate vision' of verificationist methodology that dominated American sociology at the time of the development of grounded theory (p. 300).

In short, grounded theory involves the rejection of simple deductive theorising. Theory should not be generated by logical argument from general laws. Rather, it should result from the building up of observations and insights from concrete empirical research. However, a sophisticated understanding of grounded theory also rejects simple inductive theory building. Theory building occurs in an ongoing dialogue between pre-existing theory and new insights generated as a consequence of empirical observation.

Lindesmith (1968), in his study of addiction to opiates, provides an excellent description of his method of qualitative data analysis. Lindesmith describes how he came to the study with an explicitly formulated hypothesis that addiction was related to knowing what drug was being taken and the experience of withdrawal distress. However, after beginning his empirical research, this hypothesis was revealed as 'obviously inadequate'. Lindesmith therefore reformulated his theory, hypothesising this time that 'persons become addicts when they recognise or perceive the significance of withdrawal distress which they are experiencing' (p. 8).

The relevance of Lindesmith's methodology to qualitative data analysis technique is that he explicitly formulates his theory at the beginning of his research and then reformulates it while he is conducting his fieldwork, analysing the implications of his data for his theory concurrently with the fieldwork phase. Data analysis leading to theory formulation is an explicit process. He does not pretend that theory is developed independently of prior research and only out of the data. Nor is the theory derived deductively from prior research and simply tested against the data and verified. Lindesmith describes how his hypothesis develops from pre-existing research, and then shifts and transforms as he explores and tests it against the research data from his fieldwork: 'The final revision of the hypothesis involved a shift in emphasis from the individual's recognition of withdrawal distress to his [sic] use of the drug to alleviate the distress after this insight occurred' (Lindesmith 1968, p. 8).

Lindesmith relates how he searched for cases with peculiar characteristics for whom the theory implied a certain type of experience. In other words, he attempted to falsify the theory whenever possible by deducing what it implied for the experiences of certain groups of people and then testing this deduction against their experiences. He says that he was not interested in endlessly verifying his theory but in close examination of its implications. He explored apparent weaknesses in the theory and his confidence in his explanations grew as his search for contradictory cases failed to prove the theory wrong. As Denzin (1970, p. 197) puts it, Lindesmith's strategy was 'to sample theoretically in a continual effort to find crucial cases that would invalidate his theory'.

The practice of grounded theory

At the heart of grounded theory, and thematic analysis, is the process of coding, sorting and organising data. Whether done on paper or on a computer, analysing qualitative data involves coding pieces of text (sometimes referred to as 'chunks') and then collating all those that are coded in the same way. Coding is clearly central to the analysis process. Strauss and Corbin (1990) describe three main coding procedures: open coding, axial coding, and selective coding. Although it is not necessary to do so, these three categories of coding follow a developmental path.

Open coding

Open coding involves comparisons between events, actions and interactions. The analyst searches for differences and similarities between events, actions and interactions and applies conceptual labels to these, grouping them into categories. Normal ways of conceptualising events and interactions are put aside as the analyst attempts to conceptualise the data in a way that exposes social processes. As Strauss and Corbin (1990, p. 63) put it, 'by breaking down and conceptualizing we mean taking apart an observation, a sentence, a paragraph, and giving each discrete incident, idea, or event, a name, something that stands for or represents a phenomenon'.

Open coding could be thought of as the 'first run' at coding data. It aims to look at the data in new ways, to see new relationships between events or interactions, and to develop new ways of describing these relationships. Miles and Huberman (1994, p. 148) describe a number of coding processes that are consistent with open coding, including 'noting patterns and themes', and 'making metaphors'. Making metaphors of the processes or actions being observed is useful for several reasons. For example, to describe illness experiences as like a 'quest' (Frank 1995) suggests a new way of thinking about personal responses to the suffering experienced during illness. The following list is drawn from Miles and Huberman (1994, p. 250):

- Metaphors are suggestive of the richness and complexity of the processes.
- Metaphors are data-reducing devices. They summarise a number of different aspects.
- Metaphors are pattern-making devices. They suggest new relationships as a consequence of new imagery.
- Metaphors are decentring devices. They provide a different perspective, and suggest different questions about data.

The inherent ambiguity of metaphors is useful because it allows qualitative researchers to avoid the positivistic assumptions of a fixed world that can be understood using laws. Metaphors cannot easily be quantified, and are used as a way of understanding in everyday life: 'The social individual imposes a "metaphoric measure" on the world made of collective portrayals that give objects and events a "value" each time intertwined with symbolic structures of a certain historical or cultural era' (Lalli 1989, p. 106).

Open coding may also involve locating the properties of a particular experience along a dimension (Strauss and Corbin 1990). For example, the analyst may attempt to identify the degree of reflexivity exhibited during an illness. People who see their illness as a quest may describe constantly thinking, strategising, and talking about their experience, exhibiting high reflexivity. On the other hand, other people may attempt to avoid thinking about the future, or strategising, exhibiting low reflexivity.

Axial coding

Once initial categories and relationships have been developed during open coding, the next stage involves specifying more rigorously the codes that have been developed. If open coding attempts to break down data and reconceptualise it, 'axial coding puts those data back together in new ways by making connections between a category and its sub-categories' (Strauss and Corbin 1990, p. 97). Axial coding does not involve attempting to map the links between all the codes (this is selective coding). Rather, it involves scrutinising the codes to ensure that each one is fully elaborated and delineated.

Miles and Huberman (1994, p. 254) describe the two processes of 'partitioning variables', and 'subsuming particulars into the general', which are similar to axial coding. Sometimes as the coding proceeds, it will become clear that one of the codes, or variables, needs to be partitioned into two or three sub-categories. For example, the analyst may decide that reflexivity may involve the three sub-categories of thinking, talking and writing. Similarly, it may be that two codes that were originally separate are identified as related. For example, it may become apparent that the significance of a code for 'spending time with my partner' is an aspect of reflexivity, because this activity involves extensive discussions and strategising.

Selective coding

'Selective coding is the process by which all categories are unified around a "core" category' (Corbin and Strauss 1990, p. 14). The processes involved in selective coding are much the same as in axial coding, but at a higher level of generality. The codes, or categories, are compared and a central, or core, code may be identified that provides a theoretical point of integration for the study.

In Aristotle's *Poetics*, he argues that plot (*mythos*) and action (*praxis*) are more important than the characters (*ethos*). In tragedies, for example, it is not the characters that make the play happy or melancholy, it is the plot and the action:

> In a play accordingly they do not act in order to portray the Characters; they include the Characters for the sake of the action ... We maintain, therefore, that the first essential, the life and soul, so to speak, of Tragedy is Plot; and the Characters come second. (Aristotle, quoted in Brooks 1984, p. 11)

Why is this important or relevant to qualitative data analysis? Well, qualitative data analysis can be thought of as an attempt to tell a story about the interviews, observations or other data that have been collected. One of the most important parts of the task of analysis is working out the plot of the story to be told about the data, rather than focusing on the specific techniques to be used or on the characters in the story. Strauss and Corbin (1990, p. 116) suggest that, in qualitative research, a story consists of 'a descriptive narrative about the central phenomenon of the study'.

Some qualitative researchers reject the idea that there should be a 'core' code or category, preferring instead to encourage complexity and multiplicity of interpretations (Clough 1992; Denzin 1997). Some computer programs for qualitative data analysis encourage, although do not require, selective coding with the study unified around a core category (see the section on 'Qualitative computing' later in this chapter).

The practice of coding

Charmaz' (1991) study of the self in chronic illness and time provides an excellent example of the usefulness of grounded theory in studies of health and illness. The following points are derived from her description of how she conducted her research (Charmaz 1991, p. 276):

1 Begin by 'exploring the general research questions'.
2 Gather data, and code for respondents' meanings, feelings and actions.
3 Look for processes and relationships between specific events and general processes.
4 Coding leads to new categories.
5 Collect more data on the developing categories.
6 Go back and read earlier data for the new categories and to formulate new questions.
7 Constantly compare individuals, different events, and the categories.
8 Write memos all the time about categories, processes and ideas.
9 Move towards memos that are more conceptual and codes that are more abstract.

Box 10.1 provides an example of coding using thematic analysis that was done manually on a printed transcript. We have found that printing the transcript on the left-hand side of a 'landscape' page leaves ample room on the right-hand side for notes and coding (if you are left-handed you may want to print the interview on the right-hand side). The first column is part of the text of one of Douglas' interviews from his study of mental health and job loss (Ezzy 1996). The second column includes some of the notes that were made while reading through the interview. The final column lists the final codes used in the analysis. The notes in the second column were gradually refined and combined across various interviews to develop the general codes in the last column.

A partial listing of the final coding scheme also appears in Box 10.1. As should be clear, it is a hierarchical scheme. Each coding 'stem' (such as 'Ending') is followed by several different 'tails' that provide further detail. For example, the first code in the extract is 'Ending'. This indicates that this section of the transcript is about the ending of a job, or a job-loss event. However, there is no tail attached, as the type of ending is not yet clear. Later in the extract, the code 'Ending-sacked' appears, and this specifies the type of job loss. The codes listed in the coding scheme cover the type of Ending, various general aspects of the meaning of Work, the level of Satisfaction that relates specifically to their last Job, and the level of Self-Esteem.

Orona (1990) provides an excellent description of how she went about analysing and coding her data using grounded theory. She describes how her analysis developed through interactions in the field, a careful reading of the literature, discussions with her colleagues, and detailed reading and rereading of her interview notes and transcripts. Discussing coding, Orona says that 'coding each line is the guts of [grounded theory]' (p. 1249). It takes time, but if it is done thoroughly, it can provide excellent results. Coding often involves reading through a manuscript for 'first impressions', as with the notes in the second column above. In subsequent readings, the qualitative researcher attempts to develop concepts and codes on a higher level of abstraction, similar to those in the third column.

I found that if I worked quickly, without too much ruminating, I could come to some 'first impressions'. This seemed to be an important first step for me. I then went back and more slowly re-read the interviews to see if my 'impressions' fit and to conceptualize the data … after several runs I began to see definite conceptual categories emerging. (Orona 1990, p. 1250)

Box 10.1 Coding: a worked example

Interview text	Notes	Final Codes
D: 1990 you were diagnosed with Hep C, is that right?	Hepatitis C	
M: Yep.		
D: What were the jobs that you have done since then?		
M: First, with the Bank.	Bank Job	
D: How long did you work there?		
M: I worked there for just over a year, for about 18 months.		Ending
D: And how was that?		
M: It was horrible.	Last job	
D: Why?	horrible	
M: I guess the most obvious thing was they treated us like shit, and they treated us like we were stupid. And I don't like being treated that way. The worst thing was that was the part where I broke down, at the end of 1991, December, they brought in a new shift roster and the shift roster was something like you worked 2 days, 2 mornings, 2 afternoons and 3 nights. So the shift would finish say at 7.00 on a Monday morning, they considered that your day off and then you'd	Treated like shit Broke down Shift work	Sat.job-lo-mngmnt Self.esteem-lo

go back to work on the Tuesday. And they made		
us do that and they kept saying, if you don't want	Threat of	Work-security
to do this there's other people out there who want	sacking	
this job. But I was very much in a fear space so I		
did it. And I ended up quite chronically ill. And	Fear	
we worked by ourselves on the shift, and so when	→illness	
you were doing an afternoon or a night shift you		
were the only person in the building. By yourself,	Worked	
no breaks, and they turned the ventilation off,	alone	
there were no windows to open and you were in		
this little room in the dark and it wore me down	Bad	Sat.job-lo
and I became very ill. I hated it. And then, it's like,	conditions	task
look what are we going to be paid for this, because		Sat.job-lo-
you can't get paid normal rate for this. Oh well,		illness
we'll give you an extra 20 bucks a week. And it's	Bad pay	Work-money
like, no that's not good enough, it's just not good		
enough. They knew about my illness, they sent me		
to their doctor, their doctor said, no, she shouldn't	Management	
do this sort of rotational shift, a set shift yes, but	ignored	Sat.job-lo-
not a rotational shift. And they wouldn't show me	doctor's	mngmnt
the report, and they made me do it. And as I said,	advice	
I became very, very ill. The Hepatitis just went wild		
and I had to take some time off before I went back	Hepatitis	Sat.job-lo-
to work, and it was, well sorry, we don't want you		illness
here any more. And I had been told to put in a	Sacked	Ending-sacked
workers comp form, put it in. And I thought, no I		
can't do that, it's just too hard, everything's too		
hard. And then they fired me, which they really	No right to	
didn't have a right to do. But they did anyway.	fire her	

Coding scheme

Ending-contract	Work-skill.dev
Ending-gradual.finishing	Sat.job-hi-mngmnt
Ending-left	Sat.job-hi-task
Ending-sacked	Sat.job-lo-mngmnt
Work-valued	Sat.job-lo-task
Work-devalued	Sat.job-lo-illness
Work-money	Self.esteem-hi
Work-social.life	Self.esteem-mid
Work-security	Self.esteem-lo

The value of reflecting or 'ruminating' should not be underestimated. The best examples of qualitative research using grounded theory typically describe periods of reflection and struggle as the researcher attempts to 'make sense' of their data, developing new understandings and reconstructing coding schemes. An important part of this process involves keeping a journal and writing researcher memos.

Keeping a journal or research memos

> Throughout the analysis, I wrote memos to define and examine implicit ideas and processes that I saw in the data. These memos helped me to synthesize data and to define patterns within it. As the research ensued, my memos become more conceptual and abstract. (Charmaz 1991, p. 276)

We have found it very useful to keep a journal of our experiences, theoretical ideas, analytical insights, and diagrams of relationships. This journal is separate from, and additional to, other files and forms of record keeping, such as field-notes, interview transcripts, or files used in coding the data. We often have ideas about a new code, or a question that should be asked, or a piece of theoretical literature that might relate to the study. We record these ideas in the journal, to be developed more fully at the appropriate time. It can sometimes be extremely frustrating trying to recall an idea that seemed very clear two days ago but, because it was not written down, is now vague and unclear in its relevance. Writing ideas down in a journal as they happen helps to record and develop ideas as the occur. We also use the journal to write longer accounts and analyses of the research process and data analysis.

Keeping a journal facilitates thinking about, and beginning to write about, the analysis and interpretation of qualitative data. Lofland and Lofland (1984, p. 135) refer to the potential importance of memos written while the research is being conducted. Memos are small pieces of analysis that derive from 'the interaction of the raw material with your creative and social scientific sensitivities'. Minichiello and his associates (1995, p. 218) suggest keeping an 'analytic file' that 'includes a detailed examination of the research questions asked and ideas emerging as the study progresses'. This process may be referred to as keeping a 'journal', or 'memos', or an 'analytic file'. The different titles suggest different ways of record keeping: the journal is typically a single large book, memos may be kept as part of a computer program used to assist in qualitative data analysis, and an analytic file may be a folder with loose sheets of paper. Each researcher will have different preferences, depending on their distinctive research style and practice.

Some researchers have developed quite complex and formalised classifications of the different types of memos and journals that should be kept (Strauss and Corbin 1990). We have found that a more flexible approach was more suited to our research, and have used only one or two types of journals. However, Strauss and Corbin's (1990) classification of types of memos is useful because it suggests some aspects of the research that should be reflected upon through journalling or memos. For example, Strauss and Corbin (1990, p. 220) provide a useful discussion of the importance and relevance of trying to draw diagrams of processes identified in the research, for example, to conceptualise the relationships between various codes or processes.

COMPUTER-ASSISTED QUALITATIVE DATA ANALYSIS

Weber (1971) was deeply ambivalent about the consequences of new technology. He recognised its usefulness, particularly the value of increased efficiency and productivity. However, he also highlighted the problems associated with new technology, including the loss of autonomy, freedom and creativity.

We take a Weberian approach to computer-assisted analysis of qualitative data; we have an *ambivalent* attitude to it. Computers are useful, they are more efficient in completing some tasks, and they can improve productivity. However, it is important to be aware of the difficulties associated with using them in qualitative data analysis. It may not always be appropriate to use them for some research projects. We argue that researchers should make an informed choice about whether to use computers to assist data analysis and to do so requires a good understanding of qualitative data analysis, the nature of the research project, and the various computer packages available.

Some people seem to think that qualitative computer packages will do the data analysis for them. On some of the grant applications that we have assessed, we have seen qualitative researchers suggest that they will 'analyse their data using The Ethnograph (or Nud*ist, or Atlas/ti)'. Such a statement indicates that the researcher does not really understand either the methods of qualitative data analysis, or the use of computers in assisting qualitative data analysis. The epidemiological equivalent of this statement would be something along the lines of 'the survey results will be analysed with SPSS'. Computer packages do not analyse data. Qualitative data analysis techniques such as content analysis, grounded theory and thematic analysis can all be assisted through the use of a computer. A research proposal, or grant application, should first specify how the data is to be analysed, and then that this analysis will be assisted through the use of a computer package.

Our ambivalent approach is captured succinctly in one user's comment about The Ethnograph, a popular early package for computer-assisted qualitative data analysis: 'I've always had a love/hate relationship with computers and I think that's partly my feeling towards The Ethnograph' (Lee and Fielding 1995, p. 33).

The following analysis of computer-assisted qualitative data analysis has three aims. First, we suggest some criteria to use in making a decision about whether to use a computer program to assist in analysis. Second, we review the sorts of questions that should be asked before deciding which program to use. Computer programs are currently changing rapidly and, rather than reviewing a limited number of them superficially, we provide a guide to the process of choosing one. Finally, we describe some general issues that will facilitate the use of a computer program to assist data analysis.

Why computer-assisted qualitative data analysis?

As should be evident from the above discussion of coding, one of the main tasks in qualitative data analysis is 'code and retrieve'. This involves attaching codes to all relevant data, and then retrieving these sections so that they can be examined together. For example, a set of interviews about living with HIV/AIDS might be coded for the person's description of when they were first diagnosed. These sections may then be retrieved and placed together to write a section in the analysis, titled 'Being diagnosed with HIV/AIDS'. A more complex use of the code-and-retrieve process may involve retrieving these coded chunks along with other chunks coded 'choosing treatments' to decide whether the two codes could be combined into a more general one called 'interactions with doctors'.

Lee and Fielding (1995, p. 31) report that many researchers begin to think about using a computer to assist in their qualitative research as a response to the realisation that they would have 'data management problems arising from the size and/or complexity of the data to be analysed'. Before computers, data analysis typically took the form of cutting and filing. For example, Lofland and Lofland (1984, p. 134) recommended: 'At a very concrete level, all of this means that eventually you will be disassembling copies of your notes and splitting them up into various categories ... you can literally take scissors to your notes, cutting them into small bits of paper and placing them into file folders.' Other techniques include the use of index cards, coloured pens and paper-clips. These work reasonably well when the data set is small, and the advent of photocopiers has allowed multiple copies of data. However, the larger the data set, the more difficult it is to manage using these manual systems. 'Data overload' was a serious problem (Kelle 1995).

Computers allow for data to be stored, coded and retrieved more efficiently and flexibly than is possible using the techniques of cut and paste and the filing of bits of paper. Following Kelle (1995), we list some of the benefits, and disadvantages, associated with computer-assisted data analysis:

Benefits
- Coded segments can be placed back in the context of the whole text from which they have been taken.
- Electronic codes are more flexible, being more easily combined, reworded or divided.

- Memos can be electronically linked to either codes or text segments.
- Relationships between codes can be mapped electronically.
- Text segments can be linked in a variety of ways other than through codes, such as through hypertext.
- Selective retrieval is more easily performed. For example, in a study of HIV/AIDS, it may be possible to retrieve the segments relating to being diagnosed with HIV for females infected through sexual transmission.
- Complex searches can be performed. For example, computers can easily manage a search for 'co-occurring codes' (Kelle 1995, p. 8). In a study of HIV/AIDS, all segments coded both 'diagnosis' and 'afraid' could be retrieved.
- Finally, statistical counts can also be performed on the frequency of codes.

Disadvantages
- Additional time and energy is required for entering codes. This can be particularly tedious if coding has already been performed on a printed transcript.
- Computers encourage a particular form of code-and-retrieve analysis that is not very conducive to some qualitative approaches such as narrative analysis or semiotics.
- Computer-assisted analysis may require additional resources in the form of computer hardware, software, technical support, and training.
- Computer-based analysis tends to support modernist assumptions about texts being representative of people, and also tends to disembody interviews even further than physical transcripts.

Choosing a computer program

The first question that needs to be answered is: Should a computer package be used to assist in the data analysis? It is important to consider whether the research may benefit from using available technology. Some people avoid computers out of fear or from a lack of understanding of the benefits of computer-assisted analysis of qualitative data. However, the contrary point should also be considered. It may be more efficient not to use a computer program to assist the analysis, particularly if the research has tight timelines and a limited budget.

Some researchers are very enthusiastic about particular pieces of software and will advocate them widely and indiscriminately. As Mason (1996, p. 127) observes: 'For enthusiasts, you should ask yourself whether you are placing too great an emphasis on what the software can do, to the point where this is driving your analytical activity and epistemology rather than being driven by them.' Most computer programs, for example, are best suited to coding chunks of texts and comparing them across cases. If computer-assisted data analysis is chosen without careful prior consideration of the data analysis methodology, it may restrict the possibilities of methods of data analysis, excluding, for example, the possibility of narrative analysis. Some computer programs also encourage quantification, through providing percentages and statistics on text that is coded in particular ways. As Mason (1996, p. 127) notes, these may be 'entirely inappropriate both for your overall methodological stance, and for the specific nature of the project which you have conducted'.

Agar (1991) suggests that two common responses to computers are technophilia and technophobia. Technophilia, or 'extreme computer lust' (p. 187), may be positive if it motivates people to explore the potential benefits of new technology. However, there is a common danger of goal displacement, where the means become confused with the ends. Some people become so interested in the 'features' and technical aspects of the program that they lose sight of the goal of carefully analysing the qualitative data for its meanings and interpretations. On the other hand, technophobia, or the fear of technology, may lead to the avoidance of computer packages. Computers can be dangerous, particularly at the novice-with-important-data stage. The combination of inexperienced qualitative researcher and inexperienced computer user is an invitation to problems. However, fear is not a good reason for avoiding computers. Inexperience, and fear, can be resolved through learning, and there are many good training courses that will introduce a researcher both to using computers and to specific programs designed to assist in qualitative data analysis.

The first step, before computer programs are even looked at, is to decide on the data analysis method. The reason for this is that there is a wide variety of computer programs and some are more suited to content analysis, others to grounded theory; some are more suited to a hierarchical coding scheme, others will make a hierarchical coding scheme difficult. The researcher should first decide how the analysis should be conducted, and then review the available software. Weitzman and Miles (1995) identify five different types of computer programs that can be used to assist in qualitative data analysis:

1 Text Retrievers: specialise in *finding* all instances of words or phrases in a data set. For example, Metamorph is a powerful search program that uses artificial intelligence techniques to find not only words, but forms of words and even words that mean the same thing (synonyms).

2 Textbase Managers: *systematically organise*, sort and make subsets of data. Some use fields and records, others allow free-form databases. For example, AskSam is a textbase manager that handles a mixture of free-form text and structure records and fields. It combines database-field manipulation with word processing.

3   Code-and-Retrieve Programs: are typically specially designed for qualitative research. They divide text into chunks (words, lines, paragraphs), code these, and retrieve coded chunks. Neither text retrievers nor textbase managers will do this. The Ethnograph was one of the first and widely used code-and-retrieve programs.

4   Code-based Theory-builders: perform the same functions as a code-and-retrieve program, but they also allow the user to explore connections between codes. Both Nud*ist and Atlas/ti have sophisticated code-and-retrieve facilities, along with features that allow codes to be linked and built into a model.

5   Conceptual Network Builders: are not very useful for storing and coding data, and typically cannot perform the search-and-retrieve function. However, they provide a sophisticated graphical display of the relationships between codes. SemNet, for example, is a semantic network builder that can graphically represent even very large nets, based on definitions of concepts and the relations among them.

The first point to be drawn from this classification is that not all programs do the same thing. Even within the above categories there is considerable variation. In the same way that qualitative data analysis involves a wide range of methodologies, computer programs to assist in qualitative data analysis embody a wide range of methodologies. The above classification also suggests that different programs may be more or less useful for different parts of the research process. If a project begins with a content analysis, a text retriever may be the most appropriate. A second phase may involve inductive thematic analysis, so a code-based theory-builder may be useful. Finally, a conceptual network builder may assist in mapping the conceptual analysis.

Once the broad classification of program required has been identified, the next task is to identify the specific features of the data analysis to be conducted. Weitzman and Miles (1995) list a number of processes for which computer programs may be more or less useful. We have rewritten their list as a series of questions to be asked of the methodology of a particular qualitative research project. The researcher should consider the importance of these aspects for their project and then scrutinise available programs to see if they adequately perform the required functions. The following list draws on Weitzman and Miles (1995), but includes several new points:

•   Coding: would coding be performed 'on screen'? What size 'chunks' are required? What are the maximum possible number of codes per chunk? Will there be one coding run, or will there be multiple readings and codings of the data. If the latter is the case, flexibility and ease of coding will be important.

•   Search and retrieval: what sort of searches will be performed? For example, are complex or Boolean searches required? Search and retrieval is an important part of exploratory research to inductively identify categories.

- Database management: what options are provided for data entry and manipulation? For example, would fixed fields be useful? Will records be revised and added to during the analysis? Are there different kinds of data sources, such as video and interviews, and can these be easily managed?
- Data display: how important is it to see the context of a coded chunk? Do you want to be able to see your coding scheme on screen with the data? What sort of output will best facilitate the next stage of the research?
- Memoing: will the computer also be used to write and store comments and memos about both data and codes?
- Data linking: how important is it to provide hypertext-type links between data independent of codes? Do you want to be able to export statistical summaries to a statistics program?
- Matrix building: matrices are used in some forms of qualitative data analysis to develop analyses of the relationships between codes (Strauss and Corbin 1990). Is this a potentially important procedure?
- Network display: how important is it to be able to map pictorially the relationships between codes on the computer screen?
- Theory building: how important is it to be able to explore the relationships between codes to facilitate theory building? Confirmatory data analysis is best facilitated by programs that provide theory testing features.
- User friendliness: how important is it for a novice computer user or novice qualitative researcher to be able to easily learn the program? More experienced computer users may be able to make better use of programs with advanced features.
- Team use: will the project involve multiple researchers all working on the same data? Will these researchers be in the same location?
- Hardware and costs: do you use a Macintosh, Windows, or some other platform? What hard disk space and memory are available? Are there funds to purchase additional disk space or memory if these are required?

Once these points have been addressed, the researcher should then scrutinise available programs. Weitzman and Miles (1995) provide a useful summary of many programs, but their text is now out of date and a new edition is planned. Perhaps more useful than textbooks is to examine sites on the world wide web that introduce or provide demonstration versions of some of these programs. A very useful non-profit information website is located at the University of Surrey in the United Kingdom. The Computer Assisted Qualitative Data Analysis Software (CAQDAS) networking project 'aims to disseminate an understanding of the practical skills needed to use software which has been designed to assist qualitative data analysis (eg field research, ethnography, text analysis)' (see <http://www.soc.surrey.ac.uk/caqdas/>). This page provides links to other related websites, including many devoted to particular programs, often maintained by the developers. For example, Thomas Muhr maintains a website on Atlas/ti (see

<http://www.atlasti.de/>), and there is a website on The Ethnograph (see <http://www.QualisResearch.com>). Demonstration versions of various programs can be downloaded from either the CAQDAS website or directly from the developers. We strongly recommend that people selecting software to assist with qualitative data analysis explore these versions before making a decision.

Some of the most useful sources of information about a particular program are other users of that package. It may be useful to enquire whether other researchers in the local area have any experience with particular software packages. Further, there are several email discussion lists devoted to general discussions about using computers to assist in qualitative data analysis, and some that focus on specific programs. Once a program has been selected, it may be useful to subscribe to one of these lists (details can be obtained at the CAQDAS site).

Learning to use a computer program as an aid to qualitative data analysis requires considerable time, resources and money. It may involve attending training courses and learning specific procedures. Given this investment, researchers should look beyond their current project to projects they may conduct in the future. While some programs may suit the requirements of a specific project, it may be more efficient to select a program that could also meet the requirements of future projects.

In summary, our argument is that researchers should first select carefully the shape, form and details of their data analysis methodology. If these issues are not carefully addressed prior to selecting a computer program, the computer program may decide them for you. Two of the most useful techniques that will assist in the selection of an appropriate program are to enquire about the experiences of other researchers, and to experiment with demonstration versions. Also, these computing packages are changing rapidly, so it is important to keep up with recent developments, as many of the changes provide significant improvements in the usefulness and applicability of the available packages.

However, it could also be argued that many of the advanced features of the code-based theory-builders, for example, may not be required. From this perspective, an established program such as The Ethnograph with its limited, but clear and well-documented, set of features may be more useful. We encourage researchers to consider their own requirements, skills and resources and, on this basis, select a program best suited to their needs.

Coding and computers

Coding on qualitative data analysis packages is time-consuming and sometimes tedious. This is particularly the case if a two-step process has been adopted: coding manually on the transcripts, and then entering the codes into the computer. Coding directly onto the computer is faster, although many people express concern that this distances them from their data (Lee and Fielding

1995). Coding, either one-step or two-step, typically requires more time and energy when computer packages are utilised. However, as noted by Kelle (1995), the benefit lies in the speed and ease of retrieval. The problems of coding are compounded as the size of the data set increases, with greater numbers of researchers involved, and when the coding categories are extremely exploratory. Lee and Fielding (1995, p. 34) observe that those researchers who were best able to use computer packages to assist their analysis were 'individual researchers who had small- to medium-sized data sets which they approached with a fairly delimited theoretical interest'.

Given that coding typically requires more energy when using a computer, we recommend that researchers not begin coding their data on the computer until their coding scheme is relatively established. While it is relatively easy to combine, rename and refine codes on most computer packages, in our experience it is easier still if most of the experimenting and focusing of codes occurs before they are entered onto the computer.

A 'chunk' is a segment of data that is coded, such as a word, phrase, line, sentence, paragraph, or whole document (Miles and Huberman 1994). 'Chunking' involves segmenting data into chunks. Some programs require that chunks be identified in advance, and codes can only be applied to chunks as a whole. Other programs allows significant freedom in chunking. 'In these, your data all appear on screen and you can drag the mouse over the precise chunk of text you want to code, determining the start and end points of the chunk to the letter' (Miles and Huberman 1994, p. 19).

Two common coding mistakes are either too many codes or too few codes. As the number of codes increases, so does the time consumed by coding. Codes should be carefully scrutinised as to their relevance for the particular project. It is important to include codes for processes that appear 'interesting', but cannot be clearly justified, in order to facilitate new discoveries. However, too many of these types of codes will result in frustration and inefficient use of time and resources. On the other hand, it is important to code with sufficient detail to allow for a sufficiently complex analysis. Codes that are too general will be difficult to use and to summarise in reports. Many programs will allow codes to be reviewed, and chunks recoded in more detail. This is, of course, time-consuming, and the earlier the right number of codes is established, the better.

Some people seem to expect computers to do the work of coding and analysis for them. This can be particularly problematic when automatic coding options are present. Some programs will allow searches to be performed for specific words and these segments to be coded automatically. For example, in a study of unemployment a search could be performed for every occurrence of the word 'package' and this could be automatically coded 'redundancy payment'. The problem with such automated coding is that words that express similar ideas are missed. A person who talks about being 'paid out', for example, will not be picked up in this automated coding search. While computers will assist in the analysis process, they do not replace hard work and careful thought by the researcher.

We have heard several stories of colleagues who have worked for some months, or even longer, on coding qualitative data using a computer package. Then, suddenly, an act of God (or the Goddess?), such as a fire or theft, destroys all their work. One colleague regularly backed up her work, but the thief also stole the floppy disk backups. When a computer is used to assist with data analysis, the entire investment is in the electronic data on the computer. It is therefore important to regularly back up these documents, and preferably to do so to a different location, either via the internet or by physically transporting backup disks to other locations.

Concluding comments about computer-assisted data analysis

Henry Ford (1923, p. 281) finishes his book *My Life and Work* with a quote from the Bible: 'Everything is possible ... "faith is the substance of things hoped for, the evidence of things not seen".' Ford is not, however, referring to heaven or eternal life, but to his faith in the promise of modern industry and business. Ford had a religious-like faith in technology and business that he thought would solve the problems of the world, including the elimination of dangerous jobs, poverty, environmental degradation and crime. He was wrong!

When computer packages began to become widely available to qualitative researchers, many researchers, particularly those trying to sell their programs, argued 'that the use of computers would make qualitative analysis more systematic and transparent, thus enhancing its trustworthiness ... and also [enhancing] the creativity of the researcher' (Kelle 1995, p. 9). Other researchers warned of the dangers of being distanced from their data. We have found that computers can be extremely useful as adjuncts to qualitative research. Through a process of exploration and discovery, computer-assisted qualitative data analysis can provide worthwhile results and significant efficiencies. However, in our judgment, computer programs are not always required, nor do they solve many of the central problems of qualitative research. With Weber, we remain much less certain and more ambivalent about the role of technology.

POSTSTRUCTURALISM AND SEMIOTICS

The textual analysis of meanings requires the implementation of a variety of reading strategies (feminist, semiotic, hermeneutic, deconstructive, psychoanalytic) which examine how a text constitutes (hails) an individual as a subject in a particular ideological moment and site. (Denzin 1992, p. 82)

Poststructuralist authors fundamentally challenge the epistemology, ontology and method of traditional qualitative research (Clough 1992). That is to say, they argue for a different form of knowledge, and for different assumptions about the nature of the world. The methods and approaches of one type of poststructuralist theory were discussed in Chapter 1. However, there is a large variety of other approaches, as indicated by the quote above, and some of these are reviewed in detail in Denzin's (1997) *Interpretive Ethnography*.

One way of summarising the arguments of research influenced by these research methods is to suggest that there are three main strategies of analysis (Potter 1996). First, themes and interpretations in a text are not interpreted in isolation, but with reference to other themes in the text and the text as a whole. Second, these methods typically explore themes omitted or repressed and hidden behind other themes. Third, these methods also often analyse the social and political context of text. To deconstruct, or decode, is to uncover these hidden messages and themes behind the obvious or up-front message. Theories such as feminism, Marxism, psychoanalysis and critical or discourse theory are often important influences, suggesting themes that may have been omitted.

Beyond the analysis of the content, themes, grammar and metaphors of the text that is used in traditional qualitative research methods, semiotics and poststructuralism examine the production and reception of texts, often with particular attention to political dimensions. The content of a text is often not the focus of analysis. Rather, the focus is on the way that it is produced and received.

This can be illustrated through a provocative example, which is appropriate because poststructuralists are often deliberately provocative. Imagine conducting a thematic analysis of Australian case law about theft. The research might come up with various interesting dimensions, such as the observation that greater punishments are handed out for the theft of things of greater value. The analysis may suggest that at the heart of the law is a belief in the statement: 'You shall not steal.' However, a poststructuralist would be interested in how the law was constructed, and how it operates in the Australian political context. The poststructuralist researcher might locate the development of case law in a history of relations between Europeans and Aborigines in Australia. When Europeans first arrived in Australia, they said to the Aborigines, if you steal from a white person, you will be punished under white people's law. Europeans only accept European law. However, from an Aboriginal perspective, it could be argued that white people stole the land, the wages, the children, the culture and the language of the Aboriginal people of Australia, and they do not seem to have been punished for this. Poststructuralists refuse to accept that there is only one correct way of looking at the world (in this case, a European view of theft), and point to other possible understandings. If Australian case law about theft is located in this historical context, it could be suggested that the simple statement 'You shall not steal' actually means 'You shall not steal from a white person'.

A content analysis of Australian law focusing on theft would never come up with this conclusion. The political overtones of the text become apparent only when the text is placed in a historical context that considers how it has been applied and received, and that 'decentres' a view of the world that assumes that a European understanding is the only possible interpretation.

As should be clear from this example, these forms of analysis can be emotionally and politically charged. Advocates of these forms of research argue that qualitative research must 'embrace moral criticism' (Denzin 1997, p. 252). This is because, they argue, it is no longer possible to pretend that qualitative research does not have political and moral implications intertwined with its method.

ETHICS, POLITICS AND QUALITATIVE DATA ANALYSIS

> Albert Namatjira painted
> Not so much the things he saw
> But what he felt inside
> And how he loved the Flinders Range.
> (Roach 1990)

Archie Roach's 'Native Born', which includes the above quotation, is a nostalgic and tragic song that mourns the loss of traditional Australian Aboriginal culture, and the transformation of the Australian bush under the influence of the European invaders. Roach discerns this same experience in the art of Albert Namatjira, an Aboriginal artist who painted landscapes, mainly from around the Flinders Ranges. How does this relate to qualitative research? After we have read postmodernists, poststructuralists, feminists, and hermeneutics, it is impossible to pretend that qualitative research, or quantitative research for that matter, is an objective enterprise uninfluenced by the feelings, desires and theories of the observer (Clough 1992; Denzin 1997; MacIntyre 1981; Mishler 1986; Taylor 1989). The results of qualitative data analysis clearly exhibit and represent the desires, hopes and theories of the researcher. Archie Roach is not arguing that Albert Namatjira's paintings do not give us a picture of the Flinders Ranges. Rather, he points out that the picture is both a representation and a moral message that derives from the emotions, memories, joys, hopes, pain and sadness of Albert Namatjira. In the same way, the results of a qualitative research project are integrally influenced by the theories, emotions, morals and politics of the researcher. The positivist utopia of independent objectivity is unrealisable. As Lalli (1989, p. 103) puts it, 'in fact the assumptions that social phenomena may be treated objectively, that they are value-free in themselves, and that their identification is unproblematic, have been revealed to be inadequate in fully accounting for a social world'.

How is the qualitative researcher to deal with the influence of pre-existing theory and understandings on a qualitative research project? Our contention is that the most useful response is to embrace it, rather than try to avoid it. This is best done through being explicit about the influence, right from the beginning of the project. This operates at a number of levels, depending on whether the focus is on the influence of politics, culture or theories. In the earlier discussion of 'the theory of grounded theory', we examined in detail the role of pre-existing theory in qualitative studies.

The significance of theoretical movements, such as poststructuralism and postmodernism, is still being absorbed by qualitative researchers. With Denzin (1997), we suspect that they will become more influential on the practices of qualitative researchers in the future. As any good qualitative researcher knows, meanings and interpretative practices are always changing. This insight applies as much to the interpretative practices of qualitative researchers as it does to the interpretative practices used in everyday life, or during health and illness. However, this does not mean that the older traditions of qualitative research, many of which are discussed in this chapter, should be dismissed as no longer relevant. They are part of the tradition of qualitative research that is dominant at present, but that is, and will always be, changing. 'The good stories are always told by those who have learned well the stories of the past, but who are unable to tell them any longer because those stories no longer speak to them, or to us' (Denzin 1994, p. 513).

Tutorial exercise

Imagine you have recently been employed as a new researcher, joining a team of people working on an ongoing research project studying women recovering from a heart attack. A previous researcher completed a set of focus groups and some in-depth interviews with these women. Your first task is to analyse this data. The previous researcher has left no documentation, apart from transcriptions of the interviews, and a conference paper they gave describing the project. Draw up a list of tasks, decisions, and information you require, in order to begin analysing the data. While you may take longer if you wish, you are given the option of working to a very short deadline, with the help of two research assistants, in order to present a paper at an important conference. How would your plans differ for these two options?

Further reading

Charmaz, K., 1991, *Good Days, Bad Days: The Self in Chronic Illness and Time*, Rutgers University Press, New Brunswick.

Computer Assisted Qualitative Data Analysis Software (CAQDAS) networking project <http://www.soc.surrey.ac.uk/caqdas/> (November 1998).

Denzin, N., 1997, *Interpretive Ethnography*, Sage, Thousand Oaks.

Dey, I., 1993, *Qualitative Data Analysis*, Routledge & Kegan Paul, London.

Kelle, U. (ed.), 1995, *Computer-Aided Qualitative Data Analysis*, Sage, London.

Lofland, J. and Lofland, L., 1971, *Analyzing Social Settings*, Wadsworth, Belmont, CA.

Miles, M. and Huberman, A., 1994, *Qualitative Data Analysis*, 2nd edn, Sage, Thousand Oaks.

Orona, C., 1990, 'Temporality and Identity Loss due to Alzheimer's Disease', *Social Science and Medicine*, vol. 30, pp. 1247–56.

Strauss, A. and Corbin, J., 1990, *Basics of Qualitative Research*, Sage, Newbury Park.

11

Writing a Qualitative Research Proposal

Proposal writing is not a mechanical process that follows a specific scientific procedure. But like research itself, it is a creative, conceptual process of asking the right questions, operating with partial information, following leads down blind alleys, and making difficult decisions. (Attig and Winichagoon 1993, p. 3)

INTRODUCTION

Research proposals have always been an important part of conducting research. A proposal sets forth the exact nature of the issue to be examined, a detailed description of the procedures and methods to be employed, and a time frame to keep the process on schedule (Locke et al. 1989). Writing a research proposal is therefore essential prior to undertaking a piece of research. Not only that, writing an excellent proposal has become important in recent years as obtaining the necessary funding has become highly competitive among researchers. As Neuman (1991) points out, proposal writing can be done relatively well if we follow the suggestions of those who have successfully obtained funding.

In this chapter we will outline some of the important points in writing a qualitative research proposal *in order to be funded*. This is not a guarantee, of course, that the proposal will be successful; we cannot promise that. We do, however, hope that if readers follow most of the suggestions in this chapter, they may have a better chance of obtaining funding. (Further useful information on writing research proposals can be found in Attig and Winichagoon 1993; Krathwohl 1988; Lefferts 1982, 1990; Locke et al. 1989; and Pequegnat and Stover 1995.)

WHAT IS A RESEARCH PROPOSAL?

> In its simplest sense, a proposal is a plan presented for acceptance or rejection. In its entirety, it is a positive statement, which sets forth a program, based on specific objectives and a carefully designed set of activities. (Attig and Winichagoon 1993, p. 6)

However, Lefferts (1982) points out that a research proposal is a specialised kind of proposal for financial support to undertake certain tasks to describe and explain a particular problem, issue, subject or question:

> Research proposals may be for basic research aimed at advancing knowledge, or they may be for applied research to examine behavior, attitudes, policies, programs ... or processes. Such research may contribute to a better understanding of specific phenomena or may be used to provide guidance for making decisions about policies, programs ... (p. 69)

According to Lefferts (1990, p. 5), a research proposal has five important functions:

- A proposal is a written representation of a program or a project that a researcher seeks to conduct. Part of the research development process includes telling other people about plans and intentions for the research.
- A proposal is a request for the allocation of resources from funding agencies.
- A proposal is an instrument of persuasion. It intends to persuade some funding agencies to allocate some resources to support the research and hence legitimate the proposed research.
- A proposal is a promise and a commitment that the researcher gives to the funding agencies about what he or she intends to do in a specific time period and at a given cost.
- A proposal is a plan for action that 'serves as a set of guidelines for the organization and implementation of the program'.

Attig and Winichagoon (1993) point out another important function of research proposals. Proposals have a long-term purpose in that they are a beginning to the reporting process in terms of preparing reports, journal articles and monographs (see Chapter 12).

THE STRUCTURE OF A RESEARCH PROPOSAL

A qualitative research proposal usually contains several sections (Attig and Winichagoon 1993), as summarised in Box 11.1.

Box 11.1 The sections of a research proposal

- synopsis or summary
- significance of the proposed project
- background and rationale
- research questions
- suppositions
- objectives
- theoretical/conceptual framework
- research design
- dissemination of research findings
- time frame
- budget and justification
- organisational structure and resources
- curriculum vitae of the researcher

The synopsis or summary

A research proposal should always have a synopsis or summary, sometimes called an abstract, which is normally provided in a one-page format. It should contain brief statements of only the most important aspects of the proposal, such as: the problem and its significance; the purpose and objectives; reference to any major prior research; the overall research method, scope, major procedure and analytical approach which will be used; the expected outcomes; and the benefit. In our experience, the synopsis should be written carefully. It is the first part to be read; sometimes, it is the only part read by reviewers. Locke and colleagues (1989, p. 121) state that by the time the reader/reviewer reaches the bottom of the synopsis page, they must have a clear idea about the study. In addition, the reader may want to read further if the synopsis 'contains something of special interest, something that will sustain the reader's attention through the pages that follow'. The synopsis should use some key words that reflect funding agencies' research scope. These will lead readers to the most important themes of the proposal. Since the synopsis tends to be read first and is a one-way communication, clarity is essential. If the body of the proposal is well written, but the content and language of the synopsis confuse the reader, the chance of success in obtaining some funding may be less or even lost (Locke et al. 1989).

One simple but important point about writing a synopsis is that it should be written after all other sections of the proposal have been constructed. Lefferts (1982) has warned us that writing a summary before writing the proposal is like naming a baby prior to its birth; we may end up with a girl's name for a boy.

This is true for writing a synopsis. If we prepare the synopsis first, we may leave out details that arise during the writing process (Attig and Winichagoon 1993).

The significance of the proposed project

What is the value of the proposed research project? Why bother with it? What will the funding agency obtain from the research that may assist them in attaining their goals? This has to be stated clearly and convincingly in the proposal. Most funding agencies require a statement about the significance of the proposed research. They want to see the usefulness and importance of the information to be gained from the project. Most qualitative studies aim to provide new information to fill gaps in our understanding. This section is particularly essential if a researcher wants to convince the reviewers that what is being proposed is of value and worthy of being funded. The best way to do this is to show how the findings might be applied to human services or how they might enable development of other kinds of research that have been previously impossible (Locke et al. 1989).

The background and rationale

The section on background and rationale indicates the importance and urgency of the project. The emphasis here is typically on relevant previous research. It also emphasises the situation and factors which prompt the proposed project. Attig and Winichagoon (1993, p. 68) suggest that this section should consist of at least four sub-sections: introduction, needs, rationale and purpose.

In the 'introduction' sub-section, the proposal should start with an introductory statement about the broad concept upon which the proposal is based. It needs to be concise, but adequate in leading into the problem statement. Evidence from a literature review should be used to explain the exact nature and extent of the health issue, which has led to the development of the proposed research. This sub-section is important since it demonstrates how much the researcher understands and is familiar with the literature. This in turn will be used to assess the grant application.

The 'needs' sub-section should be relatively brief but should indicate why the project is important and to whom it is important (Attig and Winichagoon 1993, p. 69). This sub-section is usually used to introduce the rationale of the proposed project.

The 'rationale' sub-section provides readers/reviewers with the reasons for the proposed research. It should include the proposal's guiding philosophy and assumptions and its relevance to problems identified in existing literature. Some researchers may include here the theoretical or conceptual framework. However, the most important issue in this sub-section is how the proposed project will help to fill a gap in existing knowledge or will solve some urgent problems. Tripp-Reimer and Cohen (1991, p. 231) point out that a literature review is essential when addressing the needs and rationale of a proposal. Major relevant studies are reviewed and 'critically analysed, noting how the proposed study builds, expands, or highlights areas that have previously been neglected or approached inadequately'. Thus, this sub-section should include a review of literature to argue why a qualitative approach is justified.

Lastly, the 'purpose' sub-section needs to point to the overall goal of the proposed project. It should also indicate how the project may build upon itself and how it may link with other studies.

Pranee's research proposal for a study of miscarriage among Hmong women in Melbourne provides an example of a background and rationale section (Box 11.2).

Box 11.2 An example of a background and rationale section

A miscarriage, or 'spontaneous abortion' in biomedical terms, has received some attention from psychologists and medical professionals (e.g. Black 1991; Cordle and Prettyman 1994; Frideman 1989; Frideman and Gath 1989; Janseen and Van-Minnen 1992; Neugebauer et al. 1992; Prettyman et al. 1993; Slade 1994; Statham and Green 1994). These studies focus mainly on the individual, although some attempt to examine the experience of pregnancy loss with social differences such as level of education and marital status. There have been some social scientists who have examined this issue (e.g. Cecil 1994; Cecil and Leslie 1993; Lovell 1983; Oakley et al. 1990; Reinharz 1988). In addition, there are a few studies which look at miscarriage from a feminist perspective (Hey 1989; Letherby 1993; Simonds 1988). One study examines miscarriage from the perspective of men whose wives have experienced it (Puddifoot and Johnson 1997). However, these studies have largely dealt with women from Anglo-Celtic backgrounds.

Very little research has examined miscarriage from a cultural point of view (Cecil 1996; Layne 1990; Sobo 1996). Some anthropological studies in the past have neglected the issue of miscarriage or only touched on it a little. Layne (1990) argues that this may in part be due to its sensitive and taboo nature. Most recently, however, there have been some studies—in Cameroon, India, Jamaica, Papua New Guinea and Tanzania—examining pregnancy loss from a cultural perspective.

As Madden (1994) and Cecil (1996) argue, the issue of miscarriage among immigrant women in Western societies has been largely neglected, with the exception of Chalmers and Meyer's study (1992a, 1992b). We do not know how immigrant women see miscarriage, what their feelings are about the loss of their pregnancies, what mechanisms they adopt to prevent or to cope with this loss, and the role of culture in protecting or reinforcing their emotional well-being. This proposal attempts to fill this gap.

In this study, I attempt to explore in detail traditional Hmong explanations about miscarriage and the ethnomedical knowledge and practices which pertain to it. In particular, because, as Cecil (1996) argues, how a miscarriage is seen, experienced and managed rests upon social and cultural factors, I set out to examine the role of cultural beliefs and practices in the response to miscarriage in Hmong society.

Research questions

A research question emerges from the need and rationale of the proposed research. It is the immediate objective, which is addressed in the proposal. The answer to the research question hence helps to fulfil the purpose and the objectives of the research. Wilkinson (1991) points out that the research question can be seen as a successive focusing from the general literature to the general problem and its potential causes to the particular research question. It is essential in this section to state as clearly as possible what the proposed research will look for.

Suppositions

In a qualitative research proposal, a supposition section is typically used instead of hypotheses. The section contains suppositions upon which the proposed project is grounded. Similar to hypotheses, suppositions usually contain statements about the relationship between two or more variables. However, suppositions are not subject to testable assertions, as in quantitative research. They seek information for clarification, and not for verification. Suppositions are usually written as declarations and without the predictive statements of hypothesis; for example, 'Dissatisfaction with hospital care leads to underutilisation of health services in a maternity hospital among women from non-English speaking background communities', or 'There is a correlation between employment outside the home and a decline in breastfeeding status among working mothers in the community'. Some qualitative researchers include suppositions in the research question section instead of having a separate section as such. Usually it appears at the end of that section and prior to the statement of the objectives of the research.

Objectives

Research objectives are the 'essence of the proposal' (Tripp-Reimer and Cohen 1991, p. 231). According to Attig and Winichagoon (1993, p. 76), research objectives are 'specific statements about exactly what the proposed project will accomplish'. They should be specified, as clearly as possible, in terms of what end results the proposed project is expected to achieve, not how these results will be achieved. The reviewer likes to see objectives which are 'specific, concrete, and achievable' (Krathwohl 1988, p. 43). Important questions to be answered in the objectives section include:

- What is the researcher planning to do (what will be done, with whom, why and where)?
- What will the researcher achieve in conducting the proposed project?

Good objectives start with concrete verb phrases such as 'to determine', 'to identify', 'to examine', 'to formulate', and so on. Such phrases show exactly what the researcher will realistically do, not what they hope to do. If there are several objectives, state them in logical order, either with the most important first or in the sequence of accomplishment (Tripp-Reimer and Cohen 1991).

The theoretical/conceptual framework

In a social science research proposal, a theoretical framework needs to be made explicit. Theories interrelate with individual findings and allow greater generalisation (Krathwohl 1988). There are many theories that qualitative research proposals can use. As Wilkinson (1991) points out, a researcher may select any theory to suit their proposed research. However, they must set the problem explicitly within the chosen framework. This will assist reviewers to see what main variables will be considered, what the relationships are between the variables, and how information about them comes together to answer the research question of the proposal. In health sociology, for example, we may find that some research proposals apply 'critical theory' and then set their theory within the framework of class, gender and ethnicity. Within these frameworks, some researchers may find the answers to improving utilisation of health care in some population groups. It is essential to discuss the theoretical and conceptual framework in detail in the proposal, particularly when the theory and concepts used are not well known among reviewers who are outside the social science discipline (Krathwohl 1988; see also Chapter 1 in this volume).

The research design

A research design is 'the logical and systematic planning and directing of a piece of research' (Attig and Winichagoon 1993, p. 85). Research designs emerge from 'translating a general scientific model into varied research procedures'. However, in qualitative research proposals, one must remember that, although a series of guidelines is useful, it needs to be flexible to allow for unforeseen problems that may arise during the research process. Attig and Winichagoon argue that, 'as the study progresses, new aspects, new conditions, and new connecting links in the data come to light, and it might become necessary to change the plan as circumstances demand' (p. 85). Therefore, some modification may be needed during the research process. This should not be seen as due to a researcher's poor performance, but as an integral part of rigorous qualitative research.

When writing a research design section, several points require special attention. At a more basic level, the researcher needs to gear the design towards available time, energy, facilities and money. The research design must also correspond with the availability of data from participants. One important consideration is the extent to which it is desirable or possible to impose upon the persons and/or social organisation that is to supply the participants and, therefore, the data.

There are several sub-sections that can be included in a research design section: research population, research method(s), and data analysis. The proposal needs to specify clearly the research population, and their social demography should be described as precisely as possible. The proposal should also state where and how this population will be selected. Usually, some sampling theoretical frameworks will be cited. In qualitative research, it is not always feasible to state clearly the number of people to be included in the sample. Sample size may be guided by 'saturation' or other non-numeric criteria (see Chapter 2 for sampling techniques). Hence, in some qualitative research proposals, the researchers may not specify the size of the samples to be recruited. If the number is to be specified, evidence to justify the sample size is essential (Minichiello et al. 1995; Strauss and Corbin 1990).

The research method is one of the most important parts of the research design. Reasons for selecting a particular method(s) should be discussed. The proposal also needs to show that the method is appropriate, adequate and feasible (Tripp-Reimer and Cohen 1991). For example, if the researcher needs to discover and understand the illness experience of people in great depth, then in-depth interviewing, life history or ethnography may be chosen as a method. The proposal must describe clearly and precisely the method to be used in order to achieve the proposal's objectives (see Chapters 3 to 9 on qualitative methods).

Data analysis should also be discussed in detail in the research design section. It is usually not enough just to state that the data will be analysed using a particular method, as can be done in quantitative research where the analysis relies on statistical packages. Qualitative research proposals need to provide some details about the analysis process so that the reviewers can clearly see how the researcher intends to manage the data, and what analytic techniques will be employed (see Chapter 10 on data analysis).

Dissemination of the findings

According to Locke and others (1989, p. 129), the final step in conducting a research enquiry is to disseminate the findings in the public domain. If researchers want their findings to be useful, they must reach those who can use them. Most funding agencies, which have to justify their investment in research, want to see that changes in practices can occur, impacts happen and new knowledge be produced (Hall 1971; Krathwohl 1988). They require, therefore, that plans for the dissemination of findings be included in a proposal. Some of the most common means of dissemination are as follows:

- papers delivered at national and international conferences;
- conferences or seminars organised for other professionals;
- newsletters or brochures distributed to selected institutions and individuals in the field;
- final reports widely circulated;
- findings published in journals (refereed and non-refereed);
- use of professional media, such as newsletters and press releases;
- visits by the research staff to agencies that would be interested in the findings and that are likely to apply them in their practices; and
- production of audiovisual material, such as slides, videos or films, for circulation in the field and for teaching.

Whatever the means chosen, there are some useful points suggested by Locke and colleagues (1989, p. 129) for planning the dissemination of research:

- specify which audiences you intend to reach, such as health professionals, academic or community members; and
- be specific about the plan, such as presenting the findings at particular conferences, workshops, publications in refereed and non-refereed journals, media releases, and reporting back to the community concerned.

The time frame

Most research projects take a considerable time to complete. Even a small pilot project may take at least twelve months, and almost every proposal submitted to major funding agencies would ask for at least two to three years' funding. A time frame is essential, therefore, for several reasons (Locke et al. 1989, p. 125):

- It keeps the researcher and other personnel on schedule throughout a long period of research.
- It helps to justify the need for two to three years of funding for the project, particularly if the researcher can show that every month is filled with what has to be done to complete the project.
- A well-planned time frame will help reviewers to understand the nature of the proposed project, and this, in turn, can prevent criticism from the reviewers that the project cannot be completed in the time proposed.

Each step in the research process must be carefully worked out for time needed. Murphy's law states that things will take longer than planned, and this is our experience too. It is necessary, therefore, to have each stage extended appropriately, to be realistic about the time needed. In presenting the time frame, the researcher may use various means, depending on the complexity of the project. However, the simplest way is to make a time schedule, with the list of dates for completion of the various activities necessary to the project (Krathwohl 1988). Box 11.3 provides an example of a time frame, taken from Pranee's research proposal relating to childbearing among women from the north of Thailand.

Box 11.3 An example of a time frame for a research project

Preparation: September–November 1998
Training of research assistants: December 1998
Data collection: January–July 1999
Data analysis: February–October 1999
Writing of reports: November 1999–June 2000
Dissemination of findings: July–August 2000

The budget and its justification

The budget is not a part of the research plan, but it is a central component in a grant application (Locke et al. 1989). The budget provides reviewers with the project's monetary requirements in terms of the estimated expenses needed to carry out the proposed research to its term (see budget example in Table 11.1). Some funding agencies may set the ceiling of the amount requested and usually a researcher cannot ask for more than what is specified. However, agencies are more concerned about whether the proposed budget is realistic and well justified. Therefore, in requesting a certain amount, the researcher needs to specifically explain why a budget item is necessary and how its estimation has been made. As Mucha (1995, p. 161) argues, a research budget needs to clearly reflect the resources required for the proposed project, and it should be 'reasonable, believable, and superbly justified'. A researcher should justify everything in the budget that may not be clear since the reviewers will be better able to judge the merit of the proposal if 'they do not have to solve mysteries'.

It is important to prepare the budget items according to details in the proposal. For example, if travelling expenses for home interviews are requested, then the methodology section must contain statements about home interviews. In addition, it is important to itemise the budget as much as possible so that reviewers can do their own estimates to confirm that the requests are sensible and realistic. Very often, proposals are criticised and hence rejected on the grounds that the budget is not realistic; that is, it asks for too much or too little. Mucha (1995) suggests that it is helpful to justify budget items in the same sequence as they appear on the budget page.

Table 11.1 An example of a budget in a grant application

Components	$ Year 1	$ Year 2	$ Year 3
Personnel:			
Chief Investigator A: Senior Research Fellow,	25 056	25 846	26 638
Level B, 06	(0.5)	(0.5)	(0.5)
3 Bicultural Research Assistants,			
Level A, 01	44 310	46 839	39 498
	(3x0.5)	(3x0.5)	(3x0.5)
Equipment:			
3 audio tape recorders, at $400 each	1200		
480 cassettes, at $5 each	2400		
3 transcribers, at $800 each	2400		
Maintenance:			
Travel	3000	3000	500
Postage, stationery, telephone	250	250	100
Production and dissemination of report			500
Total funding requested	74 616	81 737	73 197

Organisational structure and resources

Most researchers, either as a researcher or as an academic, are usually attached to an organisation or institution which provides facilities for undertaking a research project. This section demonstrates to funding agencies that the organisation and its personnel have the capability to conduct the proposed research effectively and efficiently. In particular, this section should include some information as to its expertise, experience, important programs and achievements. Future plans of the organisation and where the proposed research may fit with such plans should also be included. Other practical support from the organisation, such as facilities and personnel to assist with the running of the proposed project, should also be stated clearly in the proposal.

The curriculum vitae of the researcher

When deciding about funding, most review committees want to be sure not only that the proposal is excellent but also that the researcher is competent to conduct excellent work. The best evidence for the competence of the researcher is from prior successfully funded projects that resulted in research-based publication in refereed journals (Krathwohl 1988; Locke et al. 1989;

Tripp-Reimer and Cohen 1991). This is referred to as a 'track record' in the area of proposed study in most grant assessment criteria. Most major funding agencies require the researcher to list their relevant publications in the proposal, often allowing only one page and specifying that only publications over the last five years be included. Some agencies may also require details of past successful funding, which again assists them to determine the track record and reputation of the researcher.

Three important sections

By and large, the research proposal sections described above are those required in most funding applications, although there may be variations in format. Some may require a synopsis or summary and the benefits of the project at the beginning of the proposal; others may want them at the end. Whatever the funding agency's format, it is important that the applicant follow it strictly (Locke et al. 1989).

According to Lefferts (1982), there are three sections of a research proposal that are particularly critical: research design and procedures, problem description, and the track record of the researcher. Any weakness in these sections often leads to failure in securing funding. Lefferts argues that 'a lack of clarity, completeness, and consistency, and the presence of technical flaws are the main difficulties that arise in these sections' (p. 72). What can we do to overcome these then? The following suggestions may help:

• Be very sure that the proposal shows a high level of technical research understanding and skill. If the researcher feels that they do not have enough skills to carry out the research, they should not hesitate to seek advice from other people and/or to use consultants in the preparation of the proposal.

• The method section should explain clearly and precisely what will be done and how it will be done, although it is not necessary to provide intricate details about your particular methodology. The limitations of the methodology and how some methodological problems can be minimised should also be stated clearly. Breaking down the method section into sub-sections can be helpful in doing this.

• A 'convincing and clear' description of the problem, its significance, and a review of related work are necessary for the success of the research proposal. Therefore, as Lefferts (1982, p. 73) points out, 'selective completeness is the key to success in this section—that is, citations and the discussions of the literature (theories and other research) should be limited to those directly relevant to the research'. However, make sure that all major relevant work is referred to in order to show that the researcher is up to date and well acquainted with the area.

• The main weaknesses in the personnel section that may reduce the chances of obtaining funding include the lack of expertise, experience, training and track record of the researcher and other personnel carrying out the research. Lefferts (1982, p. 73) suggests several general ways to overcome this. First, the proposal needs to fully describe the research capabilities of the proposed personnel. Second, it should demonstrate the research competence by making all other sections as technically expert as possible. And last, it should include research consultants who have good reputations in particular areas as members of the research team. Similarly, it is valuable to have an advisory committee on the project. The expertise of such a committee can be used to strengthen the research process, from the beginning to the dissemination of the results. And this helps to strengthen the proposal.

• What about 'novice' researchers, who do not yet have a good track record? How can they convince funding agencies? Locke and others (1989) suggest that a young researcher can first try to obtain funding from local sources, particularly from the institution in which the researcher works. Obtaining several small grants will be sufficient to undertake a small pilot study. Then the findings from the pilot study can be used to write a paper for publication. Eventually, the young researcher will have enough reports or papers to use as a track record supporting a proposal for more extensive funding. Additionally, working in collaboration with a senior researcher who has good reputation in the proposed area may also help a novice researcher to secure funding from major sources (Krathwohl 1988). Later on, with some track record, they can do it on their own.

THE WRITING PROCESS

Proposals are more than simple work plans; they are the springboards by which … scientists enter the research realm. Each part of a proposal requires specific research and development skills and an understanding of how to get and put together important information. (Attig and Winichagoon 1993, p. 2)

Attig and Winichagoon (1993, p. 1) also point out that proposal writing is a process that has three key elements:
• an understanding of the proposal research and writing process;
• knowledge about different approaches and methods of writing and communicating effectively to readers; and
• a basic guideline about what goes into developing, presenting and evaluating a successful project proposal.

The first step in the proposal development process is that the researcher needs to have a firm understanding of what a proposal actually is, its different types and functions, the nature of the proposal writing and research process, as well as what characterises a good proposal. One useful strategy for developing this understanding is to read some proposals that have been successful.

In the writing process, the researcher must bear in mind that they are presenting the proposal to a group of people who may not be familiar with the nature of the proposed research and so must be made aware of the important issues in the proposal. Research proposal writing therefore needs to be clear, persuasive and convincing. Nevertheless, most people will still ask how proposal writing can be made easy but still lead to a good proposal. One way to make it more valuable and less troublesome is to make it 'an active part of the research process'. This is what Michaelson (1987) refers to as 'writing in increments' or, in Wilkinson's term (1991), 'writing concurrently with research'.

Another way to write a proposal is to write it as an article. Locke and colleagues (1989, p. 19) argue that the process of writing a research proposal is essentially the same as writing the research report. If the preparation of a proposal is well executed, 'the task of preparing the final report is more than half done'. Sometimes, a research proposal can be developed into a paper for publication. When the project is completed, the published paper can be a reference for publishing project findings. If written like a paper, the proposal will have a well-developed introduction, a review of literature, and a description of methods. This then becomes a rough draft for subsequent publications when all the results become available.

Lastly, Attig and Winichagoon (1993) suggest that the proposal writing process can be treated as a research process. They argue that proposal writing is a research, as well as a writing, process. In treating it this way, there are several points to write, in the same way as conducting a research project. Attig and Winichagoon (1993, p. 16) suggest the following points as important:
- problem identification;
- focusing the project or area of interest within a theory or body of knowledge;
- designing the study;
- collecting and recording data;
- analysing data;
- interpreting findings and drawing conclusions; and
- informing others in a report (which is the proposal).

But how do we start writing our research proposal? Each researcher has their own way of starting, which depends largely on their approach to problem solving, decision making and planning. However, there are two usual ways to begin. Some researchers may start with a general idea, theory or concept and then proceed to make it more specific. This is known as 'deductive thinking'. Others may adopt 'inductive thinking' in that they may start with very specific ideas or empirical problems and then expand them into an overall plan. Most researchers, though, tend to go back and forth between these two approaches. This means that one has to make several revisions in the process of writing a proposal.

Once the first draft has been written, it is wise to leave it for a few days before revising it. Blink and Wood (1988) say that the researcher will then see what they have written with a critical and analytical eye and be more likely to notice any weak points or mistakes. Before the proposal is submitted, it is also valuable to have someone else read it, both for content and logical composition. Tripp-Reimer and Cohen (1991) suggest two types of peer review. One reviewer should be a person who is familiar with the research area and can give feedback on the scientific merit of the proposal. Another reviewer should be someone who is not familiar with the content. This person can provide suggestions about the style, clarity and logical flow of the proposal. Most review committees consist of members who have expertise in the area and others who have little or no expertise in qualitative research. They will judge the proposal on the basis of logical arguments and clear planning. Another important point is that it usually takes several revisions before the proposal achieves its final complete form, despite feedback from other researchers, and this takes time. Therefore, the researcher needs to allow for this by beginning well before any deadline. When the proposal is eventually finalised, the process of submission to secure funding can begin.

DETERMINANTS OF A SUCCESSFUL PROPOSAL

While it is very important to carefully design a research proposal, it is equally important (if not more so) to write one that will attract funding. At a basic level, a project's 'life' depends upon a proposal's quality, since a successful proposal provides the funding necessary for a project to grow (Attig and Winichagoon 1993).

Research proposals are often subject to an intensive technical review. This is particularly true for funding agencies that are highly competitive, such as, in Australia, the National Health and Medical Research Council, and the Australian Research Council. A proposal submitted to such agencies needs therefore (following Lefferts 1982, p. 71; Neuman 1991, p. 498) to effectively:

- describe the particular problem towards which the research is directed;
- review and discuss the relevant research and literature that is pertinent to the problem being examined;
- explain the significance of the proposed research in terms of how it will further knowledge and contribute to the solution of a substantive, theoretical, methodological, policy, organisational or programmatic problem;
- define the theory or conceptual framework for the proposed research, including the basic concepts involved, their relationships, and their concrete manifestations;
- indicate the specific research objectives or questions which will be addressed;
- specify in detail the research approach, methods and procedures that will be used to obtain and analyse data;

- contain specific plans for disseminating the results;
- show well-designed planning, realistic budget and time frame; and
- show the capability of the researcher to conduct and complete the proposed work.

Essentially, as Hall (1971, p. 51) argues, it is crucial that the research proposal demonstrates that the idea for the project is important and addresses a significant need, that the researcher has done an excellent job of selecting the best approach to undertake the research, and that the researcher has the capabilities to make the proposed research a success. These points of evaluation are most commonly referred to as the 'scientific merit' of the research and the 'track record' of the researcher (Tripp-Reimer and Cohen 1991) (see the appendix to this chapter for the criteria used by the Australian Research Council for research grant assessment).

When evaluating a research proposal, most research funding agencies apply certain sets of criteria. Though there may be some variations, the following criteria proposed by Lefferts (1982, p. 13) are frequently used:

- **Clarity**. The proposal must be clearly written and structured. This will help the reviewer to easily follow the arguments and hence create a better understanding of the proposal. Writing style and organization of material need to be as simple as possible. Jargons with ambiguous meaning should also be avoided. A full explanation of each part is needed since we cannot assume that the reviewer will understand our intention. A useful question to be asked at this stage is 'Will someone unfamiliar with my research have a clear picture of what is being proposed from reading this proposal?' This can be done by asking someone outside your area to read the proposal. If the person can understand your proposal clearly, then the proposal has clarity.
- **Completeness**. The proposal must cover all relevant points so that the reviewer does not have any further queries or unanswered questions about the proposal.
- **Responsiveness**. The proposal must be responsive to the interests and purposes of the funding agency. It also needs to be responsive to the requirement of the agency. Usually, an agency has written guidelines for submitting the proposals, and it is the task of the writer to meet these guidelines as strictly as possible. Additionally, it must be responsive to the need and interests of the group of people who will be involved in the research.
- **Internal and external consistency**. All sections in the proposal must be related to and consistent with each other. The proposal needs to recognize the known and accepted ideas in the field and the methods that are believed to be effective. If there is an alternative strategy to be used, this needs to be justified in terms of a systematic critique of the dominant ideas and methods.
- **Understanding of the problem and methods**. The proposal needs to demonstrate a thorough understanding of the nature of the problem

addressed. In addition, it must include an effective plan to carry out the proposed activities. It should provide a strategy to overcome the barriers, problems, and difficulties that may occur in the process.

- **Capability.** The proposal needs to demonstrate the evidence of the capability of the researcher and his or her organization to carry out the proposed research successfully. This can be done in several ways, including: the quality of the proposal itself; the familiarity of the researcher with the problem studied; the relevant literature; and the methods used. The qualifications of the researcher and the experience and resources of his or her organizations are also important in demonstrating capability. The researcher's 'track record' is usually taken seriously in the consideration of allocating funding.
- **Efficiency.** The proposal needs to demonstrate that the project will be efficiently managed and executed. This can be done by having a clear plan of the project. Having a detailed timetable is also important in this regard.
- **Realism.** The proposal needs to be realistic. What may not be achieved in a timeline should not be promised. Realism includes the numbers of people involved, methods used, budget requested, and timeline.

Although these points are used as a formal set of criteria in assessing a research proposal, there are other specific issues frequently looked for by reviewers. Attig and Winichagoon (1993, p. 111) list the following items as important:

- Does the proposal identify the project's importance or significance to a documented need? How will it meet this need?
- Exactly who or what will the project examine, and what are their characteristics?
- Does the project involve the community's cooperation and their resources? How will the project obtain such cooperation and obtain such resources?
- To what extent does the project duplicate or overlap with other studies? Is the duplication or overlapping necessary?
- Are the objectives specifically identified? Can they be realistically achieved? Will the methodology and procedures lead to the attainment of the objectives?
- Are the proposal's tasks clearly described? Are the researchers competent in carrying out the tasks successfully?
- Can the project be related to other local, national or international programs?
- Is the budget reasonable? Is it presented accurately? What is the possibility of continuing support?

To prepare a good and successful research proposal, a researcher should try to answer all of these questions. All these requirements may seem overwhelming. However, they are important issues, which need to be addressed, and the researcher should not feel discouraged. Perhaps we should see this process as a real challenge. The better the proposal, the higher the chance that we will be able to communicate with funding agencies and hence obtain their financial support. Research funding is a prize sought after by most qualitative researchers in many competitive societies, like Australia.

Nevertheless, it is important to point out that, even though a researcher may consider that they have prepared a good quality research proposal and hence should obtain some funding, in reality this may not happen. As Lorion (1995, p. 39) points out, it is important to realise that funding opportunities are influenced by both political and scientific processes:

> Funding limitations necessitate the establishment of priorities. The process by which priorities are set, promising issues identified, and 'cutting edge' opportunities selected involves a merging of scientific knowledge and systematic debate and input from multiple sources.

The latter, Lorion argues, obviously represents a political process in the sense that reviewers differ in their estimations of the 'heuristic potential of areas of inquiry' (p. 39). Funding priorities among different funding agencies are also political in the sense that they reflect 'a balance among scientific and theoretical emphases, social concerns, and public health issues' (p. 40). Lastly, Lorion argues that it is important to recognise the human element in the grant review process. The submission of a proposal for funding is a communication between one researcher and other knowledgeable researchers. Respect, openness, acceptance and compromise are important components of this communication. Lorion also points out that it is important to appreciate the diversity of people who are involved in the grant process. These people commit themselves to achieving the balance between maximising the competitiveness for funding of each application with the scientific and public health benefits of funding decisions. In the end, a process of reviewing grant applications involves many people setting aside their time and making difficult decisions. These are important points to consider when designing and submitting a research proposal to a funding agency.

Our experiences have also taught us that the chance of obtaining funding for qualitative research can be improved through the inclusion in the proposal of a component on quantitative methods. Adding quantitative methods to the main qualitative project tends to enhance the chance of success, at least in the Australian context. Combining qualitative and quantitative methods in the research project helps to strengthen some projects, providing a rich and more robust study than one using qualitative methods alone. Both of us have successfully used this approach in research funded by major research agencies in Australia.

It is also important to select the right funding agency for the project (Tripp-Reimer and Cohen 1991). Some funding agencies may allocate funding to quantitative, clinical-based research projects only, or at least may have a tendency to do so. In this circumstance, qualitative research proposals may have no chance of securing funding, even though they are excellent. Our suggestion is that a researcher needs to do some homework on the patterns of funding allocation and the research committees of each funding agency. Try to submit the proposal to agencies that have a history of supporting qualitative research projects, and with research committees including at least some qualitative researchers who will understand the nature of qualitative research. In addition, one needs to look at the sorts of research projects that the agency may wish to support. Some funding agencies specify certain areas of research, and if any project seems to be outside the boundary, it will be rejected in the first round.

What if the research proposal is not successful? This is not the end of it. Criticisms from reviewers are excellent sources for a revision. Try to address all of these criticisms in the reconstructed proposal and then resubmit it. The persistent researcher who does so will eventually secure funding.

CONCLUSION

A research proposal is an important part of how to design research projects from the very beginning. Writing a proposal is therefore an important part of the research process. It is also relevant in the present political situation when funding is essential for a project to grow and for a researcher to obtain academic recognition in a highly competitive environment in Western and contemporary societies.

Proposal writing is not difficult. All it takes is a good knowledge of the subject material, sound writing skills, and an understanding of who is to receive the proposal and the correct techniques for approaching them (Attig and Winichagoon 1993). Most researchers have the ability to write fundable proposals. A bit of artful technique, skill and persistence may be required to refine it and make it into an effective and convincing proposal. This in turn may help to secure research funding.

Grant gathering, like any other intellectual skill, improves with practice. You may never find yourself regarding the process as enjoyable, but the challenges are always fresh and the sense of satisfaction in completing a good presentation can be a significant reward. *Better still, of course, is obtaining the money!* (Locke et al. 1989, p. 138, emphasis added)

Tutorial exercises

1 Write a small research proposal using a method or methods of your choice. Make sure that it contains all important components discussed in this chapter.
2 Obtain a funding agency application form, from the Research Office within your organisation or directly from the agency, and try to fit your proposal into the form. Make sure you fill in all sections of the form. How does it look?

Further reading

Attig, G.A. and Winichagoon, P., 1993, *Effective Proposal Writing: From Ideas to Projects*, Institute of Nutrition, Mahidol University at Salaya, Salaya.

Krathwohl, D.R., 1988, *How To Prepare a Research Proposal*, 2nd edn, Syracuse University Press, New York.

Lefferts, R., 1990, *Getting a Grant in the 1990s: How To Write Successful Grant Proposals*, Prentice-Hall, New York.

Pequegnat, W. and Stover, E. (eds), 1995, *How To Write a Successful Research Grant Application: A Guide for Social and Behavioral Scientists*, Plenum Press, New York.

Appendix: Australian Research Council (ARC) criteria for assessing grant applications

Assessment criteria

The primary criteria used for the assessment of applications are:

• the quality of the proposed research; and
• the quality of the researcher(s).

Quality of the proposed research

Consider to what extent the proposed research is likely to lead to:

• a significant conceptual advance;
• an important discovery or innovation; and/or
• the solution of an important practical problem.

In assessing the quality of the research proposal; assessors should take particular account of:

• the soundness of the planning and methodology;
• the originality of the project;
• the scientific, theoretical or technological merit;
• the capacity of the institution to provide the necessary infrastructure;
• the time and capacity of the researcher(s) to make a serious commitment to the project, i.e. a minimum of 4 days out of 21 working days, to produce the desired outcomes; and
• the scope of the project.

Quality of the researcher(s)

In assessing the quality of the researcher, consideration should be given to the applicant's track record, covering their recent research performance relative to opportunities.

12

Writing a Qualitative Research Report

Writing, the creative effort, should come first—at least for some part of every day of your life. It is a wonderful blessing if you will use it. You will become happier, more enlightened, alive, impassioned, light hearted and generous to everybody else. Even your health will improve. Colds will disappear and all the other ailments of discouragement and boredom. I know a very great woman who makes her living by teaching violin lessons in the daytime. Then from midnight until five o'clock in the morning, she is happy because she can work on her book. This is her daily routine ... One day she came to me and had a very bad cold. 'Oh, lie down quick!' I exclaimed, 'and I will get you some hot lemonade and put a shawl over yourself'. She opened her eyes wide at me, and said almost with horror in her voice. 'Oh, that is no way to treat a cold! ... No, I slumped a little yesterday and so I caught it. But I worked all night and it is much, much better now'. (Ueland 1991, p. 14, original emphasis)

INTRODUCTION

Well, once we have conducted a beautiful piece of qualitative research in health, what shall we do with our interesting and important findings? We need to put our information down on paper, we need to write about it. *Why write about it?* Apart from helping to improve our health, as Ueland argues, we need to write in order to disseminate our research findings so that other people can read and make use of them, whether for improving current health practices or using them as the basis for developing new research projects. As Attig and colleagues (1993, p. 227) put it, 'only through the reporting process can new facts and new research questions come to light and new findings be related to the research activities of other professionals'.

In this chapter, we will discuss some of the characteristics of qualitative writing. We will outline the styles of research report commonly used to disseminate findings drawn from qualitative research projects. There are a number of techniques to observe when writing good qualitative research papers, and these are considered. Lastly, we include some discussions about writing for publication. In many cases, this not only completes the project but is also the best way to disseminate the findings to wider audiences.

THE NATURE OF QUALITATIVE RESEARCH WRITING

Qualitative writing is different from quantitative writing. A quantitative report consists of a concise presentation of the methods and results of the study. However, qualitative writing 'must be a convincing argument systematically presenting data to support the researcher's case and to refute alternative explanations' (Morse 1994a, p. 231). Richardson (1994, p. 517) argues that, unlike quantitative work which relies heavily on tables and summaries, 'qualitative work depends upon people reading it. Just as a piece of literature is not equivalent to its "plot summary", qualitative research is not contained in its abstracts. Qualitative research has to be read, not scanned; its meaning is in the reading.' For this reason, writing that is based on qualitative research, be it a report, article or book, tends to be long. The written report must contain enough details to 'tell' readers about the research and its findings. Neuman (1991, p. 491) points out that there are five reasons why qualitative papers tends to be longer than quantitative writing:

- Qualitative data are more difficult to condense. Qualitative data contain words, not numbers, and include many quotes and extended case examples.
- In a qualitative report, detailed descriptions of the research sites and the population under study.need to be provided so that readers will have a better understanding of the research setting.
- Qualitative researchers employ less standardised data collection methods, ways of developing analytic categories, and modes of organising evidence. The methods chosen depend upon the conditions of the research site and the researchers' preferences. Hence, qualitative researchers need to explain what, and why, they did what they did in greater length.
- The goals of qualitative studies are to explore new settings and construct new theories. Detailed descriptions about the development of new concepts, their relationships and the interpretations of evidence need to be provided. This adds to the length of the report.
- The nature of qualitative data (such as in the form of life histories, case studies and tales) gives the writer freedom to use literary devices to keep the reader's interest and accurately translate a meaning system for the reader. This, again, lengthens the paper.

There are other distinctive characteristics of qualitative writing. This is particularly so in the presentation of research findings. As Stapleton (1987) points out, there are three ways to present results. First, the findings are given without comments or interpretations. The interpretations can be discussed later on in the discussion section. Second, interpretations can be added up to a point in order to make some connections between lines of evidence. Further detail is again provided in the discussion section. Last, the results and discussion of each point may need to go together if an in-depth discussion is required to give meaning to the findings. Attig and Winichagoon (1993) also point out that because of the nature of qualitative research that needs some interpretations to make the findings more meaningful, qualitative writing tends to include discussion throughout (as opposed to the specific 'Discussion' section in quantitative reports). This makes the report's organisational structure more critical for ensuring clarity. Writing a qualitative report, therefore, requires careful attention to structure and meaning. Writers need to make a special effort to achieve coherence and conciseness (Stapleton 1987; Wilkinson 1991).

In qualitative reports, the language is not as objective or formal as in quantitative papers. A writer usually uses the first person (I) in describing the research processes and in discussing the findings (Neuman 1991; Wilkinson 1991; Wolcott 1990). Wolcott (1990, p. 19) argues that, since the researcher's role is an 'integral' part of qualitative study, descriptive accounts need to be made in the first person. He further points out that 'the more critical the observer's role and subjective assessment, the more important to have that role and presence acknowledged in the reporting'.

However, like quantitative reports, qualitative reports also make use of graphic representations, such as figures, pictures and illustrations. Very often tables are used in order to describe the major background characteristics of the people under study. However, the tables and graphics are used to supplement the discussion, not to replace it (Attig and Winichagoon 1993; Wolcott 1990).

WRITING FOR WHOM?

Professional writers say, Always know whom you are writing for. This is because communication is more effective when it is tailored to a specific audience. (Neuman 1991, p. 482)

The same piece of qualitative research needs to be written differently for different audiences—fellow researchers, professional social scientists, health care professionals, policy makers, research funding agencies, and publishers (Agar 1986; Hammersley and Atkinson 1995; Neuman 1991). Yin (1984) points out that, because each audience has different needs and expectations, a single piece of writing cannot serve all audiences simultaneously. Similarly, Fetterman (1989) argues that the formats, languages and levels of abstraction of qualitative writing need to be constructed according to the needs and concerns of the audiences. Research funding agencies, for example, usually want to see the results of the research as well as to assess whether the project attains its objectives. Policy makers will want to know how the findings and recommendations of the research can be implemented and applied. Health professionals may wish to use research findings to improve their health services or the health status of people they care for. Professional social scientists, however, will want to look at the research process, its scientific soundness and interpretations (Attig et al. 1993). Agar (1986, p. 15), for example, states in his book *Speaking of Ethnography* that when he presents his ethnographic work to different audiences, the same piece of ethnographic material takes different forms depending on who he is writing for. When he writes for clinicians and drug policy makers, his writing is different from that which he writes for sociologists or cognitive anthropologists.

Therefore, the first task in writing up qualitative research findings is to identify the audience: who will be reading the writing? Only then can the author construct the writing to suit. Richardson (1994, p. 523) uses the analogy of 'wet clay' for qualitative data: 'It is there for us to shape.' Qualitative researchers need to ask: What are our purposes? What are our goals? Who do we want to reach? What do we want to accomplish? This will assist them in communicating with their audiences effectively. One good example of writing different pieces of research findings to match different audiences is the work of Richardson (1990). In her *Writing Strategies: Reaching Diverse Audiences*, Richardson (1990) provides an excellent description of audience and style for qualitative work (in her case, ethnographic writing). She describes how her research project led to different versions of production to match different types of audiences: academic sociologists and a popular book aimed at the trade market. But, as Hammersley and Atkinson (1995, p. 260) argue, writing for different audiences does not simply involve describing 'the same thing in different ways. We are abruptly changing what we describe as well as how we do it.' Wolf (1992), for example, utilises different 'textual strategies' in the writing of her research findings. Wolf wrote three books based on her research in Taiwan, which have different styles, target different readers and take different perspectives.

What if we are able to write only one qualitative report because of time, budget and other limitations? An example from Wax and colleagues (1989) may give us the answer. They wrote a monograph on ethnography in education, entitled 'Formal Education in an American Indian Community'. The intention of the scholarly monograph was to reach an audience of practitioners. In their one-page 'Guide to the Reader' executive summary (p. v), they advise readers who have little time to read the whole report to 'skim the pages of the report' but to read the 'Summary and Recommendations'. Those who want to understand contemporary Indian reservations are advised to turn to the chapter entitled 'Ecology, Economy, and Educational Achievement'. However, 'skeptics and critics' need 'to read not only the first chapter, but also the Appendix before proceeding into the heart of the text'.

Note particularly the guide for 'skeptics and critics', who are asked to read the first chapter, which contains the perspective and objectives of the research, as well as the appendix, which details the research procedure. Wax and others do this because they expect that their qualitative approach is likely to be subject 'to scrutiny by methodologists, but of little concern to busy practitioners' (Wolcott 1990, p. 58).

THE STRUCTURE OF QUALITATIVE RESEARCH WRITING

In this section, we will confine our discussion to three common types of writing for the dissemination of qualitative research findings: reports, articles, and books or monographs.

Reports

According to Fetterman (1989), a report tends to be more pragmatic than an article or book and tends to focus on policy issues. It is, therefore, likely to have an immediate impact on the group under investigation. The language used tends to be bureaucratic and full of jargon (such as 'prioritisation' and 'implementation') to satisfy the expectations of policy makers or research funding agencies.

Although qualitative reports do not strictly follow the format of scientific reports (Day 1979), it does not mean that they do not have any structure. Attig and Winichagoon (1993, p. 120) point out, the structure of qualitative reports 'emerges from an interaction between the topic being studied and the researcher's own style and system of logic'. Report writing needs to have a framework or plan so that it can be developed into a complete piece of work.

There are several organisational formats and components to a qualitative report. Some qualitative writers follow the format used for quantitative reports, as suggested by Day (1979). Other qualitative writers choose other styles in structuring their reports (see Plath 1980 and Neuman 1991, for example). However, they do contain certain structures in order to make the presentation of the findings clear and easy to follow. Whatever format is used, qualitative reports usually contain certain key components that are similar to those found in qualitative proposals (see Chapter 11 for these details; see also Wolcott's excellent *Writing Up Qualitative Research*, 1990). The following list of components is taken from Attig and Winichagoon (1993, p. 121):

- Title
- Table of contents
- Executive summary
- Introduction
- Theoretical framework
- Study sites and characteristics of people under study
- Research design and methodology
- Findings

- Discussion, conclusion, and detailed discussion of recommendations for implementation, interventions and for future research

Articles

Richardson (1990) points out that collecting qualitative data is labour-intensive and much of what is collected does not fit into one article. It makes sense, therefore, to write a number of different pieces from different perspectives at different stages of the project. Very often, findings from most qualitative research projects can be split into separate sections, each of which can be made into a reasonably comprehensive paper, discussing a specific issue in depth. Morse (1994a) argues that publication in the shorter form of a paper helps to increase citations in serial indexes. Publication of short papers also leads to speedier dissemination of the research findings.

The process and structure of an article may be similar to that of a report, but in a highly condensed form. Morse (1994b) points out that some journals have regulations that limit the reporting of qualitative research. Most common is a restriction on the length of a paper. Most journals have limited page numbers or words for each paper (for example, fifteen pages or less). Therefore, each section of the paper must be condensed, but there should be enough detail to take readers through the important points. This can create difficulties in writing qualitative research papers, 'for rarely can all the requirements for the richness of descriptions be developed in a short article' (Morse 1994b, p. 70). Because of this, qualitative writers often run the risk of not being able to give readers enough background to the research, thus creating misunderstandings or resulting in criticism for not being complete. However, this can be overcome by presenting only one aspect of the findings in each paper, which allows more writing space in which to present a comprehensive article. This is what Wolcott (1990, p. 69) refers to as 'doing less more thoroughly'. He suggests that 'a strategy for accomplishing this is to look for parts, instances, or cases that can stand for the whole. Reporting parts is all you can possibly do in a journal article.'

Alternatively, a qualitative writer may choose to follow Strunk and White's suggestion in their *Elements of Style* (1979, p. xiv, emphasis added):

> Vigorous writing is concise. A statement should contain no unnecessary words, a paragraph no unnecessary sentences … This requires not that the writer make his sentences short, or that he avoid all detail and treat his subjects only in outline, but that *every word tell*.

This means that heavy editing to condense the paper is needed. Although this may create some difficulties for those who have many important details to report, as most qualitative writers do, it is not impossible if the writing is done carefully.

Another restriction in writing qualitative papers for publication is that some journals require that a certain outline be strictly followed. This outline, as Morse

(1994b, p. 70) points out, may not be conducive to the presentation of qualitative research. The requirement that a literature review be presented prior to the results, for example, makes it difficult to write a paper based on grounded theory where 'linkage to the literature is inherent within the presentation of results'. As mentioned earlier, in making sense of the findings, it is sometimes necessary to include discussion and citations of other pieces of qualitative work. Some journals do not accept this integration of literature, results and discussion. Again, this may create some difficulties in constructing a qualitative article.

However, most qualitative articles can be formatted to match a journal's requirements. Most often, a qualitative paper will have different headings, which can be labelled according to the rules of the journal, such as background, theoretical framework, methodology, the sample, findings, and discussion and conclusion. However, sometimes qualitative writers may choose to use other names for each heading. In presenting findings, for example, we tend not to use the heading 'Findings' as such, but to use 'Themes' instead. Similarly, in presenting the characteristics of 'The sample', we may use 'The women in the study' instead (see, for example, Rice 1995; Rice and Naksook 1998).

There are several books that provide excellent guidance on writing qualitative articles; for example, Attig and Winichagoon (1993), Bogdan and Biklen (1982), Denzin (1989a), Ely et al. (1997), Fox (1985), Glaser and Strauss (1967), Richardson (1990), Van Maanen (1988), van Til (1987) and Wolcott (1990). These books could prove helpful to a qualitative writer struggling to construct clear and concise articles for publication in refereed journals.

Books and monographs

Some qualitative research may be published as books or monographs. Some publishers are willing to publish entire studies, rather than splitting the research into separate sections as articles. There are normally no limitations on length and so the writer is able to portray the people under study in more detail. This type of publication is therefore very suitable for qualitative research findings.

Persell (1985) believes that it is easier and faster to publish qualitative research as a book or monograph than as an article. Because of the processes involved in obtaining acceptance of an article for publication, it may take several months to many years, depending on the nature of the process. However, Fetterman (1989, p. 113) argues that scholarly books are more difficult to write than articles, partly because of their greater length. It is also because of the larger scope of intellectual effort required to reduce 'mountains of data and pools of analysis into concise expression'. Writing a book requires much more effort than writing an article.

The structure of a book or monograph varies depending on the style of the writer, but it needs to be comprehensive. Usually, a book is broken into several chapters. From the first chapter to the last, the content must flow smoothly in order to take readers through the forest of the lives of the people we are writing about. Detailed descriptions of the community and its people should be provided. In a book based on an ethnography, for example, fundamental elements about the culture, including its structure and organisation, history, politics, religion, economy and belief systems, need to be discussed at great length (Fetterman 1989, p. 111). The methodology and research processes need to be described, as in an article, but in fuller detail. However, unlike in writing an article, every important issue emerging from qualitative research can be discussed minutely. This allows the writer to portray their research findings without constraints and hence makes the writing more comprehensible and complete.

There are many classic books based on qualitative research. Some good examples include *Street Corner Society: The Social Structure of an Italian Slum* by Whyte (1955), *You Owe Yourself a Drunk: An Ethnography of Urban Nomads* by Spradley (1970), *Yanomamo: The Fierce People* by Chagnon (1977), *Nisa: The Life and Words of a !Kung Woman* by Shostak (1981), *The New Other Woman: Contemporary Single Women in Affairs with Married Men* by Richardson (1985), *Labour Pains and Labour Power: Women and Childbearing in India* by Jeffery and others (1989), *Quest for Conception: Gender, Infertility, and Egyptian Medical Traditions* by Inhorn (1994), *Good Days, Bad Days: The Self in Chronic Illness and Time* by Charmaz (1991), and *Speaking of Sadness, Depression, Disconnection and the Meanings of Illness* by Karp (1996).

GOOD WRITING: WHAT TO LOOK FOR?

What is considered a good piece of qualitative writing? What do we look for? The task in writing research reports of any kind is to transform the data into concrete and clear thinking and then convey this to the reader. To achieve this, the writer needs to construct writing that is as 'readable' as possible, which means that it needs to be 'straightforward and understandable'. Good reports will make the reader immediately understand what is being said. As Attig and colleagues (1993) point out in a highly readable paper, readers do not have to mentally bridge gaps, make assumptions, reread passages to decode information, or even pause to interpret what the writer has written.

Like a good research proposal (see Chapter 11), a good report should be 'cogent, conceptually coherent, and comprehensive' (Fetterman 1989, p. 119). Hence (based on Attig et al. 1993; Wilkinson 1991):
- It should lead readers step-by-step through the complicated parts.
- It should provide readers with directions about where to go (follow from one idea to the next) and where to turn (when one changes ideas).
- It should not mislead, confuse, or raise false expectations among readers.
- It should not leave gaps in any part of the paper (such as unanswered questions and incomplete interpretations).

- It should not change direction totally without warning.

Apart from these, there are other practical issues that may help in the composition of a good piece of qualitative writing. Fetterman (1989, pp. 118–19) suggests the following:

- Titles must catch the reader's eye and remain honest.
- Sentences should be grammatical.
- Paragraphs must be shifted to fit in the right conceptual sequence.
- Phrases must be carefully crafted to capture the imagination of the reader, but remain scientific.
- Participles should not dangle.
- Citations should correspond to references.
- Examples must be compelling and precise.

Berger (1993, p. 31) says it clearly: 'When it doubt, leave it out.' This is useful and powerful advice for any kind of research report writing. If a writer is unsure of a statement, and cannot confirm it, it should not be in the paper. It may confuse readers and lead to negative judgments about the capability of the writer.

WRITING FOR PUBLICATION

According to Morse (1994a, p. 232), 'publication is the most important means for disseminating research findings'. Through publication, our research findings can reach wider audiences and have the chance of producing results by changing some health practices for the better. Publication may be in the form of books or articles. However, books often do not have as rigorous a review process as do papers. They are also not as easily accessed as articles through electronic retrieval services such as Medline (Morse 1994b). In the next section we will concentrate on writing papers for publication only.

How do we construct our papers in order to have them published? Which journal is less likely to reject qualitative research papers in the first instance? This is a very common question posed by many qualitative researchers. The following suggestions are adopted from Fetterman (1989), Kronenfeld (1985), Mauch and Birch (1989), and Morse (1994b). See also Nemcek and Egan (1984), for some tips for nurses about writing for publication; Richardson's *Writing Strategies* (1990), and Wolcott's *Writing Up Qualitative Research* (1990), are also excellent sources.

Writing the paper

- Decide on the form in which the content will be presented. Most professional journals usually have organisational structures of their own. However, most of them require a systematic sequence of content which will enhance communication of concepts (Mauch and Birch 1989). Therefore, the structure of the paper should reflect the organisational structures of the journal and proceed in an orderly way with the facets of the topic (Mauch and Birch 1989).

- Begin and maintain a firm fix on the paper's main theme. Every large section of the paper needs to build on the foundation of the earlier section and then move the same theme ahead. Any deviant issue should be eliminated. If it is necessary to the discussion, then it needs to be justified. Ask yourself whether the first sentence of every paragraph adheres to the core theme of the paper and if it follows sensibly the first sentence in the immediately preceding paragraph. If the answer is yes, then you have begun and maintained a firm fix on your paper's main theme.
- Ensure that all grammatical, spelling and other structural composition details reflect preferred practice in contemporary usage. An impression of sloppy and inaccurate English usage may distract reviewers from the positive qualities of the paper.
- Morse (1994b, p. 71) contends that 'a smart researcher never sends an article to a publisher without both a peer review (for content) and an editor's check (for style and format)'. When you have worked on a piece for some time, it is very difficult to pinpoint inconsistency and pick out the mistakes. Giving it to some academic friends to read is a good way to check your paper (Kronenfeld 1985; Wolcott 1990).
- Before submitting the paper, revise and edit your writing to the best possible form. This takes time.

Submitting the paper

- As Mauch and Birch (1989, p. 212) argue, to achieve publication depends not only on doing a good job of 'putting together a well-composed, tightly organized manuscript', but also on 'directing it to a periodical, the style and publishing interests of which match with the article's content'. Therefore, pick the journal to match your topic. If your purpose is to have some impact on changing health services, then journals that publish papers on health practices or policies should be the target of choice. If you write for a particular journal, it is more likely that the paper will stay within the accepted bounds and be in line with the interests of the journal (Kronenfeld 1985). Hence, it is less likely the paper will be rejected in the first instance. However, you must make sure that the journal accepts papers based on qualitative research, as some journals publish so-called 'scientific' articles only.
- Find out about the journal's guidelines. Following the rules of the publishing journal is an important part of writing a paper for publication. As Agger 1990) points out, even 'liberatory and radical messages' can be published in conservative journals if the writer follows the rules. By rules, we mean, for example, the referencing system, the number of copies to be submitted, the length of the paper, the use of headings and sub-headings, and the organisational structure.

- Pay attention to the nitty-gritty of format. Using a poor quality printer to produce the final version of the paper can make reading difficult for reviewers. As Morse (1994b) points out, reviewers must be able to read clearly what they are assessing. Also, most journals require articles to be double-spaced and to have specified margins, so that reviewers have room in which to write their comments. This needs to be strictly adhered to. Checking all the references cited in the paper and making sure that they appear in the reference section is also important.

- Be prepared to try another journal if the first one rejects the paper outright. In doing so, it is important to take into account the reviewers' reasons for the rejection. Very often, they make good suggestions for the revision of the article and hence help to improve the chances of acceptance later on.

Competition for journal space is extremely high. This is particularly the case in journals that have a good reputation, such as *Social Science and Medicine*, *American Sociological Review*, and the like. Most papers are rejected in the first instance. Few researchers have their work accepted upon first submission. However, as Agger (1990) points out, some papers that show promise will be returned for revision, with a request to resubmit. If the article is rewritten to meet the criticisms and the comments, the work may eventually be accepted for publication in these journals (see Powell 1985 for a discussion about the decision-making process in scholarly publishing).

Will it be published?

Once a (male) health researcher in a health policy domain, who promoted quantitative research, told Pranee that he was sick of a qualitative paper since it would never be accepted for publication. Why did he say this? June Stevenson writes in her letter to Meloy (1993, p. 321): 'Is qualitative research getting a "bad rap" because it is viewed as easy?' Her answer is that perhaps qualitative research is considered as not as 'rigorous' because it does not engage in statistical analysis and therefore is seen as not objective. Meloy points out that qualitative research is often seen as a story, a fiction (p. 321). The story-like quality of qualitative research 'brings it too close to the reader as a thinking, feeling human being, rather than as a detached, rational mind'. And this is seen as not objective, again from the point of view of quantitative reviewers.

Nevertheless, as Moffett (1984, p. 58) argues:

> Reading engages emotion and memory and imagination by means of the mind because it is *words* not deeds or sights or sounds that elicit response. Imagery is conjured from *words*, emotion sprung by *words* and ideas generated by *words*.

And because *words* are essential in writing qualitative reports, this may create some difficulties in writing qualitative papers for publication in journals that are based on positivist-empiricist research. This has some implications for qualitative researchers who commit to qualitative research and who want to disseminate their findings to a wider audience:

> Qualitative researchers who seek to construct text that is congruent with the purposes, grounded in the assumptions, and reflective of the processes of qualitative research are still struggling to be listened to as researchers, as a part of—not apart from—their work. (Meloy 1993, p. 321)

Very often, qualitative researchers ask themselves if their writing will ever be accepted in refereed journals, particularly those promoting quantitative research. This has stopped many qualitative writers submitting articles to these journals. Our answer is that 'we can' if we write in such a way that we can convince the reviewers of the journals that our findings are of importance; if we shape our qualitative material in a way that meets the expectations of the reviewers; and if we treat the reviewers' comments as positive criticism and take them seriously. Richardson (1990, p. 53) provides the illuminating example of her qualitative paper, on the social construction of forbidden relationships between a single woman and a married man, which was published in the *American Sociological Review*, a positivist-empiricist social science journal, after she had published her book. She tells us that she regarded the reviewers' comments as 'genuine questions generated by their empiricist discourse and/or indicators of textual faults ... rather than as attacks upon the value of the work' (p. 54). Richardson treated the reviewers 'not as rigid empiricist enemies but as audience' (p. 54). By so doing, she 'integrated' the reviewers' readings of her text when she reshaped the paper. As she said, 'their comments invited me into their discourse' (p. 54).

One of our qualitative articles, which was published in a quantitative journal in Australia, reflects a similar strategy. Rice and others (1993) wrote a paper about the importance of cultural beliefs and practices related to childbirth, using a case study of a woman from Southeast Asia to illustrate their arguments. The paper was short, but focused on one important point. It was accepted by the *Medical Journal of Australia*, a positivist-empiricist medical science journal, soon after it was submitted, because of the important nature of the paper and because its structure (including the length) carefully matched the journal guidelines.

CRITERIA FOR THE EVALUATION OF QUALITATIVE PAPERS

More than two decades ago, Lofland (1974) discussed some of the criteria that journal referees used in evaluating qualitative research papers. In this paper, Lofland identified several points of importance. First is the use of a generic conceptual framework. It is not enough to report only a particular event among a particular group of people; it has to be placed in a wider framework. Second is the novelty of the paper. It must demonstrate how an existing conceptual framework is being developed, tested, modified or extended. Hence, a new analytic framework must be provided. Third, the analytic framework and the empirical evidence need to be brought together in appropriate ways; that is, a textual arrangement needs to be adequately 'elaborated'. Last, the analytic framework and the illustrative data need to be 'interpenetrated'. There should be an interaction between the concrete and the analytic, the empirical and the theoretical.

Blaxter (1996) provides a very useful set of criteria for evaluating papers based on qualitative research. The criteria presented in Box 12.1 are taken from her suggestions, published by the British Sociology Association.

Box 12.1 Criteria for the evaluation of qualitative papers

General
- Are the methods of the research appropriate to the nature of the question of the research? That is: what does the research seek to understand? Could a quantitative method have addressed the issue better?
- Is the connection to an existing body of knowledge or theory clear? That is: is there enough reference to the literature? And does the paper cohere with, or critically address, existing theory?

Methods
- Are there clear descriptions of the criteria used for the selection of participants, the data collection and analysis?
- Is the selection of participants theoretically justified?
- Does the sensitivity of the methods match the needs of the research questions? Is there any consideration of the limitations of the methods?
- Has the relationship between fieldworkers and participants been considered?
- Is there evidence about how the research was presented and explained to the participants?
- Was the data collection and record keeping systematic and appropriate?

Analysis
- Is reference made to accepted procedures for analysis?
- How systematic is the analysis?
- Is there adequate discussion of how themes, concepts and categories were derived from the data?
- Is there adequate discussion of the evidence both for and against the researcher's arguments? In particular, are negative data given? And has there been any search for cases which might refute the conclusions?

- Have measures been taken to test the validity of the findings? That is: have methods such as feeding them back to the participants, triangulation, or procedures like grounded theory been used?
- Have any steps been taken to see whether the analysis would be comprehensible to participants? In particular, has the meaning of their accounts been explored with participants?

Presentation
- Is the research clearly contextualised? That is: is relevant information about the social context of the setting and participants provided?
- Are the data presented systematically? That is: are quotations and fieldnotes identified for readers to judge the range of evidence being used?
- Is a clear distinction made between the data and their interpretation? In particular, do the conclusions follow from the data?
- Is sufficient of the original evidence presented to satisfy the reader of the relationship between the evidence and the conclusions?
- Is the researcher's own position (such as role, possible bias and influence on the research) clearly stated?
- Are the results credible and appropriate? That is: Do they address the research question? are they plausible and coherent? are they important theoretically or practically?

Ethics
- Have ethical issues been adequately considered?

If your qualitative article can provide answers to all or most of these questions in a positive way, it is likely that your paper will be accepted for publication. Most reviewers will look for any gaps by using these questions to judge if the paper is worthy of publication or not. Filling in clear answers to these suggestions may, therefore, help to get your papers in press.

CONCLUSION

Wolcott (1990, p. 90) sums up his book on *Writing Up Qualitative Research* with 'published or not, you've written up your qualitative research. Your work wasn't completed until you did.' We also believe that writing up our research findings is an 'essential' component of the research process if we wish to complete it. Writing about our findings helps to communicate the important issues from our research to wider audiences, be they academics, health professionals or policy makers. More importantly, what we find in conducting any piece of qualitative research may prove useful in improving public health and health services for many people in the society. But how will anyone find this information if we do not write and publish it? Research dissemination through writing is therefore an important part of the research process.

Writing also helps us to grow. It teaches us something about the world we live in and hence expands our life experiences. As Sondra Perl (1983, p. 49) says about writing: 'We see in our words a further structuring of the sense we began with ... we end up with a product that teaches us something ... and that lifts out or explicates or enlarges our experiences.' And we hope that by keeping on writing about your qualitative findings, 'your health will improve ... colds will disappear and all the other ailments of discouragement and boredom'.

Happy writing!

Tutorial exercise

Now, since you have conducted a piece of research using your choice of qualitative method(s), write up your findings as a journal paper designed for submission to a refereed journal in a health area. Limit the length of the paper to fifteen pages only. Good luck!

Further reading

Attig, G.A., Winichagoon, P. and Yoddumnern-Attig, B., 1993, 'Designing and Writing Qualitative Research Reports', in B. Yoddumnern-Attig, G.A. Attig, W. Boonchalaksi, K. Richter and A. Soonthorndhada (eds), *Qualitative Methods for Population and Health Research*, Institute for Population and Social Research, Mahidol University, Salaya.

Berger, A.A., 1993, *Improving Writing Skills*, Sage, New York.

Ely, M., Vinz, R., Downing, M. and Anzul, M., 1997, *On Writing Qualitative Research: Living by Words*, Falmer Press, London.

Fox, M.F. (ed.), 1985, *Scholarly Writing and Publishing: Issues, Problems, and Solutions*, Westview, Boulder, Colorado.

Powell, W.W., 1985, *Getting into Print: The Decision-Making Process in Scholarly Publishing*, University of Chicago Press, Chicago.

Richardson, L., 1990, *Writing Strategies: Reaching Diverse Audiences*, Sage, Newbury Park.

Stapleton, P., 1987, *Writing Research Papers: An Easy Guide for Non-Native English Speakers*, Australian Centre for International Agricultural Research, Canberra.

van Til, W., 1987, *Writing for Professional Publication*, Allyn & Bacon, Newton, Mass.

Wolcott, H., 1990, *Writing Up Qualitative Research*, Sage, Newbury Park.

Conclusion

If I lived twenty more years and was able to work, how I should have to modify the Origin, *and how much the views on all points have to be modified! Well it is a beginning, and that is something. (Charles Darwin to Joseph Hooker, 1869, quoted in Stone 1980)*

In trying to conclude, what can we say about qualitative research methods in the health sphere? First, health professionals and health researchers are themselves beginning to use qualitative methods as a legitimate mode of understanding health issues from the perspective of the researched. Second, health professionals are starting to work in multidisciplinary teams with social scientists who are skilled and experienced in qualitative research to investigate a wide range of health issues. Third, there has been an increase in the publication of qualitative research in medical and science journals that have not traditionally been oriented to qualitative research. Fourth, there has been more recognition of the value of qualitative research in the health sphere on the part of funding bodies in Australia and elsewhere. However, there is still a problem in teaching qualitative research methods as a standard equal partner in the research enterprise. If one examines the course outlines of introductory research methods courses, one finds that qualitative methods are usually still allocated only two sessions in the total teaching year. Qualitative methods are typically set aside as third or fourth year program electives instead of being required or compulsory core study. This may be a reflection of history, ossification of university timetabling or the resistance to taking away time from studying 'more important' quantitative research methods.

Our view is that qualitative research methods are now being used in more creative and challenging ways and that there is more acceptance at grassroots level between members of research teams. In addition, there is a more consistent use of qualitative research methods along with quantitative methods. Also, there are more research projects and programs that adopt qualitative methods as a legitimate and central mode of research in the health sphere.

The health field itself is undergoing tremendous change. This is not only due to economic factors but also to changing relationships between participants in the field. The desire for seamless health service provision, the emphasis on preventative care, and the increased acceptance of the new public health perspective has also seen the enhanced use of qualitative research methods by health professionals and research teams. There is a recognition that action to produce better health in society requires the 'close' and detailed knowledge that qualitative research can produce. It is not just improved understandings of the perspectives of the health consumer, but also an improved understanding of the perspectives of all participants in the health sphere and beyond it. For instance, there is recognition in the new public health model that social relations throughout society can produce an unhealthy society and that investigation of the relationships and processes that impinge on one's health go beyond research just in the health sector. For example, feminist research that has relied upon qualitative research methods has focused on issues such as more general relations between men and women and this has reflected on and brought about subsequent and concurrent research examining such things as domestic violence (Doyal 1995). Also, critical and Marxist researchers in the health domain have utilised qualitative research methods to examine structural impacts on health outcomes in different societies and power relationships in the health sphere (Doyal 1981; Waitzkin 1991). It is clear that qualitative research methods have been employed to explore and critically examine the interrelationships between social structure in the larger society and the social processes that become the subject matters for investigation in the health sphere.

This does not mean that we see qualitative research methods as the only appropriate means of engaging in health research, nor do we suggest that qualitative research methods have no flaws. There are many researchers from within the qualitative methods fold who have been concerned by a number of issues and problems that are specific to the qualitative domain. For example, in team research there may be some significant problems in relation to deciding when theoretical saturation has been reached; how does one make decisions relating to theoretical and methodological domains without resorting to personal preference or the degree of dominance and power held by individual players?

We also do not suggest that qualitative research methods should be employed in all health research projects and programs. It is quite clear that research designs are influenced by specific needs that are determined by the social contexts and the questions asked. There are many situations in which qualitative research methods are highly inappropriate, such as those which require epidemiological data, when randomised-controlled trials will provide broad-based information, or when generalisation across large populations is needed. There are also situations where qualitative research methods need to be combined with quantitative methods in order to respond adequately to the research questions. Rather, our view of qualitative research methods, as stated in our introduction, is that they are valuable in trying to understand and interpret the meanings people attach to the experiences of health and illness. When it is important to know about this, then qualitative research methods need to be used.

It must be noted that we could not incorporate all that we would have wished in this one volume. It would be impossible. For instance, we have not included a substantial discussion of the relationships between literary interpretation and social sciences or health research use of qualitative methods. We discuss it only briefly in relation to visual analysis and analytical processes in general. The chapters that describe data collection methods could not hope to cover all of the issues that are inevitably raised by the actual doing of research. A focus on just one particular method to the exclusion of all others, as in a text such as *In-Depth Interviewing* (Minichiello et al. 1995), would have provided the space for an in-depth account of each method.

What we have done, we hope, is to raise your interest in engaging in research that utilises qualitative methods in a way that assists in not only understanding the world but changing it for the better. We believe that there is an increasing interest in these methods in the health sphere because they have proved to be successful in helping us to achieve a better knowledge of what can be done and, in some cases such as participatory action research (Hecker 1997), the ability to jointly participate with others in the doing. We leave you with the following thoughts:

> While qualitative studies have been conducted throughout the history of the social sciences, those who have practiced qualitative research have been few. This is an exciting time for those dedicated to qualitative research methods, for interest in the products of such methods is increasing. We have reached a point where a great many researchers are needed to go to the people. There is much to be learned and many are needed to carry out the work. (Bogdan and Taylor 1975, p. 223)

Glossary

CAQDAS

The Computer Assisted Qualitative Data Analysis Software (CAQDAS) networking project. WWW page: <http://www.soc.surrey.ac.uk/caqdas/>. The site contains demonstration versions of many software packages, a variety of useful resources, and links to other sites.

Coding

Part of the data analysis process where codes are applied to segments, or chunks, of data. Codes are labels that identify general processes and themes.

Content analysis

A form of data analysis used by both qualitative and quantitative methodologies that involves the identification of codes prior to searching for their occurrence in the data. It is a deductive methodology in comparison to the inductive methodology of thematic analysis.

Co-researchers

A group of researchers who together carry out a piece of research from the planning to the final stages. This is a unique feature in participatory action research and memory-work methods, where all those involved are acknowledged as co-researchers.

Cultural anthropology

The study of the social, symbolic and material lives of human societies.

Cultural relativism

The judgment of the behaviour and beliefs of other social and cultural groups in terms of *their own* cultural values, traditions and experiences.

Data

Raw information, in any form, collected via the research process and before the analysis process takes place.

Deductive theorising

Theory developed through logical argument from other theory. A deductive theory 'builds down' from more general theories to specific propositions. These specific propositions are then typically 'tested' through comparison with empirical data.

Epistemology

The study of how people know. A positivist epistemology assumes knowledge is obtained through objectively gathering facts. An interpretivist epistemology emphasises the role of subjective understanding in shaping our knowledge.

Ethnocentrism

The judgment of the behaviour and beliefs of other social and cultural groups in terms of *one's own* cultural values and traditions.

Ethnographer

A researcher who applies an ethnographic method in their data collection process.

Ethnography

The method used to discover and describe individual social and cultural groups. Prominent features include the use of participant observation with other qualitative methods in the fieldwork.

Fieldnotes

A record of conversations, observations, reflections, and interpretations of the data collected during a fieldwork period.

Fieldwork

A period of data collection commonly employed in the ethnographic method. Fieldwork may take a year or longer. The researcher usually stays in the community being studied throughout the period.

Focus groups

A particular method making use of group discussion. Typically, there is a moderator who acts as the leader of the group. The participants (usually between eight and ten) express their views via discussing the issues in a group.

Focused or in-depth interview

A method of qualitative data collection. The interview does not used fixed questions, but aims to engage the interviewee in conversation to elicit their understandings and interpretations.

Grounded theory

A combination of theoretical sampling and thematic analysis developed by two symbolic interactionists, Glaser and Strauss (1968). Theories are grounded in the empirical data and built up inductively through a process of careful analysis and comparisons. Grounded theory developed in opposition to positivist, deductive and 'grand theory' forms of analysis.

Group interaction
A unique feature of focus group interviews when participants interact with each other in a group discussion. The idea behind this is that group processes assist the participants to explore and clarify their points of view, which tend to be less accessible in an individual interview.

Hermeneutics
A theory of the process of interpretation. Hermeneutics is used in qualitative research to examine the way people develop interpretations of their life in relation to their life experiences.

Inductive theorising
Theory built up from empirical research through observing general patterns and relationships between concepts.

Informant
A person who provides research data, including both those who agree to participate in a study and those whom the researcher observes without their knowledge.

Informed consent
A process that precedes fieldwork, in which the people to be studied are informed of the goals and methods of the research and then asked for their consent, or otherwise, to participation in the project.

Interpretation
A researcher's view of the meaning of the data collected from the research process.

Life history
A story, or account, of a person's life as a whole. The aim of the research can either be to simply report the person's life or it can be oriented to examining particular theories.

Medical anthropology
The study of the social, symbolic and material lives of human societies in relation to health and illness.

Medicalisation
A process by which aspects of people's social lives and health come under the control of medicine. The medical professions exert their power over people's health and well-being.

Memory-work
A method that makes use of retrospective information from the informant. The researcher acts as a key informant in the process and shares equal power and tasks with other participants.

Moderator
A key person in focus groups method. A moderator leads and controls group discussions.

Narrative analysis
A research methodology that focuses on the structure and nature of the narratives, or stories, produced.

Observation
The process of collecting data by looking rather than listening.

Ontology
The study of 'being', or the fundamental nature of things. A positivist ontology emphasises that the world is objective, uninfluenced by who is looking. A postmodernist ontology suggests that the world is fluid, always changing, and fundamentally shaped by the person who is observing.

Participant
An informant who has been told about the research and has agreed to participate in the project.

Participant observation
A particular method of collecting data employed in ethnography. The researcher lives in the community under study, observes their daily activities, participates in their everyday life, learns how they view the world, and witnesses firsthand how they behave.

Participatory action research
A method in which research and action are joined in order to plan, implement and monitor change. The informants become co-researchers and hence have their voices heard in all aspects of the research. The researcher becomes a participant in the initiatives and uses his or her research knowledge and expertise to assist the informants to self-research.

Patriarchal ideology
The idea and practice in societies where men dominate women in all aspects of their social lives.

Phenomenology
A European philosophical tradition developed by Husserl and Schutz, and popularised in America by Berger and Luckmann. Phenomenologists study people's understandings and interpretations of their experiences in their own terms, emphasising these as explanations for their actions.

Population
A group, or cases, from which the sample in a research project is selected.

Positivism
An approach to research that believes social science research methods should be scientific in the same way as the physical sciences such as physics or chemistry. Qualitative researchers reject the arguments of positivism, pointing out that meanings and interpretations cannot be measured like physical objects.

Postmodernism
'The culture, including the theories, of postmodernity; any culture or theory that studies, practices, celebrates, or otherwise takes seriously the breaking apart of modernity' (Lemert 1997, p. 67).

Postmodernity
An historical period identified by some theorists to follow after modernity, beginning sometime late in the twentieth century.

Poststructuralism
A philosophical movement that rejects structuralist analysis. A person, or 'subject', is not separate from the structures of the world, as the structuralists believed, but dissolves into them. History is not a story of gradual development, rather history develops and regresses without any general trend. The meaning of something is not determined by the thing referred to; rather, meanings are arbitrary, and determined by tradition and common usage.

Purposive sampling
Sampling that selects cases with the purpose of providing a representative sample of the different processes involved. Purposive sampling does not provide a statistically representative sample.

Reflexivity
An acknowledgment of the role and influence of the researcher on the research project. The role of the researcher is subject to the same critical analysis and scrutiny as the research itself.

Research proposal
A document describing how the research will be conducted and justifying the need for the research. It is normally written prior to the commencement of the research project.

Research publication
The final product of a research project. It is used for the dissemination of research findings and may be in the form of a research report, journal article, book or monograph.

Rigour
Rigorous qualitative research is trustworthy and can be relied upon by other researchers. 'Rigour' is preferred to the terms 'validity' and 'reliability', used by

quantitative researchers, because 'rigour' indicates the different methodology involved in research that focuses on meanings and interpretations.

Semiotic analysis
A form of data analysis that examines the hidden, omitted or repressed themes in a text, typically with reference to broader social and political contexts.

Subjectivity
The awareness of oneself as a subject, as a self-conscious person.

Symbolic interactionism
An American tradition that typically uses qualitative research methods to study the way people make sense of their experiences through common symbols and symbolic processes. Its leading protagonists include G.H. Mead, M. Blumer, and more recently, N. Denzin.

Thematic analysis
The identification of themes through a careful reading and rereading of the data. The methodology is inductive, building up concepts and theories from the data, compared with the deductive methodology of content analysis.

Theme
A grouping of data emerging from the research and one to which the researcher gives a name.

Theme list
A set of topics used to guide focused or in-depth interviews.

Theoretical sampling
The sampling strategy of grounded theory. The sample evolves during the research, with sampling proceeding on theoretical grounds rather than statistical grounds. New units are selected to be part of the sample on the basis of the need to fill out particular concepts or theoretical points (Glaser and Strauss 1968; Strauss and Corbin 1990).

Thick description
Descriptions based on qualitative research, typically ethnography, where ample detail and background information are provided so that people's actions can be understood in the context of the experiences and patterns of meaning that influence them.

Track record
Usually refers to the past performance of a researcher, including success in obtaining research funding and in having published in the related area. It is typically important in obtaining research funds.

Triangulation
Refers to the use of multiple methods, researchers, data sources, or theories in a research project.

Unit of analysis

The building block of data collection and analysis. Units of analysis include people, meanings, practices, encounters, narrative structures and organisations.

Unobtrusive method

A method that does not require direct contact with the informants. It makes use of data that have been published or are available in libraries, the press, or other media. Indirect and unobtrusive observation, where the informants have no knowledge about the research, is also employed.

References

Agar, M. and MacDonald, J., 1995, 'Focus Groups and Ethnography', *Human Organization*, vol. 54, no. 1, pp. 78–86.

Agar, M.H., 1986, *Speaking of Ethnography*, Sage, Beverly Hills.

Agar, M., 1991, 'The Right Brain Strikes Back', in N. Fielding and R. Lee (eds), *Using Computers in Qualitative Research*, Sage, Newbury Park.

Agger, B., 1990, *The Decline of Discourse: Reading, Writing and Resistance in Postmodern Capitalism*, Falmer Press, Bristol, PA.

Ainlay, S., 1986, 'The Encounter with Phenomenology', in J. Hunter and S. Ainlay (eds), *Making Sense of Modern Times: Peter L. Berger and the Vision of Interpretive Sociology*, Routledge & Kegan Paul, London.

Altheide, D., 1987, 'Ethnographic Content Analysis', *Qualitative Sociology*, vol. 10, no. 1, pp. 65–77.

Altheide, D. and Johnson, J., 1994, 'Criteria for Assessing Interpretive Validity in Qualitative Research', in N. Denzin and Y. Lincoln (eds), *Handbook of Qualitative Research*, Sage, Thousand Oaks.

Anderson, H. and Goolishian, H., 1992, 'The Client Is the Expert', in S. McNamee and K. Gergen (eds), *Therapy as Social Construction*, Sage, London.

Annett, H. and Rifkin, S., 1988, *Guidelines for Rapid Appraisals To Assess Community Health Needs: A Focus on Health Improvements for Low-Income Urban Areas*, WHO (Division of Strengthening of Health Services), Geneva.

Armstrong, D., Gosling, A., Weinman, J. and Marteau, T., 1997, 'The Place of Inter-Rater Reliability in Qualitative Research', *Sociology*, vol. 31, no. 3, pp. 597–606.

Atkinson, B., Heath, A., Chenail, R., Cavell, A. and Snyder, D., 1991, 'Qualitative Research: Responses to Moon, Dillon and Sprenkle', *Journal of Marital and Family Therapy*, vol. 17, no. 3, pp. 161–71.

Atkinson, P. and Hammersley, M., 1994, 'Ethnography and Participant Observation', in N.K. Denzin and Y.S. Lincoln (eds), *Handbook of Qualitative Research*, Sage, Thousand Oaks.

Attig, G.A. and Winichagoon, P., 1993, *Effective Proposal Writing: From Ideals to Projects*, Institute of Nutrition, Mahidol University, Salaya, Thailand.

Attig, G.A., Winichagoon, P. and Yoddumnern-Attig, B., 1993, 'Designing and Writing Qualitative Research Reports', in B. Yoddumnern-Attig, G.A. Attig, W. Boonchalaksi,

K. Richter and A. Soonthorndhada (eds), *Qualitative Methods for Population and Health Research*, Institute for Population and Social Research, Mahidol University, Salaya, Thailand.

Bammer, G., Ostini, R. and Sengoz, A., 1995, 'Using Ambulance Service Records to Examine Nonfatal Heroin Overdose', *Australian Journal of Public Health*, vol. 19, no. 3, pp. 316–17.

Bart, P., 1969, 'Why Women's Status Changes in Middle Age', *Sociological Symposium*, no. 13, Fall, pp. 1–18.

Bartos, M., Ezzy, D., McDonald, K., O'Donnell, D. and de Visser, R., 1998, 'Treatments, Intimacy and Disclosure in the Sexual Practice of HIV-Infected Adults in Australia', 12th World AIDS Conference, Geneva, July.

Basch, C.E., 1987, 'Focus Group Interviews: An Underutilised Research Technique for Theory and Practice in Health Education', *Health Education Quarterly*, vol. 14, no. 4, pp. 411–48.

Batchelor, J. and Briggs, C., 1994, 'Subject, Project or Self? Thoughts on Ethical Dilemmas for Social and Medical Researchers', *Social Science and Medicine*, vol. 39, no. 7, pp. 949–54.

Baum, F., 1995, 'Researching Public Health: Behind the Qualitative–Quantitative Methodological Debate', *Social Science and Medicine*, vol. 40, no. 4, pp. 459–68.

Becker, C., 1992, *Living and Relating: An Introduction to Phenomenology*, Sage, Newbury Park.

Becker, H. and Greer, B., 1957, 'Participant Observation and Interviewing: A Comparison', *Human Organization*, vol. 16, no. 3, pp. 28–32.

Beilharz, P. (ed.), 1991, *Social Theory: A Guide to Central Thinkers*, Allen & Unwin, Sydney.

Beilharz, P., 1994, *Postmodern Socialism*, Melbourne University Press, Melbourne.

Bell, D., 1993, 'Introduction 1: The Context', in D. Bell, P. Caplan and W.J. Karim (eds), *Gendered Fields: Women, Men and Ethnography*, Routledge, London.

Bell, D., Caplan, P. and Karim, W.J. (eds), 1993, *Gendered Fields: Women, Men and Ethnography*, Routledge, London.

Bentley, M. et al., 1988, 'Rapid Ethnographic Assessment: Applications in a Diarrhoea Management Programme', *Social Science and Medicine*, vol. 27, no. 1, pp. 107–16.

Berg, B., 1989, *Qualitative Research Methods for the Social Sciences*, Allyn & Bacon, Boston.

Bergen, R., 1993, 'Interviewing Survivors of Marital Rape', in C. Renzetti and R. Lee (eds), *Research Sensitive Topics*, Sage, Newbury Park.

Berger, A.A., 1993, *Improving Writing Skills*, Sage, New York.

Berger, P., 1975, *Invitation to Sociology*, Penguin, Harmondsworth.

Berger, P., 1977, *Facing Up to Modernity*, Basic Books, New York.

Berger, P. and Luckmann, T., 1967, *The Social Construction of Reality*, Penguin, Harmondsworth.

Bernard, H., 1988, *Research Methods in Cultural Anthropology*, Sage, Beverly Hills.

Bernard, H.R., 1995, *Research Methods in Anthropology: Qualitative and Quantitative Approaches*, 2nd edn, AltaMira Press, Walnut Creek, California.

Berry, J.W., 1979, 'Unobtrusive Measures in Cross-Cultural Research', in L. Sechrest (ed.), *Unobtrusive Measures Today*, Jossey-Bass, San Francisco.

Bertaux, D. and Kohli, M., 1984, 'The Life Story Approach', *Annual Review of Sociology*, vol. 10, pp. 215–37.

Biernacki, P. and Waldorf, D., 1981, 'Snowball Sampling', *Sociological Methods and Research*, vol. 10, no. 2, pp. 141–63.

Black, R.B., 1991, 'Women's Voices after Pregnancy Loss: Couples' Patterns of Communication and Support', *Social Work in Health Care*, vol. 16, no. 2, pp. 19–36.

Blake, C.F., 1981, 'Graffiti and Racial Insults: The Archaeology of Ethnic Relations in Hawaii', in R.A. Gould and M.B. Schiffer (eds), *Modern Material Culture: The Archaeology of Us*, Academic Press, New York.

Blaxter, M., 1996, 'Criteria for the Evaluation of Qualitative Research Papers', *Medical Sociology News*, vol. 22, no. 1, supplementary.

Blink, P.J. and Wood, M.J., 1988, *Basic Steps in Planning Nursing Research: From Question to Proposal*, 3rd edn, Jones & Bartlett Publishers, Boston.

Bloor, M., 1986, 'Social Control in the Therapeutic Community: A Re-Examination of a Critical Case', *Sociology of Health and Illness*, vol. 8, no. 4, pp. 305–24.

Blumer, H., 1969, *Symbolic Interactionism, Perspective and Method*, Prentice-Hall, Englewood Cliffs, New Jersey.

Bochner, S., 1979, 'Designing Unobtrusive Field Experiments in Social Psychology', in L. Sechrest (ed.), *Unobtrusive Measures Today*, Jossey-Bass, San Francisco.

Bogardus, E.S., 1926, 'The Group Interview', *Journal of Applied Sociology*, vol. 10, pp. 372–82.

Bogdan, R., 1974, *Being Different: The Autobiography of Jane Fry*, Wiley, London.

Bogdan, R. and Taylor, S.J., 1975, *Introduction to Qualitative Research Methods: A Phenomenological Approach to the Social Sciences*, John Wiley & Sons, New York.

Bogdan, R.C. and Biklen, S.K., 1982, *Qualitative Research for Education: An Introduction to Theory and Method*, Allyn & Bacon, Boston.

Booth, T. and Booth, W., 1994, 'The Use of Depth Interviewing with Vulnerable Subjects', *Social Science and Medicine*, vol. 39, no. 2, pp. 415–24.

Borkan, J., Reis, S., Hermoni, D. and Biderman, A., 1995, 'Talking about the Pain: A Patient-Centred Study of Low Back Pain in Primary Care', *Social Science and Medicine*, vol. 40, no. 7, pp. 977–88.

Bowling, A., 1997, *Research Methods in Health*, Open University Press, Buckingham.

Boyle, J., 1991, 'Field Research: A Collaborative Model for Practice and Research', in J. Morse (ed.), *Qualitative Nursing Research: A Contemporary Dialogue*, Sage, Newbury Park, California.

Brooks, P., 1984, *Reading for the Plot*, Clarendon Press, Oxford.

Brooks, P., 1994, *Psychoanalysis and Storytelling*, Blackwell, Oxford.

Brown, B., Nolan, P., Crawford, P. and Lewis, A., 1996, 'Interaction, Language and the Narrative Turn in Psychotherapy and Psychiatry', *Social Science and Medicine*, vol. 43, 1569–78.

Brown, R., 1987, *Society as Text*, University of Chicago Press, Chicago.

Browne, A., 1987, *When Battered Women Kill*, Free Press, New York.

Bruner, E.M. and Kelso, J.P., 1980, 'Gender Differences in Graffiti: A Semiotic Perspective', *Women's Studies International Quarterly*, vol. 3, no. 2/3, pp. 239–52.

Bruner, J., 1986, *Actual Minds, Possible Worlds*, Harvard University Press, Cambridge, Mass.

Bruner, J., 1987, 'Life as Narrative', *Social Research*, vol. 54, no. 1, pp. 11–32.

Bruner, J., 1990, *Acts of Meaning*, Harvard University Press, Cambridge, Mass.

Bruner, J., 1995, 'The Autobiographical Process', *Current Sociology*, vol. 35, no. 1, pp. 161–76.

Bulmer, M. (ed.), 1982, *Social Research Ethics*, Macmillan, London.

Burgess, R., 1984, *In The Field: An Introduction to Field Research*, Allen & Unwin, London.

Burke, K., 1945, *A Grammar of Motives*, Prentice-Hall, New York.

Cadava, E., Connor, P. and Nancy, J., 1991, *Who Comes after the Subject?* Routledge, New York.

Cardador, M.T., Hazan, A.R. and Glantz, S.A., 1995, 'Tobacco Industry Smokers' Rights Publications: A Content Analysis', *American Journal of Public Health*, vol. 85, no. 9, pp. 1212–17.

Carey, M.A., 1994, 'The Group Effect in Focus Groups: Planning, Implementing and Interpreting Focus Group Research', in J. Morse (ed.), *Critical Issues in Qualitative Research Methods*, Sage, Thousand Oaks, CA.

Carey, M.A., 1995, 'Issues and Applications of Focus Groups: Introduction', *Qualitative Health Research*, vol. 5, no. 4, p. 413.

Carey, M.A. and Smith, M., 1994, 'Capturing the Group Effect in Focus Groups: A Special Concern in Analysis', *Qualitative Health Research*, vol. 4, no. 1, pp. 123–7.

Carpenter, J.P., 1977, *The Screwdriver (Does It or Doesn't It?)*, Arizona State Museum Library, University of Arizona, Tucson.

Cecil, R., 1994, ' "I Wouldn't Have Minded a Wee One Running About": Miscarriage and the Family', *Social Science and Medicine*, vol. 38, no. 10, pp. 1415–22.

Cecil, R., 1996, 'Introduction: An Insignificant Event? Literary and Anthropological Perspectives on Pregnancy Loss', in R. Cecil (ed.), *The Anthropology of Pregnancy Loss: Comparative Studies in Miscarriage, Stillbirth and Neonatal Death*, Berg, Oxford.

Cecil, R. and Leslie, J.C., 1993, 'Early Miscarriage: Preliminary Results from a Study in Northern Ireland', *Journal of Reproductive and Infant Psychology*, vol. 15, pp. 347–52.

Chagnon, N.A., 1977, *Yanomamo: The Fierce People*, Holt, Rinehart & Winston, New York.

Chalmers, B. and Meyer, D., 1992a, 'A Cross-Cultural View of the Psychosocial Management of Miscarriage', *Journal of Psychosomatic Obstetrics and Gynaecology*, vol. 13, pp. 163–76.

Chalmers, B. and Meyer, D., 1992b, 'A Cross-Cultural View of the Emotional Management of Miscarriage', *Journal of Psychosomatic Obstetrics and Gynaecology*, vol. 13, pp. 177–86.

Chambron, A., 1995, 'Life History as a Dialogical Activity', *Current Sociology*, vol. 35, no. 1, pp. 127–35.

Chapman, S. and Hodgson, J., 1988, 'Showers in Raincoats: Attitudinal Barriers to Condom Use in High-Risk Heterosexuals', *Community Health Studies*, vol. XII, no. 1, pp. 97–105.

Charmaz, K., 1990, 'Discovering Chronic Illness: Using Grounded Theory', *Social Science and Medicine*, vol. 30, no. 10, pp. 1161–72.

Charmaz, K., 1991, *Good Days, Bad Days: The Self in Chronic Illness and Time*, Rutgers University Press, New Brunswick.

Charmaz, K., 1995, 'The Body, Identity and Self: Adapting to Impairment', *Sociological Quarterly*, vol. 36, no. 4, pp. 657–80.

Chase, S., 1995, 'Taking Narrative Seriously', in R. Josselson and E. Leiblich (eds), *Interpreting Experience: The Narrative Study of Lives*, vol. 3, Sage, London.

Chirawatkul, S. Sud Lyad, Sud Luuk: The Social Construction of Menopause in North-eastern Thailand, unpublished PhD thesis, University of Queensland, Brisbane.

Chrisler, J.C. and Levy, K.B., 1990, 'The Media Construct a Menstrual Monster: A Content Analysis of PMS Articles in the Popular Press', *Women and Health*, vol. 16, no. 2, pp. 89–105.

Clark, P. and Bowling, A., 1990, 'Quality of Everyday Life in Long Stay Institutions for the Elderly: An Observational Study of Long Stay Hospital and Nursing Home Care', *Social Science and Medicine*, vol. 30, no. 11, pp. 1201–10.

Clough, P., 1992, *The End(s) of Ethnography*, Sage, Newbury Park.

Clough, P., 1994, *Feminist Thought*, Blackwell, Oxford.

Cohen, A.B., Greenwood, D.J. and Harkavay, I., 1992, 'Social Research for Social Change: Varieties of Participatory Action Research', *Collaborative Inquiry*, no. 7, pp. 2–8.

Cole, J.W., 1977, 'Anthropology Comes Part Way Home: Community Studies in Europe', *Annual Review of Anthropology*, vol. 6, pp. 349–78.

Collins, P., 1991, *Black Feminist Thought*, Routledge, New York.

Colquhoun, D. and Kellehear, A. (eds), 1993, *Health Research in Practice: Political, Ethical and Methodological Issues*, Chapman & Hall, London.

Colquhoun, D. and Kellehear, A. (eds), 1996, *Health Research in Practice, Volume 2: Personal Experiences, Public Issues*, Chapman & Hall, London.

Corbin, J. and Strauss, A., 1990, 'Grounded Theory Research', *Qualitative Sociology*, vol. 13, no. 1, pp. 3–21.

Cordle, C.J. and Prettyman, R.J., 1994, 'A 2-Year Follow-Up of Women Who Have Experienced Early Miscarriage', *Journal of Reproductive and Infant Psychology*, vol. 12, pp. 37–43.

Coreil, J., Augustin, A., Holt, E. and Halsey, N.A., 1989, 'Use of Ethnographic Research for Instrument Development in a Case-Control Study of Immunization Use in Haiti', *International Journal of Epidemiology*, vol. 18, no. 4 (suppl. 2), pp. S33–7.

Corin, E. and Lauzon, G., 1992, 'Positive Withdrawal and the Quest for Meaning: The Reconstruction of Experience among Schizophrenics', *Psychiatry, Interpersonal and Biological Processes*, vol. 55, no. 3, pp. 266–79.

Cornwall, A., 1996, 'Towards Participatory Practice: Participatory Rural Appraisal (PRA) and the Participatory Process', in K. de Koning and M. Martin (eds), *Participatory Research in Health: Issues and Experiences*, Zed Books, London.

Cortazzi, M., 1993, *Narrative Analysis*, Falmer Press, London.

Crawford, J., Kippax, S., Onyx, J., Gault, U. and Benton, P., 1992, *Emotion and Gender: Constructing Meaning from Memory*, Sage, London.

Dalrymple, L. and Preston-Whyte, E.M., 1992, 'A Drama Approach to AIDS Education: An Experiment in "Action Research"', *AIDS Bulletin*, vol. 1, no. 1, pp. 9–11.

Daly, J., 1996, *Ethical Intersections: Health Research, Methods and Researcher Responsibility*, Allen & Unwin, Sydney.

Daly, J., Kellehear, A. and Gliksman, M., 1997, *The Public Health Researcher: A Methodological Approach*, Oxford University Press, Melbourne.

Daly, J. and McDonald, I., 1992, 'Introduction: The Problem as We Saw It', in J. Daly, I. McDonald and E. Willis (eds), *Researching Health Care: Designs, Dilemmas, Disciplines*, Routledge, London.

Daly, J., McDonald, I. and Willis, E., 1992, 'Why Don't You Ask Them? A Qualitative Research Framework for Investigating the Diagnosis of Cardiac Normality', in J. Daly, I. McDonald and E. Willis (eds), *Researching Health Care: Designs, Dilemmas, Disciplines*, Routledge, London.

Danziger, S.K., 1979, 'On Doctor Watching: Fieldwork in Medical Settings', *Urban Life*, vol. 7, no. 4, pp. 513–32.

Davies, B., 1990, 'Menstruation and Women's Subjectivity', paper presented at the Australian Sociological Association (TASA) Conference, Brisbane.

Davis, D.L., 1997, 'Blood and Nerves Revisited: Menopause and the Privatization of the Body in a Newfoundland Postindustrial Fishery', *Medical Anthropology Quarterly*, vol. 11, no. 1, pp. 3–20.

Dawson, S., Manderson, L. and Tallo, V.L., 1993, *A Manual for the Use of Focus Groups*, International Nutrition Foundation for Developing Countries (INFDC), Boston.

Day, R.A., 1979, *How To Write and Publish a Scientific Paper*, ISI Press, Philadelphia.

de Koning, K. and Martin, M. (eds), 1996, *Participatory Research in Health: Issues and Experiences*, Zed Books, London.

de Roux, G.I., 1991, 'Together against the Computer', in O. Fals-Borda and M.A. Rahman (eds), *Action and Knowledge: Breaking the Monopoly with Participatory Action-Research*, Apex Press, New York.

Denzin, N., 1970, *The Research Act*, Aldine, Chicago.

Denzin, N., 1978, *The Research Act: A Theoretical Introduction to Sociological Methods*, 2nd edn, Aldine, Chicago.

Denzin, N., 1986, 'Interpreting the Lives of Ordinary People: Sartre, Heidegger and Faulkner', *Life Stories/Recits de Vie*, vol. 2, no. 1, pp. 6–20.

Denzin, N., 1989a, *Interpretive Biography*, Sage, Newbury Park.

Denzin, N., 1989b, *Interpretive Interactionism*, Sage, Newbury Park.

Denzin, N., 1991, *Images of Postmodern Society*, Sage, London.

Denzin, N., 1992, *Symbolic Interactionism and Cultural Studies*, Blackwell, Cambridge, Mass.

Denzin, N., 1994, 'The Art and Politics of Interpretation', in N. Denzin and Y. Lincoln (eds), *Handbook of Qualitative Research*, Sage, Thousand Oaks.

Denzin, N., 1997, *Interpretive Ethnography*, Sage, Thousand Oaks.

Denzin, N. and Lincoln, Y. (eds), 1994a, *Handbook of Qualitative Research*, Sage, Thousand Oaks.

Denzin, N. and Lincoln, Y., 1994b, 'Introduction: Entering the Field of Qualitative Research', in N. Denzin and Y. Lincoln (eds), *Handbook of Qualitative Research*, Sage, Thousands Oaks.

Denzin, N. and Lincoln, Y., 1995, 'Transforming Qualitative Research Methods', *Journal of Contemporary Ethnography*, vol. 24, no. 3, pp. 349–58.

Dey, I., 1993, *Qualitative Data Analysis: A User Friendly Guide for Social Scientists*, Routledge & Kegan Paul, London.

Dockery, G., 1996, 'Rhetoric or Reality?: Participatory Research in the National Health Service, UK', in K. de Koning and M. Martin (eds), *Participatory Research in Health: Issues and Experiences*, Zed Books, London.

Douglas, J., 1976, *Investigative Social Research*, Sage, Beverly Hills.

Douglas, J., 1985, *Creative Interviewing*, Sage, Beverly Hills.

Dowdall, G.W. and Golden, J., 1989, 'Photographs as Data: An Analysis of Images from a Mental Hospital', *Qualitative Sociology*, vol. 12, no. 2, pp. 183–213.

Doyal, L., 1981, *The Political Economy of Health*, Pluto Press, London.

Doyal, L., 1995, *What Makes Women Sick: Gender and the Political Economy of Health*, Macmillan, London.

Duhl, L. and Hancock, T., 1988, *A Guide to Assessing Healthy Cities*, WHO Healthy Cities Papers No. 3., FADL Publishers, Copenhagen.

Edwards, J. and Lampert, M. (eds), 1993, *Talking Data: Transcription and Coding in Discourse Research*, Lawrence Erlbaum, Hillsdale, NJ.

Ely, M., Vinz, R., Downing, M. and Anzul, M., 1997, *On Writing Qualitative Research: Living by Words*, Falmer Press, London.

Emerson, R.M., Fretz, R.I. and Shaw, L.L., 1995, *Writing Ethnographic Fieldnotes*, University of Chicago Press, Chicago.

Englemann, G.J., 1882, *Labor among Primitive Peoples*, J.H. Chambers, St Louis.

Ezzy, D., 1996, Job Loss, Narrative-Identity and the Meaning of Working, PhD thesis, La Trobe University, Melbourne.

Ezzy, D., 1998, 'Lived Experience and Interpretation in Narrative Theory', *Qualitative Sociology*, vol. 21, no. 1, pp. 169–80.

Ezzy, D., Bartos, M., de Visser, R. and Rosenthal, D., 1998, 'Antiretroviral Uptake in Australia: Medical, Attitudinal and Cultural Correlates', *International Journal of STD and AIDS*, vol. 9, pp. 579–86.

Ezzy, D., de Visser, R. and Bartos, M., 1999, 'Poverty, Disease Progression and Employment among People Living with HIV/AIDS in Australia', *AIDS Care*, vol. 11, no. 1, pp. 112–33.

Faberman, H., 1992, 'The Grounds of Critique', *Symbolic Interaction*, vol. 15, no. 3, pp. 375–9.

Fals-Borda, O. and Rahman, M.A. (eds), 1991, *Action and Knowledge: Breaking the Monopoly with Participatory Action Research*, Apex Press, New York.

Farrar, P., 1994, 'Memory Work as Method', unpublished seminar paper, University of Technology, Sydney.

Fernandes, W. and Tandon, R., 1981, *Participatory Research and Evaluation: Experiments in Research as a Process of Liberation*, Indian Social Institute, New Delhi.

Fetterman, D., 1989, *Ethnography: Step by Step*, Sage Publications, Newbury Park.

Fielding, N., 1993, 'Ethnography', in N. Gilbert (ed.), *Researching Social Life*, Sage, London.

Fitzclarence, L., 1991, 'Remembering the Reconceptualist Project', paper presented at Bergamo Conference, Dayton, Ohio, 16–19 October.

Flick, U., 1992, 'Triangulation Revisited: Strategy of Validation or Alternative?', *Journal for the Theory of Social Behaviour*, vol. 22, no. 2, pp. 175–97.

Folch-Lyon, E. and Trost, J.F., 1981, 'Conducting Focus Group Sessions', *Studies in Family Planning*, vol. 12, no. 2, pp. 443–9.

Fontana, A. and Frey, J., 1994, 'Interviewing: The Art of Science', in N. Denzin and Y. Lincoln (eds), *Handbook of Qualitative Research*, Sage, Thousand Oaks.

Ford, H., 1923, *My Life and Work*, Angus & Robertson, Sydney.

Foucault, M., 1967, *Madness and Civilization*, Routledge, London.

Fox, M.F. (ed.), 1985, *Scholarly Writing and Publishing: Issues, Problems and Solutions*, Westview, Boulder, Colorado.

Frank, A., 1995, *The Wounded Storyteller*, University of Chicago Press, Chicago.

Frank, G., 1996, 'Life History in Occupational Therapy Clinical Practice', *American Journal of Occupational Therapy*, vol. 50, no. 2, pp. 251–6.

Freire, P., 1972, *Pedagogy of the Oppressed* (trans. M.B. Ramos), Penguin, Harmondsworth.

Frideman, T., 1989, 'Women's Experiences of General Practitioner Management of Miscarriage', *Journal of the Royal College of General Practitioners*, vol. 39, pp. 456–8.

Frideman, T. and Gath, D., 1989, 'The Psychiatric Consequences of Spontaneous Abortion', *British Journal of Psychiatry*, vol. 155, pp. 810–13.

Fuller, T.D., Edwards, J.N., Vorakitphokatorn, S. and Sermsri, S., 1993, 'Using Focus Groups To Adapt Survey Instruments to New Populations: Experience from a Developing Country', in D.L. Morgan (ed.), *Successful Focus Groups: Advancing the State of the Art*, Sage, Newbury Park.

Furin, J.J., 1997, ' "You Have To Be Your Own Doctor": Sociocultural Influences on Alternative Therapy Use among Gay Men with AIDS in West Hollywood', *Medical Anthropology Quarterly*, vol. 11, no. 4, pp. 498–504.

Gadamer, H., 1975, *Truth and Method*, Seabury, New York.

Gartner, L.M. and Stone, C., 1994, 'Two Thousand Years of Medical Advice on Breastfeeding: Comparison of Chinese and Western Texts', *Seminars in Perinatology*, vol. 18, no. 6, pp. 532–6.

Gaventa, J. and Horton, B., 1981, 'A Citizen's Research Project in Appalachia', *Convergence*, vol. 14, no. 1, pp. 30–40.

Gee, J., 1986, 'Units in the Production of Narrative Discourse', *Discourse Processes*, vol. 9, no. 3, pp. 391–422.

Geertz, C., 1973, *The Interpretation of Cultures*, Basic Books, New York.

George, A., 1996, 'Methodological Issues in the Ethnographic Study of Sexuality: Experiences from Bombay', in K. de Koning and M. Martin (eds), *Participatory Research in Health: Issues and Experiences*, Zed Books, London.

Gergen, K. and Gergen, M., 1988, 'Narrative and the Self as Relationship', *Advances in Experimental Social Psychology*, vol. 21, pp. 17–56.

Gergen, K. and Kaye, J., 1993, 'Beyond Narrative in the Negotiation of Therapeutic Meaning', in K. Gergen (ed.), *Refiguring the Self and Psychology*, Aldershot, Dartmouth.

Gergen, M., 1992, 'Life Stories: Pieces of a Dream', in G. Rosenwald and R. Ochberg (eds), *Storied Lives*, Yale University Press, London.

Gergen, M. and Gergen, K., 1993, 'Narratives of the Gendered Body in Popular Autobiography', in R. Josselson and A. Lieblich (eds), *The Narrative Study of Lives*, Sage, Newbury Park.

Gerson, E., 1991, 'Supplementing Grounded Theory', in D. Maines (ed.), *Social Organization and Social Process*, Aldine de Gruyter, New York.

Giddens, A. (ed.), 1974, *Positivism and Sociology*, Heinemann Educational Books, London.

Glaser, B. and Strauss, A., 1968, *The Discovery of Grounded Theory*, Aldine, Chicago.

Goffman, E., 1961, *Asylums*, Penguin, Harmondsworth.

Goffman, E., 1967, *Interaction Ritual*, Penguin, Harmondsworth.

Goffman, E., 1989, 'On Fieldwork', *Journal of Contemporary Ethnography*, vol. 18, no. 2, pp. 123–32.

Goode, E., 1996, 'The Ethics of Deception in Social Research', *Qualitative Sociology*, vol. 19, no. 1, pp. 11–33.

Goodwin, L. and Goodwin, W., 1984, 'Are Validity and Reliability "Relevant" in Qualitative Evaluation Research?', *Evaluation and the Health Professions*, vol. 7, no. 4, pp. 413–26.

Gorter, A., Miranda, E., Smith, G.D., Ortells, P. and Low, N., 1993, 'How Many People Actively Use Condoms? An Investigation of Motel Clients in Managua, *Social Science and Medicine*, vol. 36, no. 12, pp. 1645–7.

Grafanaki, S., 1996, 'How Research Can Change the Researcher: The Need for Sensitivity, Flexibility and Ethical Boundaries in Conducting Qualitative Research in Counselling/Psychotherapy', *British Journal of Guidance and Counselling*, vol. 24, no. 3, pp. 329–38.

Greenwood, D.J., Whyte, W.F. and Harkavay, I., 1993, 'Participatory Action Research as Process and as Goal', *Human Relations*, vol. 46, no. 2, pp. 175–92.

Grund, J.-P.C., Kaplan, C.D. and Adriaans, F.P., 1991, 'Needle Sharing in The Netherlands: An Ethnographic Analysis', *American Journal of Public Health*, vol. 81, no. 12, pp. 1602–7.

Guba, E. and Lincoln, Y., 1994, 'Competing Paradigms in Qualitative Research', in N. Denzin and Y. Lincoln (eds), *Handbook of Qualitative Research*, Sage, Thousand Oaks.

Hahn, R.A., 1987, 'Divisions of Labour: Obstetrician, Woman and Society in Williams Obstetrics, 1903–1985', *Medical Anthropology Quarterly*, vol. 1, no. 3, pp. 256–81.

Hall, B., 1981, 'Participatory Research, Popular Knowledge and Power: A Personal Reflection', *Convergence*, vol. XIV, no. 3, pp. 6–17.

Hall, B, 1993, 'Participatory Research', in *International Encyclopedia of Education*, Pergamon, London.

Hall, M., 1971, *Developing Skills in Proposal Writing*, 2nd edn, Continuing Publications, Portland, Oregon.

Hammersley, M., 1992a, *What's Wrong with Ethnography*, Routledge, London.

Hammersley, M., 1992b, 'Deconstructing the Qualitative–Quantitative Divide', in J. Brannen (ed.), *Mixing Methods: Qualitative and Quantitative Research*, Aldershot, Avebury.

Hammersley, M. and Atkinson, P., 1995, *Ethnography: Principles in Practice*, 2nd edn, Routledge, London.

Hart, E. and Bond, M., 1995, *Action Research for Health and Social Care: A Guide to Practice*, Open University Press, Buckingham.

Harvey, D., 1989, *The Condition of Postmodernity*, Blackwell, Oxford.

Hassin, J., 1994, 'Living a Responsible Life: The Impact of AIDS on the Social Identity of Intravenous Drug Users', *Social Science and Medicine*, vol. 39, no. 3, pp. 391–400.

Haug, F. (ed.), 1987, *Female Sexualization: A Collective Work of Memory*, Verso, London.

Haug, F., 1992, *Beyond Female Masochism: Memory-Work and Politics*, Verso, London.

Hazan, A.R., Lipton, H.L. and Glantz, S.A., 1994, 'Popular Films Do Not Reflect Current Tobacco Use', *American Journal of Public Health*, vol. 84, no. 6, pp. 998–1000.

Hecker, R., 1997, 'Participatory Action Research as a Strategy for Empowerment of Aboriginal Health Workers', *Australian and New Zealand Journal of Public Health*, vol. 21, no. 7, pp. 784–8.

Heidegger, M., 1962, *Being and Time* (trans. J. Macquarie and E. Robinson), Blackwell, London.

Helling, I., 1988, 'The Life History Method', *Studies in Symbolic Interaction*, vol. 9, no. 2, pp. 211–43.

Herzlich, C. and Pierret, J., 1989, 'The Construction of a Social Phenomenon: AIDS in the French Press', *Social Science and Medicine*, vol. 29, no. 11, pp. 1235–42.

Hey, V., 1989, 'A Feminist Exploration', in V. Hey, C. Itzin, L. Saunders and M. Speakman (eds), *Hidden Loss: Miscarriage and Ectopic Pregnancy*, The Woman's Press, London.

Hill, J. and Radiner, K., 1996, 'Health and Nutrition Messages in Food Advertisements: A Comparative Content Analysis of Young and Mature Australian Women's Magazines', *Journal of Nutrition Education*, vol. 28, pp. 313–21.

Hohnen, R., 1996, 'Women and Holidays: Memory-Work Research Project', unpublished research paper, University of Technology, Sydney.

Holman, H.R., 1993, 'Qualitative Inquiry in Medical Research', *Journal of Clinical Epidemiology*, vol. 46, no. 1, pp 29–36.

Holmes, W., Thorpe, L. and Phillips, J., 1997, 'Influences on Infant-Feeding Beliefs and Practices in an Urban Aboriginal Community', *Australian and New Zealand Journal of Public Health*, vol. 21, no. 5, pp. 504–10.

Holstein, J. and Gubrium, J., 1995, *The Active Interview*, Sage, Thousand Oaks.

Hornsby-Smith, M., 1993, 'Gaining Access', in N. Gilbert (ed.), *Research Social Life*, Sage, London.

Howard, M.C., 1996, *Contemporary Cultural Anthropology*, 5th edn, HarperCollins College Publishers, New York.

Hughes, D. and Dumont, K., 1993, 'Using Focus Groups To Facilitate Culturally Anchored Research', *American Journal of Community Psychology*, vol. 21, no. 6, pp. 775–806.

Hull, V., Widyantoro, N. and Fetters, T., 1996, 'No Problem: Reproductive Tract Infections in Indonesia', in P.L. Rice and L. Manderson (eds), *Maternity and Reproductive Health in Asian Societies*, Harwood Academic Publishers, Amsterdam.

Hyden, L., 1997, 'Illness and Narrative', *Sociology of Health and Illness*, vol. 19, no. 1, pp. 48–69.

Inhorn, M., 1994, *Quest for Conception: Gender, Infertility and Egyptian Medical Traditions*, University of Pennsylvania Press, Philadelphia.

Irwin, K., Bertrand, J., Mibandumba, N., Mbuyi, K. and Muremeri, C., 1991, 'Knowledge, Attitudes and Beliefs about HIV Infection and AIDS among Healthy Factory Workers and Their Wives', *Social Science and Medicine*, vol. 32, no. 8, pp. 17–30.

Jackson, M., 1989, *Paths toward a Clearing, Radical Empiricism and Ethnographic Inquiry*, Indiana University Press, Bloomington.

Janseen, H.J. and Van-Minnen, A., 1992, 'Prediction of Grief Intensity after Miscarriage', *Journal of Psychological Medicine*, vol. 20, pp. 226–35.

Jarrett, R.L., 1993, 'Focus Group Interviewing with Low-Income Minority Populations: A Research Experience', in D.L. Morgan (ed.), *Successful Focus Groups: Advancing the State of the Art*, Sage, Newbury Park.

Jarrett, R.L., 1994, 'Living Poor: Family Life among Single Parent, African-American Women', *Social Problems*, vol. 41, no. 1, pp. 30–49.

Jayaratne, T. and Abibail, S., 1991, 'Quantitative and Qualitative Methods in Social Sciences', in M. Fonow and J. Cook (eds), *Beyond Methodology*, Indiana University Press, Bloomington.

Jeffery, P., Jeffery, R. and Lyon, A., 1989, *Labour Pains and Labour Power: Women and Childbearing in India*, Zed Books, London.

Jones, J., 1997, Vietnamese Women and Cervical Screening: How To Encourage Them To Present, masters thesis, Monash University, Melbourne.

Joseph, J.G., Emmons, C.A., Kessler, R.C., Wortman, C.B. and O'Brien, K., 1984, 'Coping with the Threat of AIDS: An Approach to Psychosocial Assessment', *American Journal of Psychology*, vol. 39, no. 11 pp. 1297–1302.

Karger, T., 1987, 'Focus Groups Are for Focusing and for Little Else', *Marketing News*, 28 August, pp. 52–5.

Karp, D., 1996, *Speaking of Sadness: Depression, Disconnection and the Meanings of Illness*, Oxford University Press, New York.

Kaye, B.H., 1995, *Science and the Detective*, VCH Publishers, New York.

Kelle, U. (ed.), 1995, *Computer-Aided Qualitative Data Analysis: Theory, Methods and Practice*, Sage, London.

Kellehear, A., 1993a, *The Unobtrusive Researcher: A Guide to Methods*, Allen & Unwin, Sydney.

Kellehear, A., 1993b, 'Unobtrusive Research in Health Social Sciences', *Annual Review of Health Social Sciences*, vol. 3, pp. 46–59.

Kellehear, A., 1993c, 'Unobtrusive Methods in Medical Practice Research', in Proceedings of 1993 Work-In-Progress Conference on Methodological Aspects of General Practice Evaluation, General Practice Evaluation Program, Canberra.

Kemmis, S. and McTaggart, R. (eds), 1988, *The Action Research Reader*, 3rd edn, Deakin University Press, Geelong.

Khan, M.E., Anker, M., Patel, B.C., Barge, S., Sadhwani, H. and Kohle, R., 1991, 'The Use of Focus Groups in Social and Behavioural Research: Some Methodological Issues', *World Health Statistics Quarterly*, vol. 44, pp. 145–9.

Khan, M.E. and Manderson, L., 1992, 'Focus Groups in Tropical Diseases Research', *Health Policy and Planning*, vol. 7, no. 1, pp. 56–66.

Khanna, R., 1996, 'Participatory Action Research (PAR) in Women's Health: SARTHI, India', in K. de Koning and M. Martin (eds), *Participatory Research in Health: Issues and Experiences*, Zed Books, London.

Khanna, S.K., 1997, 'Traditions and Reproductive Technology in an Urbanizing North Indian Village', *Social Science and Medicine*, vol. 44, no. 2, pp. 171–80.

Kippax, S., 1990, 'Memory Work: A Method', in J. Daly and E. Willis (eds), *The Social Sciences and Health Research*, Public Health Association of Australia, Canberra.

Kippax, S., Crawford, J., Benton, P. and Gault, U., 1988, 'Constructing Emotions: Weaving Meaning from Memories', *British Journal of Social Psychology*, vol. 27, pp. 19–33.

Kippax, S., Crawford, J., Waldby, C. and Benton, P., 1990, 'Women Negotiating Heterosex: Implications for AIDS Prevention', *Women's Studies International Forum*, vol. 13, no. 2, pp. 533–42.

Kirk, J. and Miller, M., 1986, *Reliability and Validity in Qualitative Research*, Sage, Beverly Hills.

Kitzinger, J., 1994, 'The Methodology of Focus Groups: The Importance of Interaction between Research Participants', *Sociology of Health and Illness*, vol. 16, no. 1, pp. 103–21.

Kitzinger, J., 1995, 'Introducing Focus Groups', *British Medical Journal*, vol. 311, 29 July, pp. 299–302.

Kleinman, D.L. and Cohen, L.J., 1991, 'The Decontextualization of Mental Illness: The Portrayal of Work in Psychiatric Drug Advertisements', *Social Science and Medicine*, vol. 32, no. 8, pp. 867–74.

Kline, A., Kline, E. and Oken, E., 1992, 'Minority Women and Sexual Choice in the Age of AIDS', *Social Science and Medicine*, vol. 34, no. 4, pp. 447–57.

Knodel, J., 1994, 'Conducting Comparative Focus-Group Research: Cautionary Comments from a Coordinator', *Health Transition Review*, vol. 4, no. 1, pp. 99–104.

Knodel, J., 1995, 'Focus Group Research on the Living Arrangements of Elderly in Asia', *Journal of Cross-Cultural Gerontology*, vol. 10, pp. 1–162 (special issue).

Knodel, J., Chamratrithirong, A. and Debavalya, N., 1987, *Thailand's Reproductive Revolution: Rapid Fertility Decline in a Third-World Setting*, University of Wisconsin Press, Madison.

Knodel, J., Havanon, N. and Pramualratana, A., 1984, 'Fertility Transition in Thailand: A Qualitative Analysis', *Population and Development Review*, vol. 10, no. 2, pp. 297–315.

Konde-Lule, J.K., Musagara, M. and Musgrave, S., 1993, 'Focus Group Interviews about AIDS in Rakai District of Uganda', *Social Science and Medicine*, vol. 37, no. 5, pp. 679–84.

Koutroulis, G., 1990, 'The Orifice Revisited: Women in Gynaecological Texts', *Community Health Studies*, vol. 14, no. 2, pp. 73–84.

Koutroulis, G., 1993, 'Memory Work: A Critique', in B.S. Turner, L. Eckermann, D. Colquhoun and P. Crotty (eds), *Annual Review of Health Social Sciences: Methodological Issues in Health Research*, vol. 3, pp. 76–96.

Koutroulis, G., 1996, Memory-Work and Menstruation, unpublished PhD thesis, La Trobe University, Melbourne.

Krathwohl, D.R., 1988, *How To Prepare a Research Proposal*, 2nd edn, Syracuse University Press, New York.

Kroeber, A.L., 1919, 'On the Principle of Order in Civilization as Exemplified by Changes in Women's Fashions', *American Anthropologist*, vol. 21, no. 2, pp. 235–63.

Kronenfeld, J.J., 1985, 'Publishing in Journals', in M.F. Fox (ed.), *Scholarly Writing and Publishing: Issues, Problems and Solutions*, Westview, Boulder, Colorado.

Krueger, R., 1988, *Focus Groups: A Practical Guide for Applied Research*, Sage, London.

Krueger, R., 1994, *Focus Groups: A Practical Guide for Applied Research,* 2nd edn, Sage, London.

Kuhn, M. and McPartland, T., 1954, 'An Empirical Investigation of Self-Attitudes', *American Sociological Review*, vol. 19, pp. 68–76.

Kumar, K., 1987, *Conducting Group Interviews in Developing Countries*, US Agency for International Development, Washington, DC.

Labov, W. and Waletzky, J., 1997, 'Narrative Analysis', *Journal of Narrative and Life History*, vol. 7, pp. 3–38.

Lalli, P., 1989, 'The Imaginative Dimension of Everyday Life: Towards a Hermeneutic Reading', *Current Sociology*, vol. 37, no. 1, pp. 103–14.

Lammerink, M. and Wolffers, I. (eds), 1994, *Some Selected Examples of Participatory Research: Special Program on Research (DGIS/DST/SO)*, Ministry of Foreign Affairs, The Hague, The Netherlands.

Larson, E. and Franchiang, S., 1996, 'Life History and Narrative Research: Generating a Humanistic Knowledge Base for Occupational Therapy', *American Journal of Occupational Therapy*, vol. 50, no. 2, pp. 247–50.

Lather, P., 1993, 'Fertile Obsession: Validity after Poststructuralism', *Sociological Quarterly* vol. 34, no. 4, pp. 673–93.

Lather, P. and Smithies, C., 1997, *Troubling the Angels: Women Living with HIV/AIDS*, HarperCollins, Boulder.

Laurell, A.C., Noriega, M., Martinez, S. and Villegas, J., 1992, 'Participatory Research on Worker's Health', *Social Science and Medicine*, vol. 34, no. 6, pp. 603–13.

Layne, L.L., 1990, 'Motherhood Lost: Cultural Dimensions of Miscarriage and Stillbirth in America', *Women & Health*, vol. 17, pp. 69–98.

Lederman, L., 1983, 'High Apprehensives Talk about Communication Apprehension and Its Effects on Their Behaviour', *Communication Quarterly*, vol. 31, no. 3 pp. 233–7.

Lee, R. and Fielding, N., 1995, 'Users' Experiences of Qualitative Data Analysis Software', in U. Kelle (ed.), *Computer-Aided Qualitative Data Analysis*, Sage, London.

Lefferts, R., 1982, *Getting a Grant in the 1980s: How To Write Successful Grant Proposals,* 2nd edn, Prentice-Hall, Englewood Cliffs, NJ.

Lefferts, R., 1990, *Getting a Grant in the 1990s: How To Write Successful Grant Proposals*, Prentice-Hall, New York.

Lemert, C., 1997, *Postmodernism Is Not What You Think*, Blackwell, Oxford.

Lengua, L., Roosa, M.W., Schupak-Neuberg, E., Michaels, M.L., Berg, C.N. and Weschler, L.F., 1992, 'Using Focus Groups To Guide the Development of Parenting Program for Difficult-to-Reach, High Risk Families', *Family Relations*, vol. 4, no. 2, pp. 163–8.

Letherby, G., 1993, 'The Meanings of Miscarriage', *Women's Studies International Forum*, vol. 16, no. 2, pp. 165–80.

Lettenmaier, C., Langlois, P., Kumah, O.M., Kiragu, K., Jato, M., Zacharias, J., Kols, A. and Piotrow, P.T., 1994, 'Focus-Group Research for Family Planning: Lessons Learned in Sub-Saharan Africa', *Health Transition Review*, vol. 4, no. 1, pp. 95–9.

Levinson, D. (ed.), 1978, *A Guide to Social Theory: Worldwide Cross-Cultural Tests*, HRAF Press, New Haven, CT.

Lewin, K., 1946, 'Action Research and Minority Problems', *Journal of Social Issues*, vol. 2, no. 1 pp. 34–46.

Lewins, A., 1998, Basic Text Transcription Guidelines, <http://www.soc.surrey.ac.uk/caqdas/>.

Lincoln, Y., 1992, 'Sympathetic Connections between Qualitative Methods and Health Research', *Qualitative Health Research* , vol. 2, no. 4, pp. 375–91.

Lincoln, Y. and Guba, E., 1985, *Naturalistic Inquiry*, Sage, Beverly Hills.

Linde, C., 1993, *Life Stories*, Oxford University Press, New York.

Lindesmith, A., 1968, *Addiction and Opiates*, Aldine, Chicago.

Locke, L.F., Spirduso, W.W. and Silverman, S.J., 1989, *Proposals That Work: A Guide for Planning Research*, Teachers College Press, New York.

Lofland, J., 1974, 'Styles of Reporting Qualitative Field Research', *American Sociologist*, vol. 9, August, pp. 101–11.

Lofland, J. and Lofland, L., 1971, *Analyzing Social Settings*, Wadsworth, Belmont, CA.

Lofland, J. and Lofland, L., 1984, *Analyzing Social Settings*, 2nd edn, Wadsworth, Belmont, CA.

Lorion, R.P., 1995, 'Grantmanship: A View from Inside and Out', in W. Pequegnat and E. Stover (eds), *How To Write a Successful Research Grant Application: A Guide for Social and Behavioural Scientists*, Plenum Press, New York.

Lovell, A., 1983, 'Some Questions of Identity: Late Miscarriage, Stillbirth and Perinatal Loss', *Social Science and Medicine*, vol. 17, pp. 755–61.

Lucchini, R., 1996, 'Theory, Method and Triangulation in the Study of Street Children', *Childhood* vol. 3, no. 1, pp. 167–70.

Lucy, N., 1997, *Postmodern Literary Theory*, Blackwell, Oxford.

Lupton, D., 1992, 'Discourse Analysis: A New Methodology for Understanding Ideologies of Health And Illness', *Australian Journal of Public Health*, vol. 16, no. 2, pp. 145–50.

Lupton, D., 1994, 'Femininity, Responsibility and the Technological Imperative: Discourse on Breast Cancer in the Australian Press', *International Journal of Health Services*, vol. 24, no. 1, pp. 73–89.

Lupton, D., 1995, 'The Medical and Health Stories on the Sydney Morning Herald's Front Page', *Australian Journal of Public Health*, vol. 19, no. 5, pp. 501–8.

Macann, C., 1993, *Four Phenomenological Philosophers: Husserl, Heidegger, Sartre, Merleau-Ponty*, Routledge, London.

MacDonald, K. and Tipton, C., 1993, 'Using Documents', in N. Gilbert (ed.), *Researching Social Life*, Sage, London.

MacDougall, C. and Baum, F., 1997, 'The Devil's Advocate: A Strategy To Avoid Group Thinking and Stimulate Discussion in Focus Groups', *Qualitative Health Research*, vol. 7, no. 4, pp. 532–41.

MacIntyre, A., 1981, *After Virtue*, 2nd edn, Duckworth, London.

Mackie, F., 1985, *The Status of Everyday Life*, Routledge & Kegan Paul, London.

Madak, P., 1994, 'Ethical Considerations When Using Qualitative Methods in Evaluation', *Canadian Journal of Program Evaluation*, vol. 9, no. 1, pp. 1–13.

Madden, M.E., 1994, 'The Variety of Emotional Reactions to Miscarriage', *Women & Health*, vol. 21, no. 2/3, pp. 85–104.

Magill, R.S., 1993, 'Focus Groups, Program Evaluation and the Poor', *Journal of Sociology and Social Welfare*, vol. 20, no. 1, pp. 103–14.

Maguire, P., 1987, *Doing Participatory Research: A Feminist Approach*, Centre for International Education, School of Education, University of Massachusetts, Amherst, Mass.

Maguire, P., 1996, 'Proposing a More Feminist Participatory Research: Knowing and Being Embraced Openly', in K. de Koning and M. Martin (eds), *Participatory Research in Health: Issues and Experiences*, Zed Books, London.

Maines, D., 1991a, 'Introduction', in D. Maines (ed.), *Social Organization and Social Process: Essays in Honor of Anselm Strauss*, Aldine de Gruyter, New York.

Maines, D. (ed.), 1991b, *Social Organization and Social Process: Essays in Honor of Anselm Strauss*, Aldine de Gruyter, New York.

Maisano, C., 1996, The Aesthetics of Melbourne Hospitals' Birth and Delivery Rooms, unpublished masters thesis, La Trobe University, Melbourne.

Malinowski, B., 1922, *Argonauts of the Western Pacific*, Routledge, London.

Manderson, L. and Aaby, P., 1992, 'Can Rapid Anthropological Procedures Be Applied to Tropical Diseases?', *Health Policy and Planning*, vol. 7, no. 1, pp. 46–55.

Manderson, L. and Mark, T., 1997, 'Empowering Women: Participatory Approaches in Women's Health and Development Projects', *Health Care for Women International*, vol. 18, pp. 17–30.

Marindo-Ranganai, R., 1996, 'A Zimbabwean Case', in K. de Koning and M. Martin (eds), *Participatory Research in Health: Issues and Experiences*, Zed Books, London.

Martin, M., 1996, 'Issues of Power in the Participatory Research Process', in K. de Koning and M. Martin (eds), *Participatory Research in Health: Issues and Experiences*, Zed Books, London.

Mason, J., 1996, *Qualitative Researching*, Sage, London.

Mattingly, C., 1994, 'The Concept of Therapeutic Emplotment', *Social Science and Medicine*, vol. 38, no. 6, pp. 811–22.

Mauch, J.E. and Birch, J.W., 1989, *Guide to the Successful Thesis and Dissertation: Conception to Publication*, Marcel Dekker, New York.

Mauksch, H.O., 1970, 'Studying the Hospital', in R.W. Habenstein (ed.), *Pathways to Data*, Aldine, Chicago.

Mavalankar, D.V., Satia, J.K. and Sharma, B., 1996, 'Experiences and Issues in Institutionalizing Qualitative and Participatory Research Approaches in a Government Health Programme', in K. de Koning and M. Martin (eds), *Participatory Research in Health: Issues and Experiences,* Zed Books, London.

McCraken, G., 1988, *The Long Interview*, Sage, Newbury Park.

McDonald, I. and Daly, J., 1992, 'Researching Methods in Health Care: A Summing Up', in J. Daly, I. McDonald and E. Willis (eds), *Researching Health Care: Designs, Dilemmas, Disciplines,* Routledge, London.

McEwan, P., 1993, 'Editorial', *Social Science and Medicine* vol. 37, no. 12, pp. vii–viii.

McLaren, P. and Leonard, P., 1993, *Paulo Freire: A Critique Encounter*, Routledge, London.

McTaggart, R., 1993, 'Dilemmas in Cross-Cultural Action Research', in D. Colquhoun and A. Kellehear (eds), *Health Research in Practice: Political, Ethical and Methodological Issues*, Chapman & Hall, London.

Mead, G., 1934, *Mind, Self and Society*, University of Chicago Press, Chicago.

Meloy, J.M., 1993, 'Problem of Writing and Representation in Qualitative Inquiry', *International Journal of Qualitative Studies in Education*, vol. 6, no. 4, pp. 315–30.

Menegoni, L., 1996, 'Conceptions of Tuberculosis and Therapeutic Choices in Highland Chiapas, Mexico', *Medical Anthropology Quarterly*, vol. 10, no. 3, pp. 381–401.

Merton, R. and Kendall, P., 1946, 'The Focused Interview', *American Journal of Sociology*, vol. 51, no. 6, pp. 541–57.

Merton, R.K., Fiske, M. and Kendall, P.L., 1990, *The Focused Interview,* 2nd edn, Free Press, New York.

Michaelson, H.B., 1987, 'How To Write and Publish a Dissertation', *Journal of Technical Writing and Communication*, vol. 17, no. 3, pp. 265–74.

Mies, M., 1991, 'Women's Research or Feminist Research?', in M. Fonow and J. Cook (eds), *Beyond Methodology*, Indiana University Press, Bloomington.

Miles, M. and Huberman, A.M,. 1984, *Qualitative Data Analysis*, Sage, Beverly Hills.

Miles, M. and Huberman, A., 1994, *Qualitative Data Analysis,* 2nd edn, Sage, Thousand Oaks.

Miller, D., 1988, 'Approaching the State on the Council Estate', *Man*, vol. 23, no. 4, pp. 353–72.

Mills, C.W., 1959, *The Sociological Imagination*, Penguin, Harmondsworth.

Minichiello, V., Aroni, R., Timewell, E. and Alexander, L., 1990, *In-Depth Interviewing: Researching People*, Longman Cheshire, Melbourne.

Minichiello, V., Aroni, R., Timewell, E. and Alexander, L., 1995, *In-Depth Interviewing: Principles, Techniques, Analysis,* 2nd edn, Longman, Melbourne.

Mishler, E., 1986, *Research Interviewing: Context and Narrative*, Harvard University Press, Cambridge, Mass.

Mishler, E., 1990, 'Validation in Inquiry-Guided Research: The Role of Exemplars in Narrative Studies', *Harvard Educational Review*, vol. 60, no. 2, pp. 415–42.

Mishler, E., 1995, 'Models of Narrative Analysis', *Journal of Narrative and Life History*, vol. 5, no. 2, pp. 87–123.

Mitchell, P., 1991, 'Memory-Work: A Primary Health Care Strategy for Nurses Working with Older Women', in Proceedings of National Nursing Conference on Science, Reflectivity and Nursing Care: Exploring the Dialectic, December, Melbourne, pp. 48–53.

Moffett, J., 1984, *Active Voices IV*, Boynton/Cook, Upper Montclair, NJ.

Montell, F.B., 1995, 'Focus Group Interviews: A New Feminist Method', paper presented at Annual Meeting of American Sociological Association, Washington, DC.

Moore, D., 1993, 'Social Controls, Harm Minimisation and Interactive Outreach: The Public Health Implications of and Ethnography of Drug Use', *Australian Journal of Public Health*, vol. 17, no. 1, pp. 58–67.

Morgan, D.L., 1988, *Focus Groups as Qualitative Research*, Sage, Newbury Park.

Morgan, D.L., 1995, 'Why Things (Sometimes) Go Wrong in Focus Groups', *Qualitative Health Research*, vol. 5, no. 4, pp. 516–23.

Morgan, D.L., 1996, 'Focus Groups', *Annual Review of Sociology*, vol. 22, pp. 129–52.

Morgan, D.L., 1997, *Focus Groups as Qualitative Research,* 2nd edn, Sage, Newbury Park.

Morgan, D.L. and Krueger, R.A., 1993, 'When To Use Focus Groups and Why', in D.L. Morgan (ed.), *Successful Focus Groups: Advancing the State of the Art*, Sage, Newbury Park.

Morse, J. and Field, P., 1995, *Qualitative Research Methods for Health Professionals*, 2nd edn, Sage, Thousand Oaks.

Morse, J.M. (ed.), 1992, *Qualitative Health Research*, Sage, Newbury Park.

Morse, J.M., 1994a, 'Designing Funded Qualitative Research', in N.K. Denzin and Y. S. Lincoln (eds), *Handbook of Qualitative Research*, Sage, Thousand Oaks.

Morse, J.M., 1994b, 'Disseminating Qualitative Research', in E. Dunn, P.G. Norton, M. Stewart, F. Tudiver and M.J. Bass (eds), *Foundation of Primary Care Research: Disseminating Research Findings*, Sage, Newbury Park.

Moustakas, C., 1994, *Phenomenological Research Methods*, Sage, Thousand Oaks.

Mucha, F., 1995, 'Developing a Budget and Financial Justification', in W. Pequegnat and E. Stover (eds), *How To Write a Successful Research Grant Application: A Guide for Social and Behavioural Scientists*, Plenum Press, New York.

Naish, J., Brown, J. and Denton, B., 1994, 'Intercultural Consultations: Investigation of Factors that Deter Non-English Speaking Women from Attending Their General Practitioners for Cervical Screening', *British Medical Journal*, vol. 309, 29 October, pp. 1126–8.

Naruemon, S., 1988, *Nang Ngam Tuu Krachok*, Institute of Thai Study, Thammasart University, Bangkok [in Thai].

Nemcek, M. and Egan, P.B., 1984, 'Steps to Publication: A Quick Reference for Nurses', *Occupational Health Nursing*, August, pp. 425–27.

Neugebauer, R., Kline, J., O'Connor, P., Shrout, P., Johnson, J., Skodol, A., Wicks, J. and Susser, M., 1992, 'Determinants of Depressive Symptoms in the Early Weeks after Miscarriage', *American Journal of Public Health*, vol. 82, no. 10, pp. 1332–9.

Neuman, W.L., 1991, *Social Research Methods*, Allyn and Bacon, Boston.

Nichols-Casebolt, A. and Spakes, P., 1995, 'Policy Research and the Voices of Women', *Social Work Research*, vol. 19, no. 1, pp. 49–55.

Nichter, M., 1984, 'Project Community Diagnosis: Participatory Research as a First Step toward Community Involvement in Primary Health Care', *Social Science and Medicine*, vol. 19, no. 3, pp. 237–252.

O'Connor, B., 1995, *Healing Traditions: Alternative Medicine and Health Professional*, University of Pennsylvania Press, Philadelphia.

Oakley, A., 1981, 'Interviewing Women: A contradiction in terms', in H. Roberts (ed.) *Doing Feminist Research*, Routledge and Kegan Paul, Boston.

Oakley, A., McPherson, A. and Roberts, H., 1990, *Miscarriage*, Penguin, Harmondsworth.

Orona, C., 1990, 'Temporality and Identity Loss due to Alzheimer's Disease', *Social Science and Medicine*, vol. 30, pp. 1247–56.

Palca, D., 1981, *The Language of Clothes*, Random House, New York.

Patton, M., 1990, *Qualitative Evaluation and Research Methods,* 2nd edn, Sage, Newbury Park.

Pequegnat, W. and Stover, E. (eds), 1995, *How To Write a Successful Research Grant Application: A Guide for Social and Behavioural Scientists*, Plenum Press, New York.

Perl, S., 1983, 'Understanding Composing', in J.N. Hays, P.A. Roth, J.R. Ramsey and R.D. Foulke (eds), *The Writer's Mind: Writing as a Mode of Thinking*, National Council of Teachers of English, Urbana, Illinois.

Persell, C.H., 1985, 'Scholars and Book Publishing', in M.F. Fox (ed.), *Scholarly Writing and Publishing: Issues, Problems and Solutions*, Westview, Boulder, Colorado.

Personal Narratives Group, 1989, *Interpreting Women's Lives*, Indiana University Press, Bloomington.

Plath, D., 1980, *Long Engagements*, Stanford University Press, Stanford, CA.

Plummer, K., 1983, *Documents of Life*, George Allen and Unwin, London.

Plummer, K., 1995, *Telling Sexual Stories: Power, Change and Social Worlds*, Routledge, London.

Polkinghorne, D., 1988, *Narrative Knowing and the Human Sciences*, State University of New York Press, Albany.

Potter, J., 1996, *Representing Reality: Discourse, Rhetoric and Social Construction*, Sage, London.

Powdermaker, H., 1966, *Stranger and Friend: The Way of an Anthropologist*, W.W. Norton, New York.

Powdermaker, H., 1968, 'Fieldwork', in D.L. Sills (ed.), *International Encyclopaedia of the Social Sciences*, vol. 5, Macmillan, New York, pp. 418–24.

Powell, W.W., 1985, *Getting into Print: The Decision-Making Process in Scholarly Publishing*, University of Chicago Press, Chicago.

Pratt, B. and Loizos, P., 1992, *Choosing Research Methods: Data Collection for Development Workers*, Development Guidelines No. 7, Oxfam, Oxford.

Preston-Whyte, E. and Dalrymple, L., 1996, 'Participation and Action: Reflections on Community-Based AIDS', in K. de Koning and M. Martin (eds), *Participatory Research in Health: Issues and Experiences*, Zed Books, London.

Prettyman, R.J., Cordle, C.J. and Cook, G.D., 1993, 'A Three Month Follow-Up of Psychological Morbidity after Early Miscarriage', *British Journal of Medical Psychology*, vol. 66, pp. 363–72.

Prus, R., 1996, *Symbolic Interaction and Ethnographic Research*, State University of New York Press, Albany.

Puddifoot, J.E. and Johnson, M.P., 1997, 'The Legitimacy of Grieving: The Partner's Experience of Miscarriage', *Social Science and Medicine*, vol. 45, no. 6, pp. 837–45.

Punch, M., 1986, *The Politics and Ethics of Fieldwork*, Sage, New Delhi.

Race, K.E., Hotch, D.F. and Packer, T., 1994, 'Rehabilitation Program Evaluation: Use of Focus Groups To Empower Clients', *Evaluation Review*, vol. 18, no. 6 pp. 730–40.

Rahman, M.D.A., 1991, 'Glimpses of the "Other Africa"', in O. Fals-Borda and M.A. Rahman (eds), *Action and Knowledge: Breaking the Monopoly with Participatory Action-Research*, Apex Press, New York.

Rahman, M.D.A., 1993, *People's Self-Development: Perspectives on Participatory Action Research: A Journey through Experience*, Zed Books University Press, London.

Ramos, M., 1989, 'Some Ethical Implications of Qualitative Research', *Research in Nursing and Health*, vol. 12, no. 1, pp. 57–63.

Rao, V., 1997, 'Wife-Beating in Rural South India: A Qualitative and Econometric Analysis', *Social Science and Medicine*, vol. 44, no. 8, pp. 1169–80.

Rathje, W.L., 1979, 'Trace Measures, Garbage and Other Traces', in L. Sechrest (ed.), *Unobtrusive Measurement Today*, Jossey-Bass, San Francisco.

Rathje, W.L., 1984, 'The Garbage Decade', *American Behavioural Scientist*, vol. 28, no. 1, pp. 9–29.

Ratner, C., 1996, 'Solidifying Qualitative Methodology', *Journal of Social Distress and the Homeless* vol. 5, no. 3, pp. 319–26.

Reason, P., 1994, 'Three Approaches to Participative Inquiry', in N.K. Denzin and Y.S. Lincoln (eds), *Handbook of Qualitative Research*, Sage, Thousand Oaks.

Reinharz, S., 1988, 'Controlling Women's Lives: A Cross-Cultural Interpretation of Miscarriage Accounts', in D. Wertz (ed.), *Research in the Sociology of Health Care*, JAI Press, Greenwich, CT.

Reinharz, S., 1992, *Feminist Methods in Social Research*, Oxford University Press, Oxford.

Rice, P.L., 1993, *My Forty Days: A Cross-Cultural Resources Book for Health Care Professionals in Birthing Services*, Vietnamese Antenatal/Postnatal Support Project, Melbourne.

Rice, P.L. (ed.), 1994, *Asian Mothers, Australian Births*, Ausmed Publications, Melbourne.

Rice, P.L., 1995, 'Pog Laus, Tsis Coj Khaub Ncaws Lawm: The Meaning of Menopause in Hmong Women', *Journal of Reproductive and Infant Psychology*, vol. 13, no. 2, pp 79–92.

Rice, P.L., 1996a, 'In Quality We Trust!: The Role of Qualitative Data in Health Care', *Medical Principles and Practice*, vol. 5, pp. 51–7.

Rice, P.L., 1996b, 'My Soul Has Gone: Appropriate Methods for a Delicate Situation', in J. Daly. (ed.), *Ethical Intersections: Health Research, Methods and Researcher Responsibility*, Allen & Unwin, Sydney.

Rice, P.L., 1996c, 'Health Research and Ethnic Communities: Reflection on Practice', in D. Colquhoun and A. Kellehear (eds), *Health Research in Practice, Volume 2: Personal Experiences, Public Issues*, Chapman & Hall, London.

Rice, P.L., Ly, B. and Lumley, J., 1994, 'Childbirth and Soul Loss: The Case of a Hmong Woman', *Medical Journal of Australia*, vol. 160, no. 9, pp. 577–8.

Rice, P.L. and Manderson, L. (eds), 1996, *Maternity and Reproductive Health in Asian Societies*, Harwood Academic Publishers, Amsterdam.

Rice, P.L. and Naksook, C., 1998, 'Caesarean or Vaginal Birth?: Perceptions and Experience of Thai Women in Australian Hospitals', *Australian and New Zealand Journal of Public Health*, vol. 22, no. 5, pp. 604–8.

Richardson, L., 1985, *The New Other Woman: Contemporary Single Women in Affairs with Married Men*, Free Press, New York.

Richardson, L., 1990, *Writing Strategies: Reaching Diverse Audiences*, Sage, Newbury Park.

Richardson, L., 1994, 'Writing: A Method of Inquiry', in N.K. Denzin and Y.S. Lincoln (eds), *Handbook of Qualitative Research*, Sage, Thousand Oaks.

Richardson, L., 1997, *Fields of Play, Constructing and Academic Life*, Rutgers University Press, New Brunswick.

Ricoeur, P., 1984, *Time and Narrative*, vol. 1 (trans. K. McLaughlin and D. Pellauer), University of Chicago Press, Chicago.

Ricoeur, P., 1985, *Time and Narrative*, vol. 2 (trans. K. McLaughlin and D. Pellauer), University of Chicago Press, Chicago.

Ricoeur, P., 1988, *Time and Narrative*, vol. 3 (trans. K. Blamey and D. Pellauer), University of Chicago Press, Chicago.

Ricoeur, P., 1992, *Oneself as Another* (trans. K. Blamey), University of Chicago Press, Chicago.

Riessman, C., 1990a, 'Strategic Uses of Narrative in the Presentation of Self and Illness', *Social Science and Medicine*, vol. 30, no. 11, pp. 1195–1200.

Riessman, C., 1990b, *Divorce Talk*, Rutgers University Press, New Brunswick, NJ.

Riessman, C., 1993, *Narrative Analysis*, Sage, Newbury Park.

Ritchie, J.E., 1996, 'Using Participatory Research To Enhance Health in the Work Setting: An Australian Experience', in K. de Koning and M. Martin (eds), *Participatory Research in Health: Issues and Experiences*, Zed Books, London.

Rittenbaugh, C.K. and Harrison, G.G., 1984, 'Reactivity of Garbage Analysis', *American Behavioural Scientist*, vol. 28, no. 1, pp. 51–70.

Roach, A., 1990, 'Native Born', from the album *Charcoal Lane*, Mushroom Records, Melbourne.

Robinson, J. and Hawpe, L., 1986, 'Narrative Thinking as a Heuristic Process', in T. Sarbin (ed.), *Narrative Psychology*, Praeger, New York.

Rosaldo, R., 1989, *Culture and Truth*, Routledge, London.

Rosenhan, D.L. 1992, 'On Being Sane in Insane Places', in J.M. Morse (ed.), *Qualitative Health Research*, Sage, Newbury Park.

Rosenwald, G. and Ochberg, R., 1992, 'Introduction', in G. Rosenwald and R. Ochberg (eds), *Storied Lives*, Yale University Press, New Haven.

Rosenwald, G. and Wiersma, J., 1983, 'Women, Career Changes and the New Self', *Psychiatry*, vol. 46, pp. 213–29.

Rubin, H. and Rubin, I., 1995, *Qualitative Interviewing: The Art of Hearing Data*, Sage, Thousand Oaks.

Rundell, J., 1995, 'Gadamer and the Circles of Hermeneutics', in D. Roberts (ed.), *Reconstructing Theory: Gadamer, Habermas, Luhmann*, Melbourne University Press, Melbourne.

Salazar, M.C., 1991, 'Young Laborers in Bogota: Breaking Authoritarian Ramparts', in O. Fals-Borda and M.A. Rahman (eds), *Action and Knowledge: Breaking the Monopoly with Participatory Action-Research*, Apex Press, New York.

Samson, C., 1995, 'Madness and Psychiatry', in B. Turner, *Medical Power and Social Knowledge*, 2nd edn, Sage, London.

Sands, R., 1996, 'The Elusiveness of Identity in Social Work Practice with Women', *Clinical Social Work Journal*, vol. 24, no. 2, pp. 167–87.

Sani, A.B.G., Punufimana, A.N., Seuseu, N.K.F. and Shawyer, R.J., 1990, Use of Clinical Vignettes in Rapid Ethnographic Assessment: A Folk Taxonomy of Diarrhoea in Northeast Thailand, masters thesis, University of Queensland, Brisbane.

Sarbin, T., 1986, 'The Narrative as a Root Metaphor for Psychology', in T. Sarbin (ed.), *Narrative Psychology*, Praeger, New York.

Savage, J., 1995, *Nursing Intimacy: An Ethnographic Approach to Nurse–Patient Interaction*, Scutari Press, London.

Schmoll, B.J., 1987, 'Ethnographic Inquiry in Clinical Settings', *Physical Therapy*, vol. 67, no. 12, pp. 1895–7.

Schoepf, B.G., 1993, 'AIDS Action-Research with Women in Kinshasa, Zaire', *Social Science and Medicine*, vol. 37, no. 11, pp. 1401–13.

Schratz-Hadwich, B., 1995, 'Collective Memory-Work: The Self as a Re/Source for Re/Search', in M. Schratz and R. Walker (eds), *Research as Social Change: New Opportunities for Qualitative Research*, Routledge, London.

Schutz, A., 1967, *The Phenomenology of the Social World*, Northwestern University Press, Evanston, Illinois.

Scott, G.G., 1983, *The Magicians: A Study of the Use of Power in a Black Magic Group*, Irvington, New York.

Scrimshaw, S.C.M. and Hurtado, E., 1987, *Rapid Assessment Procedures for Nutrition and Primary Health Care: Anthropological Approaches To Improving Programme Effectiveness*, United Nations University, Tokyo.

Seabrook, J., 1982, *Unemployment*, Quartet Books, London.

Seamark, R. and Gaughwin, M., 1994, 'Jabs in the Dark: Injecting Equipment Found in Prisons and the Risks of Viral Transmission', *Australian Journal of Public Health*, vol. 18, no. 1, pp. 113–16.

Sechrest, L. (ed.), 1979, *Unobtrusive Measurement Today*, Jossey-Bass, San Francisco.

Sechrest, L. and Flores, L., 1969, 'Homosexuality in the Philippines and the United States: The Handwriting on the Wall', *Journal of Social Psychology*, vol. 79, October, pp. 3–12.

Seeley, J.A., Kengeya-Kayondo, J.F. and Mulder, D.W., 1992, 'Community-Based HIV/AIDS Research: Whither Community Participation? Unsolved Problems in a Research Programme in Rural Uganda', *Social Science and Medicine*, vol. 34, no. 10, pp. 1089–95.

Seidman, I., 1991, *Interviewing as Qualitative Research*, Teachers College Press, New York.

Sennet, R. and Cobb, J., 1972, *The Hidden Injuries of Class*, Vintage Books, New York.

Shaffir, W.B., 1991, 'Managing a Convincing Self-Presentation', in W.B. Shaffir and R.A. Stebbins (eds), *Experiencing Fieldwork*, Sage, Newbury Park, pp. 72–81.

Shaffir, W.B. and Stebbins, R.A., 1991, *Experiencing Fieldwork: An Inside View of Qualitative Research*, Sage, Newbury Park.

Sharp, V., 1975, *Social Control in the Therapeutic Community*, Saxon House, Farnborough.

Sherman, B.L. and Dominick, J.R., 1986, 'Violence and Sex in Music Videos: TV and Rock 'n Roll', *Journal of Communication*, vol. 36, no. 1, pp. 79–93.

Shostak, M., 1981, *Nisa: The Life and Words of a !Kung Woman*, Vintage Books, New York.

Simonds, W., 1988, 'Confessions of Loss: Maternal Grief in True Story 1920–1985', *Gender and Society*, vol. 2, no. 2, pp. 149–71.

Sittitrai, W. and Brown, T., 1990, *Training Manual on Focus Group Discussions in Human Sexuality Research*, Chulalongkorn University, Bangkok.

Skolbekken, J.-A., 1995, 'The Risk Epidemic in Medical Journals', *Social Science and Medicine*, vol. 40, no. 3, pp. 291–305.

Slade, P., 1994, 'Predicting the Psychological Impact of Miscarriage', *Journal of Reproductive and Infant Psychology*, vol. 12, pp. 5–16.

Sliverman, M., Ricci, E. and Gunter, M., 1990, 'Strategies for Increasing the Rigor of Qualitative Methods in Evaluation of Health Care Programs', *Evaluation Review*, vol. 14, no. 1, pp. 57–74.

Small, J., 1997, *Memory-Work: A Feminist Social Constructionist Method for Researching Tourist Behaviour*, Working Paper No. 7, School of Management, University of Technology, Sydney.

Smith, D., 1987, *The Everyday World as Problematic: A Feminist Sociology*, Open University Press, Milton Keynes.

Snow, D. and Morrill, C., 1995, 'A Revolutionary Handbook or a Handbook for Revolution?', *Journal of Contemporary Ethnography*, vol. 24, no. 3, pp. 341–9.

Sobo, E.J., 1996, 'Cultural Explanations for Pregnancy Loss in Rural Jamaica', in R. Cecil (ed.), *The Anthropology of Pregnancy Loss: Comparative Studies in Miscarriage, Stillbirth and Neonatal Death*, Berg, Oxford.

Spradley, J.P., 1970, *You Owe Yourself a Drunk: An Ethnography of Urban Nomads*, Little, Brown, Boston.

Spradley, J.P., 1979, *The Ethnographic Interview*, Holt, Rinehart & Winston, New York.

Spreen, M. and Zwaagstra, R., 1994, 'Personal Network Sampling, Outdegree Analysis and Multilevel Analysis', *International Sociology* vol. 9, no. 4, pp. 475–91.

Stapleton, P., 1987, *Writing Research Papers: An Easy Guide for Non-Native English Speakers*, Australian Centre for International Agricultural Research, Canberra.

Statham, H. and Green, J., 1994, 'The Effects of Miscarriage and Other "Unsuccessful" Pregnancies on Feelings Early in a Subsequent Pregnancy', *Journal of Reproductive and Infant Psychology*, vol. 12, pp. 45–54.

Stein, H.F., 1991, 'The Role of Some Non-Biomedical Parameters in Clinical Decision Making: An Ethnographic Approach', *Qualitative Health Research*, vol. 1, no. 1, pp. 6–26.

Stevens, P. and Doerr, B., 1997, 'Trauma of Discovery: Women's Narratives of Being Informed They Are HIV-Infected', *AIDS Care*, vol. 9, no. 5, pp. 523–38.

Stewart, D.W. and Shamdasani, P.N., 1990, *Focus Groups: Theory and Practice*, Sage, Newbury Park.

Stone, I., 1980, *The Origin: A Biographical Novel of Charles Darwin*, Doubleday & Co. Inc., New York.

Story, M. and Faulkner, P., 1990, 'The Prime Time Diet: A Content Analysis of Eating Behavior and Food Messages in Television Program Content and Commercials', *American Journal of Public Health*, vol. 80, no. 6, pp. 738–40.

Strauss, A., 1970, 'Discovering New Theory from Previous Theory', in T. Shibutani (ed.), *Human Nature and Collective Behavior*, Prentice-Hall, New Jersey.

Strauss, A., Becker, H., Geer, B. and Hughes, E., 1961, *Boys in White*, University of Chicago Press, Chicago.

Strauss, A. and Corbin, J., 1990, *Basics of Qualitative Research: Grounded Theory Procedures and Techniques*, Sage, Newbury Park.

Strunk, W. Jr. and White, E.B., 1979, *The Elements of Style*, 3rd edn, Macmillan, New York.

Stycos, J.M., 1981, 'A Critique of Focus Group and Survey Research: The Machismo Case', *Studies in Family Planning*, vol. 12, no. 12, pp. 450–6.

Styles, J., 1979, 'Outsider/Insider: Researching Gay Baths', *Urban Life*, vol. 8, no. 2, pp. 135–52.

Tagg, S., 1985, 'Life Story Interviews and Their Interpretations', in M. Brenner, J. Brown and D. Conater (eds), *The Research Interview*, Academic Press, London.

Tandon, R., 1988, 'Social Transformation and Participatory Research', *Convergence*, vol. 21, no. 2/3, pp. 5–14.

Tandon, R., 1996, 'The Historical Roots and Contemporary Tendencies in Participatory Research: Implications for Health Care', in K. de Koning and M. Martin (eds), *Participatory Research in Health: Issues and Experiences*, Zed Books, London.

Tandon, R. and Brown, L.D., 1981, 'Organization Building for Rural Development: An Experiment in India', *Journal of Applied Behavioral Science*, vol. 17, no. 2, pp. 172–98.

Taylor, B., 1993, 'Phenomenological Method in Nursing', in D. Colquhoun and A. Kellehear (eds), *Health Research in Practice*, Chapman & Hall, London.

Taylor, C., 1989, *Sources of the Self*, Cambridge University Press, Cambridge.

Taylor, S. and Bogdan, R., 1998, *Introduction to Qualitative Research Methods*, John Wiley & Sons, New York.

Tesch, R., 1990, *Qualitative Research: Analysis Types and Software Tools*, Falmer Press, New York.

Thomas, E.M., 1958, *The Harmless People*, Random House, New York.

Thomas, W., 1928, *The Child in America*, Knopf, New York.

Thomas, W. and Znaniecki, F., 1918–20, *The Polish Peasant in Europe and America*, Dover, New York.

Thompson, J.L., 1991, 'Exploring Gender and Culture with Khmer Refugee Women: Reflections on Participatory Feminist Research', *Advanced Nursing Science*, vol. 13, no. 3, pp. 30–48.

Threlfall, T.J., 1992, 'Sunglasses and Clothing: An Unhealthy Correlation?', *Australian Journal of Public Health*, vol. 16, no. 2, pp. 192–6.

Tolley, E.E. and Bentley, M.E., 1996, 'Training Issues for the Use of Participatory Research Methods', in K. de Koning and M. Martin (eds), *Participatory Research in Health: Issues and Experiences*, Zed Books, London.

Toolan, M., 1988, *Narrative: A Critical, Linguistic Introduction*, Routledge, London.

Toulmin, S. and Gustavsen, B., 1996, *Beyond Theory: Changing Organizations through Participation*, John Benjamins Publishing Co., Amsterdam.

Trinh, T. Minh-ha, 1991, *When the Moon Waxes Red: Representation, Gender and Cultural Politics*, Routledge, New York.

Tripp-Reimer, T. and Cohen, M.Z., 1991, 'Funding Strategies for Qualitative Research', in J.M. Morse (ed.), *Qualitative Nursing Research: A Contemporary Dialogue*, Sage, Newbury Park.

Trost, J., 1986, 'Statistically Nonrepresentative Stratified Sampling: A Sampling Technique for Qualitative Studies', *Qualitative Sociology*, vol. 9, no. 1, pp. 54–7.

Tyler, S., 1986, 'Postmodern Ethnography: From Document of the Occult to Occult Document', in J. Clifford and G. Marcus (eds), *Writing Culture: The Poetics and Politics of Ethnography*, University of California Press, Berkeley.

Ueland, B., 1991, *If You Want To Write: Releasing Your Creative Spirits*, Element, Shaftesbury, Dorset.

Van Esterik, P., 1988, 'To Strengthen and Refresh: Herbal Therapy in Southeast Asia', *Social Science and Medicine*, vol. 27, no. 8, pp. 751–9.

Van Maanen, J., 1982, 'Fieldwork on the Beat', in J. Van Maanen, J. Babbs and R. Faulner (eds), *Varieties of Qualitative Research*, Sage, Beverly Hills.

Van Maanen, J., 1988, *Tales of the Field: On Writing Ethnography*, University of Chicago Press, Chicago.

Van Til, W., 1987, *Writing for Professional Publication*, Allyn & Bacon, Newton, MA.

Vecchiato, N.L., 1997, 'Sociocultural Aspects of Tuberculosis Control in Ethiopia', *Medical Anthropology Quarterly*, vol. 11, no. 2, pp. 183–201.

Vidich, A. and Lyman, S., 1994, 'Qualitative Methods: Their History in Sociology and Anthropology', in N. Denzin and Y. Lincoln (eds), *Handbook of Qualitative Research*, Sage, Thousand Oaks.

Wadsworth, Y., 1991, *Everyday Evaluation on the Run*, Action Research Issues Association, Melbourne.

Waitzkin, H., 1991, *The Politics of Medical Encounters: How Patients and Doctors Deal with Social Problems*, Yale University Press, New Haven.

Waterston, A., 1997, 'Anthropological Research and the Politics of HIV Prevention: Towards a Critique of Policy and Priorities in the Age of AIDS', *Social Science and Medicine*, vol. 44, no. 9, pp. 1381–91.

Wax, M.L., Wax, R.H. and Dumont, R.V. Jr., 1989, 'Formal Education in an American Indian Community', *Social Problem*, vol. 11, no. 4, supplement.

Webb, E.L., Campbell, D.T., Schwartz, R.D. and Sechrest, L., 1966, *Unobtrusive Measures: Non-Reactive Research in the Social Sciences*, Rand McNally & Co., Chicago.

Weber, M., 1971, *Economy and Society* (eds G. Roth and C. Wittich), University of California Press, Berkeley.

Weber, R.P., 1990, *Basic Content Analysis,* 2nd edn, Sage, Newbury Park.

Weiler, K., 1991, 'Freire and a Feminist Pedagogy of Difference', *Harvard Educational Review*, vol. 61, no. 4, pp. 449–74.

Weitzman, E. and Miles, M., 1995, *Computer Programs for Qualitative Data Analysis*, Sage, Thousand Oaks.

Welbourn, A., 1992, 'Rapid Rural Appraisal, Gender and Health: Alternative Ways of Listening to Needs', *Institute of Development Studies Bulletin*, vol. 23, no. 1, pp. 8–18.

Whiteford, L.M., 1997, 'The Ethnoecology of Dengue Fever', *Medical Anthropology Quarterly*, vol. 11, no. 2, pp. 202–23.

Whitehead, T.L., 1997, 'Urban Low-Income African American Men, HIV/AIDS and Gender Identity', *Medical Anthropology Quarterly*, vol. 11, no. 4, pp. 411–47.

Whitehead, T.L. and Conaway, M.E. (eds), 1986, *Self, Sex and Gender in Cross-Cultural Fieldwork*, University of Illinois Press, Urbana and Chicago.

Whittaker, A., 1994, Issan Women: Ethnicity, Gender and Health in Northeast Thailand, unpublished PhD thesis, University of Queensland, Brisbane.

Whyte, W.F., 1955, *Street Corner Society: The Social Structure of an Italian Slum,* University of Chicago Press, Chicago.

Whyte, W.F. (ed.), 1991, *Participatory Action Research*, Sage, Newbury Park.

Whyte, W.F., Greenwood, D.J. and Lazes, P., 1991, 'Participatory Action Research: Through Practice to Science in Social Research', in W.F. Whyte (ed.), *Participatory Action Research*, Sage, Newbury Park.

Wiersma, J., 1992, 'Karen: The Transforming Story', in G. Rosenwald and R. Ochberg (eds), *Storied Lives*, Yale University Press, New Haven.

Wilkinson, A.M., 1991, *The Scientist's Handbook for Writing Papers and Dissertations*, Prentice-Hall, Englewood Cliffs, NJ.

Williams, R., 1976, *Keywords*, Fontana Press, London.

Williamson, J., 1986, *Consuming Passions*, Marion Boyers, London.

Willms, D., Best, J., Taylor, D., Gilber, J., Wilson, D., Lindsay, E.and Singer, J., 1990, 'A Systematic Approach of Using Qualitative Methods in Primary Prevention Research', *Medical Anthropology Quarterly*, vol. 4, no. 4, pp. 391–411.

Winch, P.J., Makemba, A.M., Kamazima, S.R., Lwihula, G.K., Lubega, P., Minjas, J.N. and Shiff, C.J., 1994, 'Seasonal Variation in the Perceived Risk of Malaria: Implications for the Promotion of Insecticide-Impregnated Bed Nets', *Social Science and Medicine*, vol. 39, no. 1, pp. 63–75.

Winefield, A., Tiggemann, M., Winefield, H. and Goldney, R., 1993, *Growing Up with Unemployment*, Routledge, London.

Wolcott, H., 1990, *Writing Up Qualitative Research*, Sage, Newbury Park.

Wolf, D.R., 1991, 'High-risk Methodology: Reflections on Leaving an Outlaw Society', in W.B. Shaffir and R.A. Stebbins (eds), *Experiencing Fieldwork*, Sage, Newbury Park, pp. 211–23.

Wolf, M., 1992, *A Trice Told Tale: Feminism, Postmodernism and Ethnographic Responsibility*, Stanford University Press, Stanford, CA.

Yach, D., 1992, 'The Use and Value of Qualitative Methods in Health Research in Developing Countries', *Social Science and Medicine*, vol. 35, no. 4, pp. 603–12.

Yelland, J. and Gifford, S., 1995, 'Problems of Focus Group Methods in Cross-Cultural Research: A Case Study of Beliefs about Sudden Infant Death Syndrome', *Australian Journal of Public Health*, vol. 19, no. 3, pp. 257–63.

Yimyam, S. and Suwanwong, B., 1995, *Culturally Appropriate Strategies for Food Supplement Promotion in Rural Northern Thailand*, Chiang Mai University School of Nursing, Chiang Mai [in Thai].

Yin, R.K., 1984, *Case Study Research: Design and Methods*, Sage, Beverly Hills.

Yule, V., 1987, 'Observing Adult–Child Interaction: An Example of a Piece of Research Anyone Could Do', in M. O'Connell (ed.), *New Introductory Reader in Sociology*, Nelson, Edinburgh.

Zeitlyn, S. and Rowshan, R., 1997, 'Privileged Knowledge and Mothers' "Perceptions": The Case of Breast-Feeding and Insufficient Milk in Bangladesh', *Medical Anthropology Quarterly*, vol. 11, no. 1, pp. 56–68.

Index